T0130825

Role of Psychologists in Pediatric Subspecialties

Editors

ROGER W. APPLE
ETHEL G. CLEMENTE

PEDIATRIC CLINICS
OF NORTH AMERICA

www.pediatric.theclinics.com

Consulting Editor
BONITA F. STANTON

October 2022 • Volume 69 • Number 5

ELSEVIER

1600 John F. Kennedy Boulevard ● Suite 1800 ● Philadelphia, Pennsylvania, 19103-2899

http://www.theclinics.com

THE PEDIATRIC CLINICS OF NORTH AMERICA Volume 69, Number 5
October 2022 ISSN 0031-3955, ISBN-13: 978-0-323-98779-0

Editor: Kerry Holland
Developmental Editor: Axell Ivan Jade M. Purificacion

The Pediatric Clinics of North America (ISSN 0031-3955) is published bimonthly by Elsevier Inc., 360 Park Avenue South, New York, NY 10010-1710. Months of issue are February, April, June, August, October, and December. Periodicals postage paid at New York, NY and additional mailing offices. Subscription prices are $263.00 per year (US individuals), $1028.00 per year (US institutions), $331.00 per year (Canadian individuals), $1074.00 per year (Canadian institutions), $395.00 per year (international individuals), $1074.00 per year (international institutions), $100.00 per year (US students and residents), $100.00 per year (Canadian students and residents), and $165.00 per year (international residents and students). To receive students/resident rare, orders must be accompanied by name of affiliated institution, date of term, and the signature of program/residency coordinator on institution letterhead. Orders will be billed at individual rate until proof of status is received. Foreign air speed delivery is included in all *Clinics* subscription prices. All prices are subject to change without notice. **POSTMASTER:** Send address changes to *The Pediatric Clinics of North America*, Elsevier Health Sciences Division, Subscription Customer Service, 3251 Riverport Lane, Maryland Heights, MO 63043. **Customer Service: 1-800-654-2452 (US and Canada). From outside of the US and Canada: 1-314-447-8871. Fax: 1-314-447-8029. For print support, E-mail: JournalsCustomerService-usa@elsevier.com. For online support, E-mail: JournalsOnlineSupport-usa@elsevier.com.**

Reprints. For copies of 100 or more, of articles in this publication, please contact the Commercial Reprints Department, Elsevier Inc., 360 Park Avenue South, New York, NY 10010-1710. Tel.: 212-633-3874; Fax: 212-633-3820; E-mail: reprints@elsevier.com.

The Pediatric Clinics of North America is also published in Spanish by McGraw-Hill Inter-americana Editores S.A., Mexico City, Mexico; in Portuguese by Riechmann and Affonso Editores, Rua Comandante Coelho 1085, CEP 21250, Rio de Janeiro, Brazil; and in Greek by Althayia SA, Athens, Greece.

The Pediatric Clinics of North America is covered in *MEDLINE/PubMed (Index Medicus), Excerpta Medica, Current Contents, Current Contents/Clinical Medicine, Science Citation Index, ASCA, ISI/BIOMED*, and *BIOSIS*.

PROGRAM OBJECTIVE

The goal of the *Pediatric Clinics of North America* is to keep practicing physicians and residents up to date with current clinical practice in pediatrics by providing timely articles reviewing the state-of-the-art in patient care.

TARGET AUDIENCE

All practicing pediatricians, physicians, and healthcare professionals who provide patient care to pediatric patients.

LEARNING OBJECTIVES

Upon completion of this activity, participants will be able to:

1. Review ways behavioral therapy, screening, and brief interventions can be used by pediatric psychologists to promote the health of pediatric patients.
2. Discuss the importance of addressing the biopsychosocial needs of pediatric patients and their families by incorporating the psychologist's role into the healthcare team.
3. Recognize the psychologist as an essential member of the multidisciplinary health care team in a variety of pediatric specialties to assist with the diagnosis, treatment, and management of pediatric health disorders.

ACCREDITATIONS

Physician Credit

The Elsevier Office of Continuing Medical Education (EOCME) is accredited by the Accreditation Council for Continuing Medical Education (ACCME) to provide continuing medical education for physicians.

The EOCME designates this journal-based activity for a maximum of 16 *AMA PRA Category 1 Credit*(s)™. Physicians should claim only the credit commensurate with the extent of their participation in the activity.

All other healthcare professionals requesting continuing education credit for this journal-based activity will be issued a certificate of participation.

ABP Maintenance of Certification Credit

Successful completion of this CME activity, which includes participation in the activity and individual assessment of and feedback to the learner, enables the learner to earn up to 16 MOC points in the American Board of Pediatrics' (ABP)

Maintenance of Certification (MOC) program. It is the CME activity provider's responsibility to submit learner completion information to ACCME for the purpose of granting ABP MOC credit.

DISCLOSURE OF CONFLICTS OF INTEREST

The EOCME assesses conflict of interest with its instructors, faculty, planners, and other individuals who are in a position to control the content of CME activities. All relevant conflicts of interest that are identified are thoroughly vetted by EOCME for fair balance, scientific objectivity, and patient care recommendations. EOCME is committed to providing its learners with CME activities that promote improvements or quality in healthcare and not a specific proprietary business or a commercial interest.

The planning committee, staff, authors, and editors listed below have identified no financial relationships or relationships to products or devices they or their spouse/life partner have with commercial interest related to the content of this CME activity:

Kanhai Amin; Roger Apple, PhD; Orhan Atay, MD; Brittany N. Barber Garcia, PhD; Nicholas Beam, MD; Katherine Tennant Beenen, PhD; Bethelhem Belachew, MA; Swati Y. Bhave, MD DCH FCPS FIAP FAAP (HON); Ayse Bulan, MD; Summer Chahin, MA; Ethel Gonzales Clemente, MD; Jennie David, PhD; Cheryl Dickson, MD, MPH; Ronald Espinal, MD, FAAP; Marissa A. Feldman, PhD; William S. Frye, PhD, ABPP; Lauren Gardner, PhD, ABPP; Mark G. Goetting, MD, FAASM, DBSM, FACLM; Jason Hangauer, PhD; Mariam Ischander, MBChB; Olga Jablonka, PhD; Judy Jasser, MBBS; Manmohan K. Kamboj, MD; Shibani Kanungo, MD, MPH; Christina Limke, PsyD; Sheryl Lozowski-Sullivan, MPH, PhD; Rajkumar Mayakrishnan, BSc, MBA; Ami Mehta, MD; Diana Milojevic, MD; Vincent J. Palusci, MD, MS; Dilip R. Patel, MBBS, MBA, MPH; Priyal Patel, BS; Keshav Patel, MD, MS; Amy Pugh, PsyD; Vimal Master Sankar Raj, MD; Samir R. Shah, MB, DCH; Anuradha V. Sovani, MA, MPhil, PhD; Doreen Thomas-Payne, MSN, BSN, RN, PMHNP-BC; Toni Whitaker, MD, FAAP; Katie White, MA; Heather L. Yardley, PhD

UNAPPROVED/OFF-LABEL USE DISCLOSURE

The EOCME requires CME faculty to disclose to the participants:

1. When products or procedures being discussed are off-label, unlabelled, experimental, and/or investigational (not US Food and Drug Administration [FDA] approved); and
2. Any limitations on the information presented, such as data that are preliminary or that represent ongoing research, interim analyses, and/or unsupported opinions. Faculty may discuss information about pharmaceutical agents that is outside of FDA-approved labelling. This information is intended solely for CME and is not intended to promote off-label use of these medications. If you have any questions, contact the medical affairs department of the manufacturer for the most recent prescribing information.

TO ENROLL

To enroll in the *Pediatric Clinics of North America* Continuing Medical Education program, call customer service at 1-800-654-2452 or sign up online at http://www.theclinics.com/home/cme. The CME program is available to subscribers for an additional annual fee of USD 324.00.

METHOD OF PARTICIPATION

In order to claim credit, participants must complete the following:

1. Complete enrolment as indicated above.
2. Read the activity.
3. Complete the CME Test and Evaluation. Participants must achieve a score of 70% on the test. All CME Tests and Evaluations must be completed online.

In order to claim MOC points, participants must complete the following:

1. Complete steps listed above for claiming CME credit
2. Provide your specialty board ID#, birth date (MM/DD), and attestation.
3. Online MOC submission is only available for the American Board of pediatrics' (ABP) Maintenance of Certification (MOC) program

CME INQUIRIES/SPECIAL NEEDS

For all CME inquiries or special needs, please contact elsevierCME@elsevier.com

Contributors

CONSULTING EDITOR

BONITA F. STANTON, MD[†]
Professor of Pediatrics and Founding Dean, Robert C. and Laura C. Garrett Endowed
Chair, Hackensack Meridian School of Medicine, President, Academic Enterprise,
Hackensack Meridian Health, Nutley, New Jersey, USA

EDITORS

ROGER W. APPLE, PhD
Associate Professor, Chief, Division of Pediatric Psychology, Director, WMed Pediatric
Autism Center, Department of Pediatric and Adolescent Medicine, Western Michigan
University Homer Stryker M.D. School of Medicine, Kalamazoo, Michigan, USA

ETHEL G. CLEMENTE, MD
Pediatric Endocrinology, Valley Children's Healthcare, Madera, California, USA; Clinical
Assistant Professor, Division of Pediatric Endocrinology, Department of Pediatric and
Adolescent Medicine, Western Michigan University Homer Stryker M.D. School of
Medicine, Kalamazoo, Michigan, USA

AUTHORS

KANHAI AMIN
Department of Molecular, Cellular, and Developmental Biology, Yale University,
New Haven, Connecticut, USA

ROGER W. APPLE, PhD
Associate Professor, Chief, Division of Pediatric Psychology, Director, WMed Pediatric
Autism Center, Department of Pediatric and Adolescent Medicine, Western Michigan
University Homer Stryker M.D. School of Medicine, Kalamazoo, Michigan, USA

ORHAN ATAY, MD
Director, Neurogastroenterology Motility Program, Division of Pediatric Gastroenterology,
Children's Hospital of The King's Daughters, Associate Professor, Eastern Virginia
Medical School, Norfolk, Virginia, USA

BRITTANY N. BARBER GARCIA, PhD
Spectrum Health Helen DeVos Children's Hospital, Pediatric Behavioral Medicine, College
of Human Medicine, Michigan State University, Grand Rapids, Michigan, USA

NICHOLAS BEAM, MD
College of Human Medicine, Michigan State University, Spectrum Health, Office of
Graduate Medical Education, Grand Rapids, Michigan, USA

KATHERINE T. BEENEN, PhD
Department of Pediatric and Adolescent Medicine, Western Michigan University Homer Stryker M.D. School of Medicine, Kalamazoo, Michigan, USA

BETHELHEM BELACHEW, MA
Division of Pediatric Psychology, Western Michigan University Homer Stryker M.D. School of Medicine, Kalamazoo, Michigan, USA

SWATI Y. BHAVE, MD, DCH, FCPS, FIAP, FAAP (HON)
Adjunct Professor in Adolescent Medicine, Dr. D.Y Patil Medical College, Pimpri, India; Dr. D.Y. Patil Vidyapeeth, Pune, India; Executive Director, Association of Adolescent and Child Care in India (AACCI), Mumbai, India

AYSE BULAN, MD
Section of Endocrinology, Department of Pediatrics, Nationwide Children's Hospital, The Ohio State University, Columbus, Ohio, USA

SUMMER CHAHIN, MA
Western Michigan University, Western Michigan University Homer Stryker M.D. School of Medicine, Kalamazoo, Michigan, USA; St. Jude Children's Research Hospital, Memphis, Tennessee, USA

JENNIE DAVID, PhD
Pediatric Psychology and Neuropsychology, Assistant Professor, Department of Pediatrics, Nationwide Children's Hospital, The Ohio State University College of Medicine, Columbus, Ohio, USA

CHERYL DICKSON, MD, MPH
Western Michigan University Homer Stryker M.D. School of Medicine, Kalamazoo, Michigan, USA

RONALD ESPINAL, MD, FAAP
University of Tennessee Health Science Center, Center on Developmental Disabilities, Memphis, Tennessee, USA

MARISSA A. FELDMAN, PhD
Department of Psychology, Johns Hopkins All Children's Hospital, St Petersburg, Florida, USA

WILLIAM S. FRYE, PhD, BCB, ABPP
Department of Psychology, Johns Hopkins All Children's Hospital, St Petersburg, Florida, USA

LAUREN GARDNER, PhD, ABPP
Johns Hopkins All Children's Hospital, St Petersburg, Florida, USA

MARK G. GOETTING, MD, FAASM, DBSM, FACLM
Associate Professor, Diplomate, Behavioral Sleep Medicine, Department of Pediatric and Adolescent Medicine, Department of Medicine, Center for Clinical Research, Western Michigan University Homer Stryker M.D, School of Medicine, Kalamazoo, Michigan, USA

JASON HANGAUER, PhD
Johns Hopkins All Children's Hospital, St Petersburg, Florida, USA

MARIAM ISCHANDER, MBChB
Department of Pediatric and Adolescent Medicine, Division of Pulmonology and Sleep Medicine, Western Michigan University Homer Stryker M.D. School of Medicine, Kalamazoo, Michigan, USA

OLGA JABLONKA, PhD
Clinical Assistant Professor, Department of Child and Adolescent Psychiatry, NYU Grossman School of Medicine, New York, New York, USA

JUDY JASSER, MBBS
Department of Pediatric and Adolescent Medicine, Western Michigan University Homer Stryker M.D. School of Medicine, Kalamazoo, Michigan, USA

MANMOHAN K. KAMBOJ, MD
Section of Endocrinology, Department of Pediatrics, Nationwide Children's Hospital, The Ohio State University, Columbus, Ohio, USA

SHIBANI KANUNGO, MD, MPH, FAAP, FACMG
Associate Professor, Department of Pediatric and Adolescent Medicine, Department of Medical Ethics, Humanities and Law, Western Michigan University Homer Stryker M.D. School of Medicine, Kalamazoo, Michigan, USA

CHRISTINA LIMKE, PsyD
Spectrum Health Helen DeVos Children's Hospital, Pediatric Behavioral Medicine, College of Human Medicine, Michigan State University, Grand Rapids, Michigan, USA

SHERYL LOZOWSKI-SULLIVAN, MPH, PhD
Department of Pediatric and Adolescent Medicine, Division of Psychology, Western Michigan University Homer Stryker M.D. School of Medicine, Kalamazoo, Michigan, USA

AMI MEHTA, MD
Pediatric Pain and Palliative Care, Children's Hospital of The King's Daughters, Norfolk, Virginia, USA

DIANA MILOJEVIC, MD
Department of Medicine, Johns Hopkins All Children's Hospital, St Petersburg, Florida, USA

VINCENT J. PALUSCI, MD, MS
Professor, Department of Pediatrics, NYU Grossman School of Medicine, New York, New York, USA

DILIP R. PATEL, MBBS, MBA, MPH
Department of Pediatric and Adolescent Medicine, Western Michigan University Homer Stryker M.D. School of Medicine, Kalamazoo, Michigan, USA

KESHAV PATEL, MD, MS
Department of Internal Medicine, University of Illinois College of Medicine, University of Illinois at Chicago, Chicago, Illinois, USA

PRIYAL PATEL, BS
Bradley University, Peoria, Illinois, USA

AMY PUGH, PsyD
Spectrum Health Helen DeVos Children's Hospital, Pediatric Behavioral Medicine, College of Human Medicine, Michigan State University, Grand Rapids, Michigan, USA

VIMAL MASTER SANKAR RAJ, MD
Associate Professor of Clinical Pediatrics, Division Head, Pediatric Nephrology, University of Illinois College of Medicine, Peoria, Illinois, USA

SAMIR R. SHAH, MB, DCH
Consultant Paediatrician, Samir Hospital & Narahari Hospital, Vadodara, India; Samir Hospital, Lakdikapul, Hyderabad, India

ANURADHA V. SOVANI, MA, MPhil, PhD (Psychology)
Professor and Head, Department of Psychology, Dean, Faculty of Humanities, SNDT Women's University, Mumbai, Maharashtra, India

TONI WHITAKER, MD, FAAP
University of Tennessee Health Science Center, Center on Developmental Disabilities, Memphis, Tennessee, USA

KATIE WHITE, MA
Division of Pediatric Psychology, Assistant Professor, Western Michigan University Homer Stryker M.D. School of Medicine, Kalamazoo, Michigan, USA

HEATHER L. YARDLEY, PhD
Department of Pediatric Psychology and Neuropsychology, Nationwide Children's Hospital, Columbus, Ohio, USA

Contents

Physicians have a lot of information to cover in a short amount of time. Over time, this creates burnout and compassion fatigue for physicians. However, psychologists are trained and have a unique skillset they can use to help decrease some of these difficulties. This article is an introduction to the general roles of psychologists and some of their unique responsibilities. The other sections in this article will dive into more specific psychological services for medical specialties.

This article addresses, in more general terms, the overarching concepts of the role of integrated psychologists and how their services are incorporated in the medical home with the use of provider consultation, administering assessments in identifying common mental health concerns, providing interventions for treatment adherence and providing short-term therapy within pediatric subspecialties.

Pediatric cancer and hematological disorders affect a significant number of children and their families each year. The most impactful and effective patient care involves collaboration of medical providers and psychosocial services. Psychologists have a significant role on a patient's care team and can provide a multitude of services including brief intervention, psychotherapy, assessments, consultation, and additional support to the rest of the team.

Adolescent Medicine addresses the health care of adolescents, young adults, and their families. Adolescent psychology constitutes an important part. The COVID-19 pandemic has given insight into adolescent needs, bringing the focus on prevention rather than mere correction. One needs to factor in the unique aspects of adolescence, their need to impress peers and gain acceptance, and their unique information processing, not calculating trade-offs between risk and reward the way adults might, in a linear, rational, logical, and verbal manner. The article focuses on the need for collaborative training among the various stakeholders in Child and Adolescent Mental Health.

Kanhai Amin and Keshav Patel

Congenital heart disease (CHD) is stressful to both pediatric patients and their caregivers. Maternal anxiety during pregnancy is associated with adverse perinatal outcomes. After birth, a prolonged hospital stay can be taxing on the infant and caregiver leading to long-term adverse effects. During adolescence, CHD continues to serve as a stressor for the child not only due to medical care but also due to social limitations and bullying. Many patients also struggle during the transition from adolescence to adult care. Psychologists may aid both the parents and child at all stages from pregnancy to the child's transition to adulthood.

Olga Jablonka and Vincent J. Palusci

This article describes the extent of the problem and the medical evaluation of child maltreatment, focusing on the outpatient interdisciplinary assessment of suspected child physical and sexual abuse. Separate from their role as clinicians, the roles of the child psychologist before, during, and after the medical assessment are highlighted. The child psychologist is an important member of the interdisciplinary team who helps the team prepare for the evaluation (before), assists in screening and determining immediate psychological safety during the medical evaluation (during), and communicating the need for further treatment and follow-up (after).

Lauren Gardner, Jason Hangauer, Toni Whitaker, and Ronald Espinal

Providing high-quality clinical services to patients with neurodevelopmental disabilities (NDDs) requires interprofessional collaboration. This article highlights the importance of collaboration between psychology and developmental-behavioral pediatrics (DBP) to promote diagnosis, treatment recommendations, and integrated care for patients and their families. Interprofessional collaboration requires health care providers to work together toward solutions, including diagnosis, treatment recommendations, and ongoing care coordination. Case examples are presented to capture collaborative practice between psychology and DBP. Several established programs for providing interprofessional collaboration are highlighted, with noted benefits and barriers to collaborative care for NDD patients.

Marissa A. Feldman, Heather L. Yardley, Ayse Bulan, and Manmohan K. Kamboj

The care of youth managed within pediatric endocrine clinics is complex and requires a multi- or interdisciplinary approach. Psychosocial aspects of chronic health conditions are well-documented. Clinical practice guidelines outline the importance of routine psychosocial screening and support for youth with diabetes and obesity. This article outlines the diverse role of psychologists in pediatric endocrinology, including screening, in-clinic intervention, outpatient psychological services, and inpatient consultation. Although research exists documenting the effectiveness of behavioral interventions to improve adherence and health-related quality of life, cost analysis research is emerging.

Irritable bowel syndrome (IBS) can have a substantial impact on the physical, academic, and psychosocial functioning of pediatric patients. As a functional gastrointestinal disorder, pediatric patients with IBS are thought to benefit from a multidisciplinary approach to target the biopsychosocial factors of this condition. In this co-authored article by a Pediatric Gastroenterologist, Pediatric Pain and Palliative Care specialist and Pediatric GI Psychologist, we present a hypothetical case of a pediatric patient who will undergo evaluation and treatment by each of these specialists demonstrating how a collaborative effort amongst multidisciplinary specialists is the ideal approach to care.

The authors review the multiple roles of the pediatric psychologist in hospital medicine practice, which is commonly referred to as pediatric consultation-liaison (CL) psychology. A brief history of development of training of CL psychologists is discussed as well as current models of practice. The authors describe specific populations that CL psychologists assist in managing when hospitalized as well as how the CL psychologist can contribute to health care systems and public policy advocacy. Physicians are encouraged to request the services of pediatric CL psychologists to help promote psychological adjustment, coping, and well-being in hospitalized youth.

Renal disease in pediatric patients tends to have a broad clinical spectrum from milder disease to severe progressive renal dysfunction requiring renal replacement therapy. Patients with chronic kidney disease (CKD) can have additional comorbidities including hypertension, diabetes, and obesity, which can add to the disease burden. The psychosocial or the mental component of the pediatric CKD patient is often overlooked by health care professionals due to a lack of resources and training in identifying psychological disorders. In addition, many components of kidney disease like fatigue from anemia and cognitive impairment make it difficult for the untrained physician to identify underlying psychological disorders. This review explores the complex psychosocial issues in patients with kidney disease and the need of more comprehensive multidisciplinary approach for treatment.

Metabolic disorders or inborn errors of metabolism (IEMs) can have a wide range of neurodevelopmental and behavioral presentations. These can vary with age and/or management or stressors from common childhood/intercurrent illnesses/procedures/interventions. Collaborative care models such as multidisciplinary metabolic clinics or colocated models with behavioral health clinics and metabolic clinics in the same location can be valuable resources in improving long-term outcomes in patients with IEM. Psychologists' expertise using behavioral interventions, screening, or adaptive/cognitive measures can help with diagnosis, treatment adherence, school performance, family support, community resources, transition to adolescence and young adulthood using health belief concepts to improve outcomes.

PEDIATRIC CLINICS OF NORTH AMERICA

SERIES OF RELATED INTEREST

Critical Care Clinics of North America
www.criticalcare.theclinics.com

THE CLINICS ARE AVAILABLE ONLINE!
Access your subscription at:
www.theclinics.com

Preface

Role of Psychologists in Pediatric Subspecialties

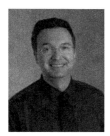 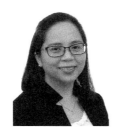

Roger W. Apple, PhD   Ethel G. Clemente, MD

Editors

Psychologists are essential in pediatric subspecialties. The COVID-19 pandemic, current mental health crisis for children and adolescents, and an abundance of data highlighting the vast amount of mental health concerns in medical practice overwhelmingly support the need for psychologists in pediatric subspecialties. In addition, for the increasing numbers of medical providers and medical centers focusing on health equity and reducing health care disparities, providing psychological care to their patients is essential. This issue of the *Pediatric Clinics of North America* takes an in-depth look at the role of psychologists across 14 pediatric subspecialties.

Patients in pediatric subspecialty clinics often experience comorbid medical and psychological conditions often requiring the expertise of specialty-trained medical providers and specialty-trained psychological providers who understand the complexities of the mind/body connection. This complexity of clinical presentation necessitates having "in-house" specialty-trained psychologists who work collaboratively with the pediatric subspecialty providers. Referring out to another location for psychological services is quite problematic for several reasons: finding specialty-trained psychologists within local communities can be very difficult, and those that are working in the community often have full caseloads and waiting lists and often do not take all insurance plans. Referring out also significantly limits the collaboration between psychologist and physician that is often critical for patients in pediatric subspecialties.

Improved outcomes can also result from psychologists working in pediatric subspecialties. For example, psychologists can help adolescents with diabetes improve treatment adherence, which can result in improved A1c and help to avoid costly hospitalizations. Patients in pediatric subspecialties also often have complex psychosocial factors impacting their medical care that the medical providers often do not have the time nor the amount of expertise as psychologists to adequately address. Having

Pediatr Clin N Am 69 (2022) xv–xvi
https://doi.org/10.1016/j.pcl.2022.08.005
0031-3955/22/© 2022 Published by Elsevier Inc.

psychologists in pediatric subspecialty clinics will provide an opportunity to address these complex needs while allowing the physician to manage the medical concerns and keep up with the pace of the clinic.

This issue of *Pediatric Clinics of North America* focusing on the role of psychologists in multiple pediatric subspecialties will provide a wealth of information that will shine a spotlight on the fact that psychologists are essential in pediatric subspecialties. Fully integrating psychologists into pediatric subspecialties will provide not only improved medical care but also whole person care. This integration will work toward providing health equity, reduce health care disparities, and lessen the bias toward psychology by improving the understanding that psychology is an essential part of medical care.

Roger W. Apple, PhD
Western Michigan University
Homer Stryker MD School of Medicine
Department of Pediatric & Adolescent Medicine
Division of Pediatric Psychology
1000 Oakland Drive
Kalamazoo, MI 49008, USA

Ethel G. Clemente, MD
2028 Waterfall Court
Modesto, CA 95355, USA

E-mail addresses:
roger.apple@med.wmich.edu (R.W. Apple)
ECLemente@valleychildrens.org (E.G. Clemente)

Helping Physicians Collaborate with Psychologists

Summer Chahin, PhD[a],*, Roger W. Apple, PhD[b],
Cheryl Dickson, MD, MPH[b]

KEYWORDS

- Psychology • Multidisciplinary • Collaboration • Communication • Interdisciplinary

KEY POINTS

- Health care goes beyond the biomedical care of an individual and includes behavioral and psychosocial factors as well, and the interaction of these factors facilitates a higher understanding of neurotypical behavior versus dysfunction.
- Psychologists have specialized training to further facilitate conversations and patient care related to behavioral, cognitive, and mood concerns.
- Collaborative multidisciplinary care is imperative for patient care, stress-reduction for physicians, and reducing mental health stigma.

INTRODUCTION

Leon Eisenberg was a leading figure in psychiatry. He believed that beyond just the inclusion of biological science and chemistry, the practice of medicine should include other factors such as psychosocial considerations and the patient-provider interactions.[1] There is a particular importance in integrating behavioral, biomedical, and psychosocial factors in the understanding of how the brain works. Further, understanding the way these factors interact helps providers better understand normal behaviors from dysfunction.[2] Thus, psychologists should play a significant role in the integrative approach. Unfortunately, for many providers in medicine, the role of psychologists is unclear. This article further aims to illustrate the many roles psychologists can play in medicine.

[a] Western Michigan University, Western Michigan University Homer Stryker M.D. School of Medicine, St. Jude Children's Research Hospital, 1000 Oakland Drive, Kalamazoo, MI 49008-1284, USA; [b] Western Michigan University Homer Stryker M.D. School of Medicine, 1000 Oakland Drive, Kalamazoo, MI 49008-1284, USA
* Corresponding author.
E-mail addresses: summer.s.chahin@wmich.edu; summer.chahin@gmail.com

Pediatr Clin N Am 69 (2022) 819–823
https://doi.org/10.1016/j.pcl.2022.06.002
0031-3955/22/© 2022 Elsevier Inc. All rights reserved.

pediatric.theclinics.com

THE ROLE OF PSYCHOLOGISTS

One potential area psychologists may be able to assist medical providers is the provision of short- or long-term therapy services. For example, a psychologist may provide individual services to treat behavioral concerns and learn emotion regulation techniques or coping strategies for a variety of concerns. In other situations, a psychologist may provide family services, which can be beneficial to help with parent–child interactions or help parents manage behavioral concerns more effectively.

Furthermore, psychologists can be helpful to medical providers in working with patients on health-related behaviors and lifestyle changes such as smoking cessation and medical adherence. Psychologists have special training in human behavior and can use these principles to work with patients to improve these areas in their life, as well as help medical providers save time in their busy day-to-day schedules. One strategy psychologists can be engaged when working with these providers is by implementing motivational interviewing (MI) strategies.

MI is a technique used to instill motivation in an individual. Originally, MI was implemented with individuals who abuse substances and other health-related concerns such as medication compliance. The principles behind MI help providers get a better sense of what is happening in their client's lives. Using this framework allows patients to have a safe space to discuss their barriers to change their behavior, which further creates a stronger patient-provider alliance. The foundational skills of MI are open-ended questions, affirmations, reflective listening, and summarizing. Another key component involves eliciting change talk from the patient. This component refers to the process of helping the patient to express thoughts and illicit behaviors that are in the direction of making positive changes, which is especially helpful when clients are ambivalent.

Chronic pain is a common presenting concern made to physicians. Psychologists can assist physicians with these presenting concerns by providing non-pharmacological pain management strategies to patients. Psychological providers are equipped to provide psychoeducation around pain and help teach patients strategies such as breathing techniques, progressive muscle relaxation, guided imagery, mindfulness, and cognitive restructuring. Physician and psychologist collaboration with this presenting concern also helps lessen the burden of adding extra medications to a patient's regimen and decreases the physician's future time spent on medication management as well.

Moreover, psychologists are also unique in the sense that they are the only profession to have training in the administration, scoring, and interpretation of behavioral and psychological assessments. Although, these assessments are time-consuming, they provide a significant amount of data and information that can help physicians make decisions about medications and psychosocial care for a patient. Psychologists also work closely with developmental–behavioral pediatricians to help assess for developmental concerns as well. One part of these longer full assessments is a clinical interview, which psychologists have special clinical training to conduct, as well as the time to conduct the interviews. This helps the care team gather more information to make better overall decisions for patient care.

However, as these full assessments can be involved and time-consuming, psychologists can also gather information more quickly through the use of shorter screeners and clinical judgment. Further, psychologists are trained to conduct full risk assessments for suicidal and homicidal ideation. Psychologists are able to step in when these thoughts are reported to conduct the assessment and create a safety plan, which also helps physicians save time by having a well-trained mental health professional focus on this aspect of patient care.

These are just some of the areas psychologists can help. Psychologists are also trained to help in areas such as sleep, pill swallowing, care of adolescents, cardiology care, child abuse, developmental–behavioral pediatrics, endocrinology concerns, gastroenterology difficulties, pediatric hospital medicine, nephrology, pulmonology, rheumatology, sports medicine, metabolic disorders, and many other areas. The following sections will dive into these areas.

ADVANTAGES TO PHYSICIAN AND PSYCHOLOGIST COLLABORATION

There are several advantages to physicians choosing to work with psychologists. This section highlights a few key advantages. Collaborative care between physicians and psychologists allows for providers to be readily accessible to each other for consultation in the moment. Additionally, having quick and easy access to the other provider allows for smooth transitions between care and for more warm handoffs to occur. Warm handoffs allow for the physician to introduce the psychologist and show their respect and trust in the psychology provider. This helps build rapport between the patient and providers and creates a stronger professional relationship between the physician and psychologist. Further, collaboration between physicians and psychologists allows all health care to be taken care of in one location and during one appointment. This saves time and space on other days as well. Among the advantages to collaborative care between physicians and psychologists is breaking down social barriers and stigma, identifying creative solutions to patient care, prevents frustration between providers, prevents physician and provider burnout, and helps reduce compassion fatigue.[3]

BARRIERS TO COLLABORATIVE CARE

Despite all of the advantages to collaboration between psychologists and physicians, there are a few barriers to be aware of that can be overcome. For example, differences in training can play a role in the success of the collaborative partnership. Recently, medical residents have had at least some interaction with psychology during their residency training. The level of exposure to the other field varies in training, so that allowing each provider the space to describe their role and the unique care they can provide is useful. Additionally, being willing to hear what providers can do can help physicians and psychologists be more effective and efficient.

Further, it is especially important to be willing to listen to feedback and engage in effective problem-solving. This can be done through perspective taking, but also by setting expectations and guidelines about communication, care, and clinic flow from the start. Another barrier that one may come across is the proximity between physicians and psychologists. There are clinics and hospitals that use more of a colocated model where psychologists are in the same building but on a different floor or in a different building. This is not as an effective model and creates barriers to access and a less efficient workflow. However, finding ways to incorporate physicians and psychologists into the same area, so that each provider is accessible helps overcome this obstacle.

Another potential barrier is the rules around reimbursement.[4] Billing codes can be difficult to understand and figure out. It helps to spend time learning which codes are the best for billing psychological services in a medical setting. Additionally, mental health can still be taboo to discuss at times. Owing to this, patients may be resistant to psychological care. However, incorporating psychological services into follow-up care, regular care visits, and specialty care visits helps decrease the stigma and normalize discussing these concerns. In creating a safe space to discuss mental health concerns, providers are increasing the care received in an appointment and decreasing additional appointments in the future and decrease time spent overall.

KEYS TO SUCCESSFUL COLLABORATION

Collaborative care is an art and can take some time to work through the barriers and challenges to a successful practice. Additionally, members of a care team receive different training and it can be difficult to communicate differences in specialties and training. However, there are several key components to a successful collaboration between physicians and psychologists. Psychologists and physicians spent many years in school learning as much as they could to be effective in their careers. Professionals should be mindful of different styles in practice and communication and find a balance in how to communicate effectively with different professionals. It helps to have open communication, willingness to ask questions, and willingness to learn and educate.

In addition, a provider in a collaborative professional relationship should be willing to expand their expertise. Professionals in the medical and allied-health fields are lifelong learners and should be open to learning from other members of the care team. This allows for trust to grow between providers on a team. In the same realm, keeping the lines of communication open on a team is important. It is particularly important for psychologists and physicians to stay in contact and provide necessary information to each other. This constant contact allows for continuity of care and decreases the amount of information that is lost. Further, providers should remember to always keep patient information confidential during these conversations. Providers should ensure they are only looping in necessary care members and speaking in private.

TRUE COLLABORATION VERSUS HIERARCHICAL PROFESSIONAL RELATIONSHIPS

True collaboration between physicians and psychologists is essential for having the most impact on patient care. A colocated model is not effective in creating a collaborative environment between providers and care team members. Rather, using a true collaborative care model allows for greater interdisciplinary and coordinated care. A fully integrated model implies that mental health is part of overall health and creates an open environment for patients to have all their needs met in one place.

SUMMARY

Overall, the integration of psychology into the medical field is beneficial. The benefits include the reduction of stress for physicians, increase in time to spend on more severe presenting concerns and other tasks, continuity of care, a colocated care for all medical needs, and the further expansion of services.

CLINICS CARE POINTS

- Advantages to interdisciplinary health care have been found to prevent burnout, create cohesive health care teams, break down barriers and stigma, foster creative solutions for patient care, and open colocated patient care.[3]
- Barriers to interdisciplinary care include difficulties with reimbursement and billing codes.[4]
- Keys to successful interdisciplinary collaboration include open communication, willingness to ask questions, willingness to teach and learning, and willingness to expand expertise.[3,4]

DISCLOSURE

The authors report no conflicts of interest or connection with any funding sources.

REFERENCES

1. Eisenberg L. Is psychiatry more mindful or brainier than it was a decade ago? Br J Psychiatry 2000;176:1–5.
2. Wahass SH. The role of psychologists in health care delivery. J Fam Community Med 2005;12:2.
3. Holleman WI, Bray JH, Davis L, et al. Innovative ways to address the mental health and medical needs of marginalized patients: Collaborations between family physicians, family therapists, and family psychologists. Am J Orthopsychiatry 2004;74: 242–52.
4. Kainz K. Barriers and enhancements to physician psychologist collaboration. Prof Res Pract 2002;33:169–75.

Role of Psychologists in Pediatric Subspecialties
Integrated Psychological Services Overarching Concepts Across Pediatric Subspecialties

Katie White, MA*, Bethelhem Belachew, MA

KEYWORDS

- Integrated psychologists • Assessment • Short-term therapy • Interventions
- Pediatric subspecialty care

KEY POINTS

- Children with chronic conditions are at an increased risk of developing mental health conditions compared with their typically developing peers.
- Comorbid psychological and behavioral symptoms can exacerbate a patient's medical concerns.
- Integrated psychologists can provide collaboration, consultation, assessment, treatment adherence, and short-term therapy to support patients in subspecialty care.
- These services can promote better quality of life and outcome for patients with chronic conditions.

INTRODUCTION

Psychologists, the services they provide, and their integration within the medical model are a critical role in the medical field as a whole and are essential in 2 areas of pediatric practice: one that encompasses children with chronic conditions and one that includes children within the primary care setting.[1] Often a child's primary care and/or pediatric subspecialty provider are the gateway to identifying several mental health concerns.[2] Studies have suggested the following: individuals with mental health conditions and substance abuse issues will likely surpass physical health problems, 50% of serious mental health disorders emerge by age 14 years, and 20% of children have a mental health condition that is diagnosable, and mental health disorders affect 1 in 5 children.[3–5]

Division of Pediatric Psychology, Western Michigan University School of Medicine, 1000 Oakland Drive, Kalamazoo, MI 49008, USA
* Corresponding author.
E-mail address: Kathryn.white@med.wmich.edu

Pediatr Clin N Am 69 (2022) 825–837
https://doi.org/10.1016/j.pcl.2022.06.003
0031-3955/22/© 2022 Elsevier Inc. All rights reserved.

Chronic conditions, injuries, and/or illness that require subspecialty care can span from children with lifelong medical conditions that have been present since birth (ie, down syndrome) to those that may develop later in childhood (ie, adolescent diabetes, cancer) to children who may require subspecialty care after a trauma (ie, substantial injuries as a result of a car crash). Children with chronic conditions have a prevailing need for the collaboration between physician and psychologist due to the complexity in the care that they require including multidimensional symptoms that in turn impair a child's overall functioning and its inevitable impact on the family system.[4] Further, those with chronic conditions have an increased risk of experiencing anxiety, depression, and suicidal ideation compared with typically developing peers, which is also true for their caregivers whom have similar elevations in trauma, anxiety, and depression when caring for a child with special needs.[6–8] In addition, when comorbid mental health symptoms exist, but go unidentified or untreated, the cost of managing a chronic condition increases significantly.[9]

These statistics that highlight the likelihood of a person developing or experiencing mental health symptoms along with the increased risk when a chronic medical condition is introduced stresses the importance of integrating psychologists across pediatric subspecialties. This article addresses, in more general terms, the overarching concepts of the role of integrated psychologists and how their services are incorporated in the medical home with the use of provider consultation and collaboration, administering assessments in identifying common mental health concerns, providing interventions for treatment adherence, and providing short-term therapy within pediatric subspecialties.

ROLE OF INTEGRATED PSYCHOLOGISTS

Psychology allows for training to incorporate expertise in not only identifying and working with individuals whom have behavior and emotional concerns but also on how to provide services to promote health, prevent disease, and work with patients with chronic conditions and neurodevelopmental disorders.[2] The role of a psychologist within a medical environment is similar across settings wherein they administer screening and assessment tools, provide interventions, consult with families and physicians, and provide education on prevention.[1] However, these roles can become medically specific to address the patient's needs within their particular subspecialty environment. For example, a psychologist can provide adherence to medical regimens, be a liaison between the family and school to ensure the child is receiving adequate academic and social interventions, and help physicians identify learning and developmental patterns that may be affected by their medical diagnosis.[1] Further, they can address behaviors that may affect outcomes, provide care that encompasses medication consistency, help with alternate ways to manage pain, and introduce ways to improve quality of life.[9]

INTEGRATED PSYCHOLOGIST CONSULTATION AND COLLABORATION

A psychologist within the pediatric population has a consulting and collaboration role that can span across many different connections: physician, patient, family, and school. Not only does this population of children with chronic conditions have an increased risk of emotional and behavioral problems than their peers but they also have unique medical needs that can place an increase strain on their caregivers.[7] This setting can be ideal for an integrated psychologist to provide consultation and co-ordination of a child's medical, mental health and access to community care resources to help the child and their family navigate the illness and all that it encompasses.[2] Further, the integrated psychologist can add a unique perspective to the medical provider by helping them understand how human factors can affect medical needs (ie, treatment adherence).[2]

Most of the children see their primary care physician each year for a variety of reasons, with estimates that nearly 20% of the childhood population has a special health care need that may require subspecialty care[10]; this provides an environment that is ideal for the assessment, identification, intervention, and/or prevention of behavioral and mental health concerns; however, in the same breath, medical providers whom they come in contact with typically lack the time, confidence, training, and expertise to address such issues.[2] Bright Futures Guidelines, which are endorsed by the American Academy of Pediatrics, were developed to address and provide procedures on ensuring physicians are providing optimal medical care and meeting the patient's needs within pediatrics with topics also encompassing ways to manage mental health concerns.[2,10] These guidelines gave credence to the need for integrated psychologists. When psychologists are integrated in the primary and/or subspecialty environment, they are available for quick consultations with providers in real time. For example, a psychologist can provide the physician with tactics on ways to clarify or gather additional information regarding concerns, provide strategies to facilitate changes in a desired behavior, provide recommendations on appropriate treatment, and collaborate with the medical team in developing a treatment plan to help manage a patient's chronic condition.[9] Lastly, incorporating psychologists into subspecialty care can decrease the cost of care by reducing the frequency of in-person visits and hospitalizations.[9]

Chronic illness can put a toll on a caregiver's mental health, and studies have shown that they tend to have higher levels of anxiety and depression than parents of typically developing children.[7] However, it is not uncommon for their needs to be overlooked and neglected, causing them to become the "invisible patient."[8] Because parents tend to accompany their child to appointments, there is ample opportunity for providers to screen for possible concerns.[8] If concerns are identified, integrated psychologists can provide information on interventions and community support for caregivers to address their own mental health concerns.[8] Providing this level of support can decrease caregiver stress and provide caregivers with tools to support their child's illness, all of which can promote positive outcomes for the patients' health and a better quality of life for all involved.[7,8]

Integrated psychologists can be a liaison with the school system to help ensure a child is obtaining the correct support to address any medical needs, academic, and/or adaptive delays in this environment. Studies suggests that anywhere between 10% and 30% of children in the educational system have a chronic condition.[11] These patients may have unique academic needs as a result of their chronic condition such as support to address intellectual disabilities, specific learning disorders, and the increase in mood and/or emotional symptoms. Further, they have unique medical needs such as medications they need to take during the school day, an increase in medical appointments, and the need to use certain medical devices to address their medical concerns. All of this can be difficult for both physicians and educators to navigate.[11] Psychologists have the training in problem solving, assessing, consulting, shared decision-making, and monitoring progress that can be a vital in the success of not only the medical needs of the child but also the academic and emotional needs by providing collaboration across and between settings.[11]

PSYCHOLOGICAL ASSESSMENT

As mentioned earlier, individuals with chronic medical conditions are at a higher risk of developing mental health symptoms, such as depression, than their peers, yet are less likely to be screened during medical appointments.[12] The foundation for delivering appropriate services comes from the ability to provide an accurate assessment of a patient's symptoms.[13] The pediatric population as a whole can be tricky to work with because in order to render an accurate diagnosis, the provider must gather data from multiple people and settings to differentiate current and prior level of functioning.[13] Psychologists have the unique training that allows them to administer and interpret assessments that can be used to identify various mental health conditions. These assessments are typically used to clarify a presenting problem by first using tools that assesses for a broad range of symptoms and then moving onto more specific ones as deemed necessary from the results to help narrow down a diagnosis, all of which can help guide treatment and intervention.[13,14] **Table 1** provides a list of assessments that psychologists can use to evaluate common mental health concerns; this can be a difficult task for physicians to complete, as they typically do not have the luxury of time within the appointment to administer the tools or in gathering and integrating information from multiple resources to aid in an accurate diagnosis and likely do not have the expertise, training, and/or comfort level to interpret the results.[5,13]

Within pediatrics the most common mental health concerns that are presented include attention deficit hyperactivity disorder, depression, anxiety, obesity, substance use, bullying, school violence, and Internet safety.[9] More concerning is that children with chronic health conditions are more likely to attempt and/or complete suicide than those without a medical problem.[15] In mental health, it is not uncommon for mental health symptoms to overlap multiple diagnoses, which can make it difficult to discern an appropriate and accurate diagnosis. Because of this, integrated psychologists can provide quick assessment tools to narrow down a diagnosis and in turn provide suggestions on appropriate interventions and services.[16]

Their ability to provider quick assessments can help clarify whether a comprehensive evaluation is needed. For example, a child may present with delays in language, which could signal concerns for autism; however, this is not always the case. Providing additional, specific screeners can help gather data to assist the psychologist and physician in making a more informed decision on whether an autism evaluation is necessary; this can help screen out false positives and inappropriate referrals that may congest the system.[16] It is possible that some of the diagnoses may allow for brief intervention that can occur within the medical setting, such as Parent Management Training to address behavior concerns, whereas other diagnosis such as Autism and Major Depressive Disorder may need more intensive services.[16] Further integrated psychologists can use assessments to monitor symptoms to determine severity, therefore giving data on the need to adapt and change level of care based on the results.[16]

TREATMENT ADHERENCE

In addition to providing consultation services and assessing for psychosocial concerns, integrated psychologists contribute to improvements in adherence to medical regimens. Generally, treatment adherence refers to the degree to which a patient's behaviors (eg, medication compliance, adopting lifestyle changes) align with medical or health recommendations.[17] Overall, treatment adherence is associated with improved health outcomes; however, studies show that only 40% to 60% of patients are adherent, which typically decreases over time.[18–20]

Lack of treatment adherence could lead to a variety of consequences. For one, poor treatment adherences could lead to inadequate disease management and negative

Table 1 Brief assessments		
Presenting Concerns	**Brief Assessments**	**Age Range**
Anxiety	• Generalized Anxiety Disorder (GAD-7) • Screen for Child Anxiety Related Disorders (SCARED) • Spence Children's Anxiety Scale (SCAS) • Multidimensional Anxiety Scale for Children—2nd edition (MASC-2) • Beck Anxiety Inventory (BAI) • Revised Children's Manifest Anxiety Scale (RCMAS-2)	• 11–17 y • ≥8 y • 2–12 y • 8–19 y • 17–80 y • 6–19 y
Depression	• Patient Health Questionnaire Adolescent (PHQ-A) • Kutcher Adolescent Depression Scale (KADS) • Children's Depression Inventory (CDI-2) • Reynolds Child Depression Scale (RCDS-2)	• 11–17 y • 12–17 y • 7–17 y • 7–13 y
Suicidal Ideation	• Suicidal Ideation Questionnaire (SIQ & SIQ-Jr)	• *Grade 7–12*
Psychosocial/Behavior Concerns	• Pediatric Symptom Checklist (PSC-17) • Strength and Difficulties Questionnaire • Behavior Assessment System for Children (BASC-3) • Beck Youth Inventories (BYI-2)	• 4–16 y • 3–17 y • 2–21:11 y • 7–18 year old
Developmental Disorders/Autism Spectrum Disorder	• Ages and Stages Questionnaire (ASQ-3) • Survey of Well-being of Young Children (SWYC) • Parents' Evaluation of Developmental Status (PEDS) • Childhood Autism Rating Scale (CARS-2) • M-CHAT & M-CHAT Follow-up • Gilliam Autism Rating Scale (GARS-3) • Adaptive Behavior Assessment System (ABAS-3)	• 4 mo–5 y • 1 month–5 years • 0–8 y • 3–22 y • 16–48 mo • 3–22 y • Birth-89:11 y
ADHD	• Brown Attention-Deficit Disorder Scales (Brown—ADD Scale) • Clinical Assessment of Attention Deficit (CAT-C) • Conner's (Kiddie) Continuous Performance (K-CPT-2 & CPT-3) • Conners 3 • Vanderbilt ADHD Diagnostic Rating Scale	• 3 year old—adult • 8–79 y • 4 y—adult • 6–18 y • 4–18 y

(*continued on next page*)

Table 1 (continued)		
Presenting Concerns	**Brief Assessments**	**Age Range**
Tobacco, Alcohol, and/or Drug Use Assessment	• CRAFFT (Car, Relax, Alone, Forget, Friends, Trouble) • CAGE-AID	• 11–21 y • Adolescent

This table offers a list of tools, but is not meant to be an exhaustive list, but merely a representation of a range of screenings available.

treatment outcomes.[19] In turn, this could increase rates of morbidity and mortality among patients with severe chronic conditions. Furthermore, lack of adherence could increase in the required amount of medical appointments. In particular, poor adherence is associated with increasing health care costs up to 25 to 100 billion dollars due to additional treatment and hospital admission costs.[21] For instance, diabetes is a complex chronic condition that requires significant lifestyle changes including changes in diet and physical activity to manage blood sugar levels. However, many patients with diabetes do not adhere to the recommended regimen, which leads to suboptimum glycemic control as well as acute and chronic complications.[22]

Despite the consequences, there are several factors that create barriers to treatment adherence.[23] Oftentimes, general recommendations are provided to patients and their families. Because of the fast-paced nature of medical care, there is limited time and opportunity to provide individualized or personalized recommendations for patients.[24] Therefore, there is a likelihood the recommendations provided are not feasible for each patient based on their sociocultural background. Unfortunately, the provider may not be aware of this issue until there is a noticeable change or lack of change to the patient's condition.

In addition to individualized care, the patient-provider relationship or the working alliance has been associated with treatment adherence and subsequent treatment outcomes.[25–27] The working alliance refers to the agreement on treatment goals, emotional bond, and trust between the patient and provider. In addition, patient perceptions of a provider empathy and cultural competence such as the provider's understanding of patient beliefs and values have been found to affect the working alliance and adherence.[25,28] However, lack of time might create challenges for medical providers to foster a strong working alliance that would have meaningful impact on patient care.

In all, there are several factors that affect health behaviors and treatment adherence such as the lack of individualized recommendation that account for the patient sociocultural background of the patient. However, the biopsychosocial model of health care, with the emphasis on integrated services, allows psychologists to support medical providers in the provision of care while addressing barriers to treatment adherence.[29,30]

Integrated psychologists are able to address the multifaceted factors affecting adherence including the patient's behavioral, psychosocial, and environmental circumstances. Three prominent strategies used to address treatment adherence include consultation, psychoeducation, and SMART goals. As discussed previously, through consultation between the patient and the health care team, an integrated psychologist is able to facilitate understanding of the treatment recommendations. Depending on the patient and the medical condition, consultation could include caregivers, family members, social workers, teachers, and other health care providers (eg, dietician, psychiatrist), which ensures the patient is receiving holistic care.[29] Lastly, consultation and the multidisciplinary approach reduces the risk of neglecting aspects of their care, which would affect long-term adherence. For instance, for patients who might be facing socioeconomic stressors, coordinating access to social services would improve their ability to adhere to a medical regimen.[31–33]

During consultation, psychoeducation is also provided to elaborate on the medical condition or diagnosis as well as the treatment recommendations to improve understanding and clarify concerns.[34] Following, to ensure patients are receiving individualized and attainable recommendations, SMART goals can be used to improve treatment adherence and efficacy.[35] Generally, SMART (Specific, Measurable, Achievable, Relevant, and Time-bound) goals create an individualized plan to successfully adhere to their recommendations. In particular, rather than broad and unattainable goals, setting SMART goals has been found to successfully support behavior change by addressing potential barriers such as lack of resources, time restrictions, lack of clarity, and more.[36]

SHORT-TERM THERAPY

In addition to aforementioned strategies used for treatment adherence, there are a variety of effective short-term interventions for a range of presenting concerns within health care settings. **Table 2** provides a list of common presenting concerns in pediatric psychology with corresponding evidence-based brief interventions. Overall, the interventions are focused on improving patient care, reducing symptoms, and improving psychosocial functioning. A prominent evidence-based intervention used in health care is motivational interviewing.[37,38] For prevention- and intervention-based services, the patient's willingness to follow treatment recommendations has a significant impact on outcomes. Motivational interviewing is client-centered approach to elicit (or motivate) change by helping patients and their caregivers explore and resolve ambivalence regarding a treatment or recommendation. The technique has support for effectively treating a range of psychology and physical health conditions including, depression, anxiety, sleep quality, weight management, smoking cessation, diabetes management, and other chronic conditions.[38–42]

Within health care, elevations in stress are typical when faced with a medical diagnosis, for the patient and their family.[43,44] Unfortunately, increased levels of stress as well as chronic stress have a negative impact on physical and mental health outcomes, which creates a coercive cycle.[45] Therefore, another prominent intervention used in integrated care is stress management. Stress management may entail assisting the patient and their family in problem solving and overcoming barriers affecting health outcomes. In addition, patients and their family might benefit from learning skills (eg, interpersonal effectiveness skills, communication skills) to foster their self-advocacy, as they continue to seek health care services. Similarly, distress tolerance skills are helpful to address short- and long-term stressors as well as comorbid anxiety symptoms following a medical diagnosis. Distress tolerance skills are adopted from dialectical behavioral therapy and include a variety of strategies used to prevent an escalation of negative emotions.[46] A widely used distress tolerance is TIPP, which is an acronym for temperature, intense exercise, paced breathing, and paired muscle relaxation. TIPP skills are able to efficiently (within a few seconds) lower the state of emotional arousal by calming the limbic system.[47] Integrated psychologists would be able to provide psychoeducation about these strategies and model them for patients and their family. Overall, the distress tolerance skills would be beneficial for managing stress during medical appointments or outside of the medical setting.

Table 2	
Brief interventions	
Presenting Concerns	**Brief Interventions**
Anxiety and depression	• Cognitive behavioral therapy (cognitive restructuring) • Behavioral activation • Dialectical behavioral therapy (distress tolerance skills) • Acceptance and commitment therapy (mindfulness; values identification)
Behavior concerns	• Parent management training (behavioral plan, reinforcements, consequences) • Parent-child interaction therapy (time out, child-directed interaction)
Coping with medical problems	• Supportive intervention • Psychoeducation • Cognitive behavioral therapy (cognitive restructuring) • Behavioral activation • Dialectical behavioral therapy (distress tolerance skills) • Motivational interviewing
Feeding/Eating/Appetite	• Behavioral intervention (successive approximation, repeated exposure) • Relaxation strategies • Parent management training (behavioral plan, reinforcements, consequences)
Life changes/Adjustment	• Supportive intervention • Solution-focused therapy • Motivational interviewing
Sleep concerns	• Sleep hygiene • Cognitive behavioral therapy for insomnia • Brief behavioral treatment for insomnia
Somatic symptoms	• Behavioral activation • Dialectical behavioral therapy (distress tolerance skills)
Stress reduction	• Behavioral activation • Dialectical behavioral therapy (distress tolerance skills) • Solution-focused therapy
Toileting concerns	• Bedwetting alarms • Parent management training (behavioral plan, reinforcements, consequences)

This table offers a list of brief interventions, but is not meant to be an exhaustive list, but merely a representation of a range of interventions available.

Generally, integrated psychologist emphasizes functional outcomes to address the biopsychosocial domains affecting patient health outcome. Hence, behavioral interventions are typically used to target behaviors affecting patient functioning in a variety of areas including education, familial relationships, social relationships, leisure, work, and other life domains. For instance, integrated psychologists frequently address sleep hygiene due to the widespread impact sleep quantity and quality have on physical, cognitive, and psychological functioning.[48,49] Similarly, an integrated psychologist is able to assist patients develop health goals related to their medical condition including changes in physical activity or eating habits. In addition, behavioral activation, an evidence-based intervention adopted from cognitive behavioral therapy, can serve as a strategy to maintain the patient's quality of life as they manage their chronic condition.[50] Behavioral activation is useful in making behavioral and environmental changes to ensure patients are engaging in activities they value and find meaningful, which improves life satisfaction and ability to manage life stress. Behavioral activation has been effective in treating depressive symptoms that are common comorbidities for a variety of chronic medical conditions such as diabetes, cardiovascular disease, and cancer.[51–53]

Lastly, among pediatric subspecialties family intervention is critical to treatment success.[54] For instance, family psychoeducation is essential in ensuring all the individuals involved in the patient's care understand the diagnosis and treatment recommendations. In addition, the family has a significant role in the patient's environment; therefore, their involvement is essential to fostering behavior change that improves treatment outcomes. For one, the integrated psychologist can assist the family in improving the patient's adherence to the medical or psychological/behavioral interventions. For instance, children and adolescents may have difficulties accepting the life changes and demands following a medical diagnosis. Among the pediatric population, the stress caused by those changes might lead to behavior problems including noncompliance. Similarly, the stress the family experiences creates challenges in effectively addressing noncompliance and managing the patient's care.[55] Therefore, parent-focused evidence-based interventions such as Parent-Management Training and Parent-Child Interaction Therapy would be beneficial.[56–58] For instance, behavioral plans can be used to implement reinforcements and consequences to improve specific "target" behaviors (eg, compliance to the treatment regimen). In addition, the interventions provide effective parenting skills (eg, effective prompts and instructions, time out strategies) that can be generalized to the home and other setting to improve general compliance as well as the parent-child relationship.[59,60]

Despite the range of effective short-term interventions, there are limitations to the scope of integrated care. Because of the short-term nature of integrated care, there are presenting concerns that would not be suitable for the service.[61] For instance, severe anxiety and depression, suicidality, and posttraumatic stress disorder are some conditions that would not be adequately addressed through brief intervention. For these circumstances, integrated psychologists can create a bridge to specialty mental health services and community resources.[62] In addition, integrated care creates an opportunity to maintain ongoing communication with the patient as they continue to seek health care services through their primary care physician. In turn, the psychologist is able to coordinate care and collaborate with community providers to ensure the patient is receiving appropriate and effective services as they continue managing their chronic condition.

SUMMARY

Based on the biopsychosocial model of health care, integrated psychologists serve on a multidisciplinary team to address psychosocial and behavioral concerns. Among pediatric patients with chronic conditions, there are increasing cases of comorbid psychological and behavioral symptoms that exacerbate their medical concerns. Integrated psychologists within the medical home can aid patients, their family, and the medical team by addressing those comorbid concerns. For one, integrated psychologist plays a significant role in identifying behavioral and emotional concerns by administrating and interpreting screening and assessment tools. Following, psychologist consult with the medical team (eg, physician, nurses, psychiatrist, dietician, and so forth), the patient, and their family to facilitate communication and coordinate care. In addition, psychologists assist the patient and their family navigate services and address their psychosocial needs to improve adherence to the recommended medical regimen as well as overall health outcomes. For instance, psychologist can provide short-term interventions to address a range of concerns to improve treatment outcomes, reduce symptoms, and improve psychosocial functioning. Overall, integrated psychologists can serve a variety of roles to ensure pediatric patients are receiving holistic care by addressing a variety of biopsychosocial factors to improve health outcomes.

CLINICS CARE POINTS

- Twenty percent of children have a chronic medical condition and are at a higher risk of developing mental health symptoms and are twice as likely to attempt and/or complete suicide.
- Poor treatment adherences and the development of a mental health symptoms can lead to inadequate disease management and negative treatment outcomes, whereas those that receive services to address these issues have a better quality of life and management of their illness.
- Integrated psychologists can support children and adolescents with chronic medical conditions in a variety of ways through short-term and brief intervention; however, there are situations where longer term or specialty mental health services outside of medical home are necessary.

DISCLOSURE

There are no conflict of interests to disclose.

REFERENCES

1. Asarnow JR, Kolko DJ, Miranda J, et al. The pediatric patient-centered medical home: Innovative models for improving behavioral health. Am Psychol 2017; 72(1):13–27.
2. Stancin T, Perrin EC. Psychologists and pediatricians opportunities for collaboration in primary care. Am Psychol 2014;69(4):332–43.
3. Campo JV, Geist R, Kolko DJ. Integration of Pediatric Behavioral Health Services in Primary Care: Improving Access and Outcomes with Collaborative Care. Can J Psychiatry 2018;63(7):432–8.
4. Samsel C, Ribeiro M, Ibeziako P, et al. Integrated Behavioral Health Care in Pediatric Subspecialty Clinics. Child Adolesc Psychiatr Clin N Am 2017;26(4): 785–94.
5. Soares N, Apple RW, Kanungo S. The role of integrated behavioral health in caring for patients with metabolic disorders. Ann Transl Med 2018;6(24):478.
6. Urban TH, Stein CR, Mournet AM, et al. Level of behavioral health integration and suicide risk screening results in pediatric ambulatory subspecialty care. Gen Hosp Psychiatry 2022;75:23–9.
7. Bennett SD, Kerry E, Fifield K, et al. A drop-in centre for treating mental health problems in children with chronic illness: Outcomes for parents and their relationship with child outcomes. JCPP Adv 2021;1(4). https://doi.org/10.1002/jcv2. 12046.
8. Kahhan NA, Junger KW. Introduction to the special interest issue on parent/ guardian interventions in pediatric psychology: The role of the pediatric

psychologist working with caregivers as the target of intervention. Clin Pract Pediatr Psychol 2021;9(2):107–11.

9. Kazak AE, Nash JM, Hiroto K, et al. Psychologists in patient-centered medical homes (PCMHs): Roles, evidence, opportunities, and challenges. Am Psychol 2017;72(1):1–12.

10. Hagan JF, Shaw JS, Duncan PM, American Academy of Pediatrics., Bright Futures. Bright Futures : Guidelines for Health Supervision of Infants, Children, and Adolescents : Pocket Guide.

11. Bradley-Klug KL, Sundman AN, Nadeau J, et al. Communication and collaboration with schools: Pediatricians' perspectives. J Appl Sch Psychol 2010;26(4): 263–81.

12. Iturralde E, Adams RN, Barley RC, et al. Implementation of Depression Screening and Global Health Assessment in Pediatric Subspecialty Clinics. J Adolesc Health 2017;61(5):591–8.

13. Sattler AF, Leffler JM, Harrison NL, et al. The Quality of Assessments for Childhood Psychopathology Within a Regional Medical Center. Psychol Serv 2018. https://doi.org/10.1037/ser0000241.

14. Beidas RS, Stewart RE, Walsh L, et al. Free, brief, and validated: Standardized instruments for low-resource mental health settings. Cogn Behav Pract 2015; 22(1):5–19.

15. Lois BH, Urban TH, Wong C, et al. Integrating Suicide Risk Screening into Pediatric Ambulatory Subspecialty Care. Pediatr Qual Saf 2020;5(3):e310.

16. White K, Stetson L, Hussain K. Integrated Behavioral Health Role in Helping Pediatricians Find Long Term Mental Health Interventions with the Use of Assessments. Pediatr Clin North Am 2021;68(3):685–705.

17. Brian H, Wayne T. Compliance in Health Care. Baltimore (MD): Johns Hopkins University Press; 1979. p. 516.

18. Dunbar-Jacob J, Mortimer-Stephens MK. Treatment adherence in chronic disease. J Clin Epidemiol 2001;54(12):S57–60.

19. Lemanek KL, Yardley H. Noncompliance and nonadherence. In: Friedberg RD, Paternostro JK, editors. Handbook of cognitive behavioral therapy for pediatric medical conditions. Switzerland: Springer Nature; 2019. p. 407–16.

20. Hommel KA, Davis CM, Baldassano RN. Objective versus subjective assessment of oral medication adherence in pediatric inflammatory bowel disease. Inflamm Bowel Dis 2009;15(4):589–93.

21. Sokol MC, McGuigan KA, Verbrugge RR, et al. Impact of Medication Adherence on Hospitalization Risk and Healthcare Cost. Med Care 2005;43(6):521–30.

22. Krass I, Schieback P, Dhippayom T. Adherence to diabetes medication: a systematic review. Diabet Med 2015;32(6):725–37.

23. Greca AM La. Issues in Adherence With Pediatric Regimens. J Pediatr Psychol 1990;15(4):423–36.

24. Bremer V, Becker D, Kolovos S, et al. Predicting Therapy Success and Costs for Personalized Treatment Recommendations Using Baseline Characteristics: Data-Driven Analysis. J Med Internet Res 2018;20(8):e10275.

25. Fuertes JN, Boylan LS, Fontanella JA. Behavioral Indices in Medical Care Outcome: The Working Alliance, Adherence, and Related Factors. J Gen Intern Med 2009;24(1):80–5.

26. Street RL, Makoul G, Arora NK, et al. How does communication heal? Pathways linking clinician–patient communication to health outcomes. Patient Educ Couns 2009;74(3):295–301.

27. Cheng AW, Nakash O, Cruz-Gonzalez M, et al. The association between patient–provider racial/ethnic concordance, working alliance, and length of treatment in behavioral health settings. Psychol Serv 2021. https://doi.org/10.1037/ser0000582.
28. Baudrant-Boga M, Lehmann A, Allenet B. Penser autrement l'observance médicamenteuse : d'une posture injonctive à une alliance thérapeutique entre le patient et le soignant – Concepts et déterminants. Ann Pharm Françaises 2012; 70(1):15–25.
29. Lemanek KL. Empirically Supported Treatments in Pediatric Psychology: Regimen Adherence. J Pediatr Psychol 2001;26(5):253–75.
30. Quittner AL, Modi AC, Lemanek KL, et al. Evidence-based Assessment of Adherence to Medical Treatments in Pediatric Psychology. J Pediatr Psychol 2008; 33(9):916–36.
31. Berardi R, Morgese F, Rinaldi S, et al. Benefits and Limitations of a Multidisciplinary Approach in Cancer Patient Management. Cancer Manag Res 2020;12: 9363–74.
32. Monteleone AM, Fernandez-Aranda F, Voderholzer U. Evidence and perspectives in eating disorders: a paradigm for a multidisciplinary approach. World Psychiatry 2019;18(3):369–70.
33. Odell S, Logan D. Pediatric pain management: the multidisciplinary approach. J Pain Res 2013;785. https://doi.org/10.2147/JPR.S37434.
34. Day M, Clarke S-A, Castillo-Eito L, et al. Psychoeducation for Children with Chronic Conditions: A Systematic Review and Meta-analysis. J Pediatr Psychol 2020;45(4):386–98.
35. Ostarello L, Wright M, Waltz TJ. Medical treatment adherence. In: Maragakis A, O'Donohue W, editors. Principle-based stepped care and brief psychotherapy for integrated care settings. Cham: Springer; 2018. p. 241–55.
36. Shaw RL, Pattison HM, Holland C, et al. Be SMART: examining the experience of implementing the NHS Health Check in UK primary care. BMC Fam Pract 2015; 16(1):1.
37. Erickson SJ, Gerstle M, Feldstein SW. Brief Interventions and Motivational Interviewing With Children, Adolescents, and Their Parents in Pediatric Health Care Settings. Arch Pediatr Adolesc Med 2005;159(12):1173.
38. Lundahl BW, Kunz C, Brownell C, et al. A Meta-Analysis of Motivational Interviewing: Twenty-Five Years of Empirical Studies. Res Soc Work Pract 2010;20(2): 137–60.
39. Westra HA, Aviram A, Doell FK. Extending Motivational Interviewing to the Treatment of Major Mental Health Problems: Current Directions and Evidence. Can J Psychiatry 2011;56(11):643–50.
40. Berhe KK, Gebru HB, Kahsay HB. Effect of motivational interviewing intervention on HgbA1C and depression in people with type 2 diabetes mellitus (systematic review and meta-analysis). PLoS One 2020;15(10):e0240839.
41. Cho JM, Lee K. Effects of motivation interviewing using a group art therapy program on negative symptoms of schizophrenia. Arch Psychiatr Nurs 2018;32(6): 878–84.
42. Geller J, Avis J, Srikameswaran S, et al. Developing and Pilot Testing the Readiness and Motivation Interview for Families in Pediatric Weight Management. Can J Diet Pract Res 2015;76(4):190–3.
43. Zehnder D, Prchal A, Vollrath M, et al. Prospective Study of the Effectiveness of Coping in Pediatric Patients. Child Psychiatry Hum Dev 2006;36(3):351–68.

44. Compas BE, Jaser SS, Bettis AH, et al. Coping, emotion regulation, and psycho-pathology in childhood and adolescence: A meta-analysis and narrative review. Psychol Bull 2017;143(9):939–91.
45. Juster R-P, McEwen BS, Lupien SJ. Allostatic load biomarkers of chronic stress and impact on health and cognition. Neurosci Biobehav Rev 2010;35(1):2–16.
46. Zeifman RJ, Boritz T, Barnhart R, et al. The independent roles of mindfulness and distress tolerance in treatment outcomes in dialectical behavior therapy skills training. Personal Disord Theory Res Treat 2020;11(3):181–90.
47. Lelonek G, Crook D, Tully M, et al. Multidisciplinary Approach to Enhancing Safety and Care for Pediatric Behavioral Health Patients in Acute Medical Settings. Child Adolesc Psychiatr Clin N Am 2018;27(3):491–500.
48. Buysse DJ, Grunstein R, Horne J, et al. Can an improvement in sleep positively impact on health? Sleep Med Rev 2010;14(6):405–10.
49. Alvarez GG, Ayas NT. The Impact of Daily Sleep Duration on Health: A Review of the Literature. Prog Cardiovasc Nurs 2004;19(2):56–9.
50. Kanter JW, Manos RC, Bowe WM, et al. What is behavioral activation?A review of the empirical literature. Clin Psychol Rev 2010;30(6):608–20.
51. Gold SM, Köhler-Forsberg O, Moss-Morris R, et al. Comorbid depression in medical diseases. Nat Rev Dis Prim 2020;6(1):69.
52. Watson LC, Amick HR, Gaynes BN, et al. Practice-Based Interventions Addressing Concomitant Depression and Chronic Medical Conditions in the Primary Care Setting. J Prim Care Community Health 2013;4(4):294–306.
53. Cuijpers P, van Straten A, Warmerdam L. Behavioral activation treatments of depression: A meta-analysis. Clin Psychol Rev 2007;27(3):318–26.
54. Vanderhout SM, Smith M, Pallone N, et al. Patient and family engagement in the development of core outcome sets for two rare chronic diseases in children. Res Involv Engagem 2021;7(1):66.
55. Neece CL, Green SA, Baker BL. Parenting Stress and Child Behavior Problems: A Transactional Relationship Across Time. Am J Intellect Dev Disabil 2012;117(1):48–66.
56. Berkovits MD, O'Brien KA, Carter CG, et al. Early Identification and Intervention for Behavior Problems in Primary Care: A Comparison of Two Abbreviated Versions of Parent-Child Interaction Therapy. Behav Ther 2010;41(3):375–87.
57. Mingebach T, Kamp-Becker I, Christiansen H, et al. Meta-meta-analysis on the effectiveness of parent-based interventions for the treatment of child externalizing behavior problems. PLoS One 2018;13(9):e0202855.
58. Pinquart M, Shen Y. Behavior Problems in Children and Adolescents With Chronic Physical Illness: A Meta-Analysis. J Pediatr Psychol 2011;36(9):1003–16.
59. Hagen KA, Ogden T, Bjørnebekk G. Treatment Outcomes and Mediators of Parent Management Training: A One-Year Follow-Up of Children with Conduct Problems. J Clin Child Adolesc Psychol 2011;40(2):165–78.
60. Cooley ME, Veldorale-Griffin A, Petren RE, et al. Parent–Child Interaction Therapy: A Meta-Analysis of Child Behavior Outcomes and Parent Stress. J Fam Soc Work 2014;17(3):191–208.
61. Buchanan GJR, Piehler T, Berge J, et al. Integrated Behavioral Health Implementation Patterns in Primary Care Using the Cross-Model Framework: A Latent Class Analysis. Adm Policy Ment Heal Ment Heal Serv Res 2022;49(2):312–25.
62. Asarnow JR, Rozenman M, Wiblin J, et al. Integrated Medical-Behavioral Care Compared With Usual Primary Care for Child and Adolescent Behavioral Health. JAMA Pediatr 2015;169(10):929.

Psychologists' Role in a Multidisciplinary Approach to Pediatric Hematology and Oncology Care

Summer Chahin, PhD

KEYWORDS

- Psychology • Multidisciplinary • Pediatric hematology • Pediatric oncology
- Psychosocial • Collaborative

KEY POINTS

- Psychologists do more than address behavioral and mood concerns including adherence, pain management, pill swallowing, sleep, and many other areas.
- Pediatric hematological and oncological diagnoses affect a child and their family beyond just biological and physiologically. Psychologists can help supplement care by attending to the various other factors that affect a child and their family.
- Collaborative multidisciplinary care is imperative to the success of a child and family throughout diagnosis, treatment, transition, and survivorship.

INTRODUCTION

Approximately 40% of children and adolescents in the United States are experiencing at least one chronic health illness.[1] In the United States, approximately 15,000 individuals under the age of 20 receive a cancer diagnosis each year.[2] Pediatric cancer deaths have decreased by 70% during the past 40 years.[3] Approximately 85% of children and adolescents diagnosed with cancer survived at least 5 years.[4] Although pediatric cancer death rates have dropped, cancer remains the leading cause of death in children and adolescents aged 14 years and younger.[2] Rates of new cancer diagnoses were higher in men than in women and in children aged younger than 4 years and 15 to 19 years. Further, the incidence rates were higher for white children and adolescents and lowest for black children and adolescents.[5] The medical needs of those with chronic and devastating health conditions can be complex, continuous, and include both daily health-care management and addressing medical emergencies that may come up.

Western Michigan University Homer Stryker M.D. School of Medicine, 1000 Oakland Drive, Kalamazoo, MI 49008-1284, USA
E-mail addresses: summer.s.chahin@wmich.edu; summer.chahin@gmail.com

Pediatr Clin N Am 69 (2022) 839–846
https://doi.org/10.1016/j.pcl.2022.06.004
0031-3955/22/© 2022 Elsevier Inc. All rights reserved.

Physicians do not receive the training necessary in medical school to conduct a comprehensive evaluation of a patient's entire biopsychosocial network. Due to the multifaceted nature of complex medical conditions, medical care teams should include other allied-health professionals to assist in gathering and assessing for the other information medical providers cannot assess, so that physicians can focus on the medical side of a patient's care. Psychologists are particularly well equipped to assess for the psychosocial aspects of an individual's life and do so as part of the rest of the psychosocial team. Individual's lives are as complex as their conditions, diagnoses, and treatments. The benefits of including psychosocial providers, especially psychologists on a multidisciplinary team are infinite.

COLLABORATION ON A MULTIDISCIPLINARY TEAM

Effective patient care can be achieved through open communication and collaboration among medical providers and other health-allied professionals. Integration of psychosocial professionals is integral to patient success in pediatric oncology care settings. Further, care team members should have trust in each care team member's role and ability to effectively help the patient as well as respect for each individual and discipline. Ideally, for a team to function, anyone on the medical or psychosocial team should have the capability to refer to psychology and to each other. This allows for cohesiveness of a team and for effective whole person-centered care.

Health-allied professionals should work together to ensure that children and adolescents are supported in all aspects of their life. For example, pediatric patients with cancer should be provided with opportunities for social interactions during their treatment and into survivorship. Care teams should collaborate on creating experiences and providing opportunities for children and adolescents to increase social interaction and enjoyed activities. Children and adolescents undergoing treatment can feel isolated at times. Further, increased social support during treatment and transitions off treatment have been found to be related to positive treatment outcomes, such as decreased depression and anxiety,[6] and easier transitions back to school and work.[7]

ROLE OF PSYCHOLOGY

Individuals who want to be successful in working with pediatric chronic illness or pediatric patient populations with cancer benefit from specialized training in pediatrics, pain management, adherence, grief and bereavement, psycho-oncology, health promotion, and decision making. Psychologists have a unique role in hematology and oncology patient care in that psychologist's skill sets are fluid, vast, and versatile. Psychologists can conduct brief interventions, psychotherapy, assessments, and consults. Additionally, psychologists also provide crisis consults for patients who present with acute needs.

Psychologists can provide services for both cancer-related treatment as well as behavioral and emotional concerns. In terms of cancer-related treatment, psychologists can assist with patient and family adjustment concerns, medical adherence problems such as pill swallowing, procedural distress, nonpharmacological pain management, and end-of-life issues. Trained psychologists can also assist with behavioral concerns, parenting difficulties, family conflict, stress management, mood and emotional disturbance, anxiety, sleep concerns, feeding concerns such as pica, and toileting difficulties as examples.

In terms of interventions, psychologists should always turn to the most up-to-date evidence-based interventions to treat the presenting concerns. There are many strategies psychological providers can implement to provide evidence-based care. For example, acceptance and commitment therapy, cognitive behavior therapy, dialectical behavior therapy, and motivational interviewing are some evidence-based treatments that have been proven to be effective in treating many of these presenting concerns in this specific population.[8]

Additionally, psychological interventions have been shown to lower pain, anxiety, distress, and physiologic arousal.[9,10] Several of the strategies that can be implemented can be used for a variety of presenting concerns as well. A few of these strategies include distraction, guided imagery, cognitive reframing, breathing techniques, relaxation strategies, positive reinforcement, coping self-statements, pill swallowing training, and behavioral activation. Furthermore, the most effective approaches combine pharmacologic and psychosocial guidance and intervention.

Techniques that have been useful in providing developmentally appropriate information to children include modeling and rehearsing procedures and treatment, use of puppets and dolls, books, and themed coloring books, as well as medical play. As previously mentioned, there are several members of multidisciplinary teams that have overlapping skillsets. For example, psychologists and child life providers are both trained to provide pill-swallowing training. Thus, it is helpful to collaborate with other providers on the medical team to ensure comprehensive care is provided to children and their families.

Comprehensive health care is crucial for the success of pediatric patients with cancer and their families. Psychologists have a major role to play in this care. Psychologists should provide psychoeducation and anticipatory guidance to help children, adolescents, and their families with decision-making related to disease, treatment, acute and long-term effects of diagnosis and treatment, adjustment to hospitalization and treatment, procedures and procedural distress, and adaptation of psychosocial factors in their lives. It is critical for providers to remember to provide information that is developmentally appropriate for children, as well as keeping information accurate and honest.

ADHERENCE

Treatment of cancer and chronic health disorders can be complex at times, and there may be many barriers to adhering to treatment requirements. Families find themselves having to manage complex medical recommendations and treatment regimens, which at times can be difficult. Nonadherence to complex medical presentations is a threat to outcomes and success of treatment. Psychologists have an important role to play in assessing patient and family adherence to medical guidelines. It is critical that psychologists conduct routine assessment and obtain self-reported and parent-reported information of adherence to their medical guidelines. Psychologists can also assist the medical team in providing psychoeducation on the purpose, administration, side effects, and reiterate the importance of adhering to medical recommendations. Additionally, psychologists can assess and discuss common and unique barriers with each family, as well as discuss strategies on how to improve adherence given their unique situation.

SLEEP

Bedtime difficulties are common in children. In the general pediatric population, 10% to 30% of children experience some form of sleep–wake difficulties.[11] In the pediatric oncology population, approximately 30% to 60% of children and adolescents experience fatigue or excessive daytime sleepiness.[12] Normal sleep patterns include repeating cycles of REM (rapid eye movement) and non-REM sleep, which has 4 stages of sleep. Developmental changes in sleep should be considered but generally, night wakings are normal.[13] In the general population, bedtime resistance and stalling, difficulty falling asleep, nighttime awakenings, feedings during the night, and parasomnias are the most common sleep problems. In the pediatric oncology population, insomnia, fatigue, prolonged sleep onset latency, abnormal sleep duration, nighttime and premature awakenings, and excessive daytime sleepiness are the most common sleep difficulties.[12,14,15]

An additional benefit of working on a multidisciplinary team is that psychologists have the training to assess pediatric sleep difficulties and help treat those concerns. Further, physicians and other psychosocial care providers look to psychologists for effective behavioral intervention recommendations. Psychologists thoroughly assess sleep and bedtime problems by assessing whether the sleep difficulties are a result of maladaptive sleep habits or more severe emotional difficulties. Additionally, psychologists are able to assess sleep routines and habits, as well as give developmentally appropriate recommendations and discuss effective sleep hygiene. Psychologists may also request parents to fill out a sleep diary during a week or 2 to gather data on current sleep habits and functioning.

In terms of effective behavioral sleep interventions, psychologists may provide guidance on sleep associations, such as helping the child connect certain conditions or routines with sleep. Psychologists may also recommend the progressive waiting approach for difficulty falling asleep,[16] the sleep shuffle,[17] and limit setting for bedtime resistance. Parents of children experiencing cancer may become more lenient on house rules and boundaries related to other health-related behaviors such as sleep. Psychologists can help parents maintain appropriate boundaries and limit setting around sleep and other important health areas to ensure maximum success in the treatment.

PAIN MANAGEMENT

Pain is a common symptom of children and adolescents undergoing treatment of cancer and hematological disorders. Typically, pain is managed with medications. However, patients and their families have reported that they do not want to add additional medications to their regimen. Psychologists can be helpful when this issue comes up because some psychologists have training in nonpharmacological pain management. Psychological providers can assist patients with strategies to cope and manage their pain without the use of medications and assist parents in how to support their child as well.

Psychologists can start with providing developmentally appropriate psychoeducation about pain. In providing psychoeducation on pain, providers should collaborate with other care team members, such as child life in these discussions, because child life specialists are trained in medical play and can further assist in this discussion. Additionally, the gate control theory of pain[18] is a great framework for discussions around pain. Moreover, discussion should revolve around different types of pain, the pain cycle and how pain may affect a person, how pain affects each person differently, the impact of pain on how one may think, how to break the cycle of pain, as well as how to manage pain.

In terms of nonpharmacological pain strategies, psychologists can teach children and adolescents deep breathing, progressive muscle relaxation, mini-relaxation, and cognitive restructuring to think about their pain differently, guided imagery, and mindfulness practices.[19]

Further, psychologists may offer additional suggestions to parents that may help with supporting their child. For example, advising a parent to remove the focus on pain and shift it elsewhere. It is helpful for psychologists to explain to parents to reduce the number of times they ask their child about pain and the child bring it up themselves. Additionally, psychologists may offer other suggestions such as encouraging normal activities during episodes of pain to not give excessive attention, providing positive reinforcement for when the child engages in activities and school, and encouraging the child to manage their pain without help and praising them for their efforts.

PILL SWALLOWING

Oral medications are a somewhat normal part of our everyday lives. Although this is a task many must engage in daily, there are some who have difficulties with oral pill swallowing. At times, children can have an especially difficult time with this task. This becomes a barrier to cancer treatment at times. Psychologists have the training to assist children in learning how to swallow pills, which can make treatment easier and more tolerable at times, because it decreases the amount of needle sticks experienced. There are a few different techniques used to teach children how to swallow pills that fall in line with other evidence-based strategies that psychologists use. These strategies include behavioral approaches, such as positive reinforcement, stimulus shaping (starting with small candy like sprinkles, small candies, and working up to sugar-based pill substitutes, and increasing in size), relaxation training, and head position training.[20]

PSYCHOSOCIAL STANDARDS OF CARE

Psychosocial risk factors should be considered whenever one interacts with their patients. Children with pediatric cancer and their families especially need collaborative and systematic assessment of their psychosocial and health-care needs. Further, screening should take place during high-stress times (eg, at diagnosis, beginning of treatment, transition off treatment, and so forth). It is necessary for psychological providers to collect information on child and family risk factors. For example, depression, anxiety, adjustment concerns, financial stressors are all common difficulties that patients and families present with. Additionally, in considering the best treatment and intervention options, providers should ask about child and family strengths and resiliencies, such as their support network and existing coping strategies. Psychologists are also in a unique position and should thoroughly assess for concerns with intelligence, attention, memory, language, executive functioning, and processing speed. These cognitive areas should be assessed before, during, and after treatment.

FAMILIES AND SIBLINGS OF PEDIATRIC PATIENTS WITH CANCER

Cancer diagnosis and treatment are significant stressors on the child. The cancer journey is also a significant stressor and can be difficult on the patient's caregivers and family. Families of children and adolescents with cancer and hematological disorders should be assessed for mental health and psychosocial needs throughout the cancer journey as well. Providing access to effective interventions for families will help optimize overall family well-being. Further, families should have access to individual therapy, crisis intervention, marital therapy, and family systems-based intervention. There is significant evidence indicating that families with these additional supports are able to solve problems more effectively and present with better mood. Additionally, patient's families benefit from education on diagnoses and planned treatment procedures as well as how to prepare for procedures and what to expect.

Siblings of children with cancer are at an increased risk of psychosocial concerns and need their own services too. Siblings are exposed to additional stress during this period in a multitude of ways. For example, deciding if they want to be a donor for their sibling can be a confusing and difficult decision. Psychosocial support is limited for siblings because the focus is typically on the patient. Beyond limited support for siblings, they can be difficult to work with because they may not be in attendance with the patient, and providers have limited access to siblings. Regardless, siblings need the opportunity to talk and receive psychoeducation on their sibling's diagnosis and treatment. Additionally, siblings would benefit from learning coping strategies for dealing with their stressors related to their sibling's health status.

LONG-TERM CANCER SURVIVORS

Pediatric cancer survivors should have continued assessment of their health care and psychosocial needs. The needs of patients after treatment change significantly and additional support is needed for continued success. Psychological providers should assess for any difficulties or stress related to adverse educational, social, and work issues. Further, mental health difficulties should be continuously assessed. At times, cancer survivors experience distress, anxiety, and depression, which could lead to adverse health outcomes too. In addition to mental health, cancer survivors should assess for risky health behaviors and help to promote behaviors consistent with a healthy lifestyle. Additionally, psychologists, in collaboration with the medical team, should provide anticipatory guidance to patients transitioning off cancer treatment about continued follow-up with their medical team throughout their lifetime.

END OF LIFE AND PALLIATIVE CARE

Psychologists are also in a position to support the medical team in helping facilitate conversations about end of life and palliative care. Typically, palliative care options should be discussed early on in diagnosis and treatment to reduce suffering. Additionally, early discussions allow children, adolescents, and their families to understand the individual's desires and to have a plan in place. Further, early conversations enable psychologists to work with the rest of the medical team, social workers, child life specialists, and chaplains to plan for transitions between care settings and come up with a plan for handling pain and other disease and treatment-related burdens. Palliative care and end of life can be difficult topics to approach for families, and psychologists have the skill set to work through difficult conversations. However, patients, especially adolescents appreciate being asked, being part of the conversation, and feeling heard. Overall, adolescents and parents feel that discussing these topics helps alleviate some of their stressors and find it beneficial.[21]

SUMMARY

The benefits of integrating psychology on a health-care team are unquestionable. Psychologists are trained in a vast variety of evidence-based interventions and assessment that can help with a slew of presenting concerns and treatment difficulties. Additionally, psychologists are capable of assisting a variety of allied-health professionals on the health-care team and can collaborate with others to provide the best care for a patient. Effective communication is a strong characteristic of psychologists, which can help during team huddles, in discussing difficult topics with patients and their families, and in talking with other professionals outside of the health-care team and organization.

Furthermore, psychologists have specialty training in nonpharmacological strategies for coping with and treating a variety of difficulties in childhood cancer. Psychologists are able to support children, their families, and the health-care team in a variety of areas such as treatment adherence, sleep, nonpharmacological pain management, pill swallowing, and other areas of concern that are unique to this population. Psychologists can also collaborate with other team members in discussing difficult topics with patients and their families. Examples of this include discussing diagnosis and treatment at a developmentally appropriate level, discussing palliative care and end of life, supporting children's parents and siblings throughout the cancer journey, and continuing to support and provide services into survivorship.

CLINICS CARE POINTS

- Health-allied professionals are pertinent to the care of a child with a hematological or oncological diagnosis, and it has been found to decrease anxiety and depression,[6] as well as improve outcomes in school and work among transitions.[7]
- Psychological interventions have been shown to lower pain, anxiety, distress, and physiologic arousal.[9,10]

DISCLOSURE

The author reports no conflicts of interest or connection with any funding sources.

REFERENCES

1. National Survey of Children's Health. NSCH 2018, 19: Number of Current or Lifelong Health Conditions, Nationwide, Age in 3 Groups website. Available at: Childhealthdata.org.
2. US Cancer Statistics Working Group. United States Cancer Statistics. 1999-2014 Incidence and mortality web-based report. Atlanta, GA: US Department of Health and Human Services, CDC; National Cancer Institute; 2017.
3. National Program of Cancer Registries. Tracking Pediatric and Young Adult Cancer Cases. 2021. CDC. online. Availabe at: https://www.cdc.gov/cancer/npcr/pediatric-young-adult-cancer.htm.
4. Howlader N, Noone AM, Krapcho M, et al, editors. Based on November 2020 SEER data submission, posted to the SEER website. SEER cancer Review, 1975-2018. . Bethesda, (MD): National Cancer Institute; 2021.
5. Siegel DA, Li J, Henley SJ, et al. Geographic Variation in Pediatric Cancer Incidence- United States, 2003-2014. MMWR Morb Mortal Wkly Rep 2018;67: 707–13.
6. Applebaum AJ, Stein EM, Lord-Bessen J, et al. Optimism, social support, and mental health outcomes in patients with advanced cancer. Psychooncology 2014;23(3):299–306.
7. Pennant S, Lee SC, Holm S, et al. The role of social support in adolescent/young adults coping with cancer treatment. Children 2019;7(2).
8. Fair C, Thompson A, Barnett M, et al. Utilization of psychotherapeutic interventions by pediatric psychosocial providers. Children 2021;8:1045.
9. Coakley R, Wihak T. Evidence-based psychological interventions for the management of pediatric chronic pain: New directions in research and clinical practice. Children 2017;4(9).

10. Barlow JH, Ellard DR. Psycho-educational interventions for children with chronic disease, parents and siblings: An overview of the research evidence base. Child Care Health Development 2004;30:637–45.
11. Ford ES, Wheaton AG, Cunningham TJ, et al. Trends in outpatient visits for insomnia, sleep apnea, and prescriptions for sleep medications among US adults: findings form the national ambulatory medical care survey 1999-2000. Sleep 2014;37(8):1283–93.
12. Kaleyias J, Manley P, Kothare SV. Sleep disorders in children with cancer. Seminarsin Pediatr Neurol 2012;19(1):25–34.
13. Galland BC, Taylor BJ, Elder DE, et al. Normal sleep patterns in infants and children: A systematic review of observational studies. Sleep Med Rev 2012;16(3):213–22.
14. Armstrong TS, Shade MY, Breton G, et al. Sleep-wake disturbance in patients with brain tumors. Neuro-oncology 2017;19(3):323–35.
15. Clanton NR, Klosky JL, Li C, et al. Fatigue, vitality, sleep, and neurocognitive functioning in adult survivors of childhood cancer: A report from the childhood cancer survivor study. Cancer 2011;117(11):2559–68.
16. Ferber R. Solve your child's sleep problems. New York: Simon & Schuster; 2006.
17. West K. The sleep lady's good night, sleep tight. New York: Vanguard Press; 2010.
18. Melzack R, Wall PD. Pain mechanisms: A New Theory. Science 1965;150(3699):971–9.
19. Wren AA, Ross AC, D'Souza G, et al. Multidisciplinary pain management for pediatric patients with acute and chronic pain: A foundational treatment approach when prescribing opioids. Children 2019;6(33).
20. Dersch-Mills D, Kaplan BJ. Giving oral medicines and supplements to children. Br Med J 2020;371.
21. Friebert S, Grossoehme DH, Baker JN, et al. Congruence gaps between adolescents with cancer and their families regarding values, goals, and beliefs about end-of-life care. J Am Med Assoc 2020;3(5).

Role of Psychologist in Adolescent Medicine

An International Perspective

Swati Y. Bhave, MD, DCH, FCPS, FIAP[a,b,c,*],
Anuradha V. Sovani, MA, MPhil, PhD (Psychology)[d,1],
Samir R. Shah, MB, DCH[e,f,2]

KEYWORDS

- Psychological assessment and interventions with adolescents
- Adolescent psychology • Adolescent mental health • Adolescent help-seeking
- Integrated behavioural health, focus on adolescent disorders, distress, development, need for team work • life skills and positive psychology
- Adolscent Counseling

KEY POINTS

- Adolescent mental health service use, supportive role of physicians for psychological issues, removing the stigma of accessing mental health services, holistic health of adolescents, involvement of family and community, teamwork by pediatricians and psychologists.

INTRODUCTION

As quoted by Shakespeare *"I would there were no age between ten and three-and-twenty, or that youth would sleep out the rest; for there is nothing in the between but getting wenches with child, wronging the ancientry, stealing, fighting."*[1]

Definition: *Adolescent psychology* is the field of psychology that focuses on the issues that are unique to adolescents. Adolescence is a time of fluctuating and rapidly changing interests and desires and many characteristics that are unique to this age.[2]

The branch of *Adolescent Medicine* addresses the health and health care of adolescents, young adults, and their families. Psychological aspects are very important in

[a] Dr D.Y Patil Medical College, Pimpri; [b] Dr D.Y. Patil Vidyapeeth, Pune; [c] AACCI, Mumbai (Association of Adolescent and Child Care in India); [d] Department of Psychology, Faculty of Humanities, SNDT Women's University; [e] Samir Hospital & Narahari Hospital, Vadodara; [f] Samir Hospital, Lakdipul

[1] Present address: OM 31 Shreesh Society, LIC Cross Road, Off Eastern Express Highway, Thane West 400604, Maharashtra, India.

[2] Present address: Dandi Bazar Main Road, Vadodara - 390001, Gujarat State, India.

* Corresponding author. 601 Alliance Shanti , Shantisheela Co-operative society Near FTII, Law College Road , Erandawane Pune 411 004 ,Maharashtra, India

E-mail address: sybhave@gmail.com

Pediatr Clin N Am 69 (2022) 847–864
https://doi.org/10.1016/j.pcl.2022.05.001
0031-3955/22/© 2022 Elsevier Inc. All rights reserved.

pediatric.theclinics.com

adolescents and a lot of aspects are preventive in nature.[3,4] Many articles cite the load of adolescent cases in a pediatrician's office as being a quarter of the total caseload. A recent JAMA publication by Trent titled *"Why Adolescent Medicine?"* addresses the question reflecting the various domains whereby this age group requires attention.[5]

Importance of Dealing with Mental Health Issues to Promote in the Well-Being of Adolescence

Mental health is an important component of an individual's overall health, affecting all domain areas of life. The COVID-19 pandemic has brought to forefront the importance and exacerbation of the mental health burden globally.[6]

World Health Organization and Adolescent Mental Health

Worldwide, 10% of children and adolescents experience a mental disorder, but most of them do not seek help or receive care. Suicide is the fourth leading cause of death in 15 to 19 years old.[7]

Pattern of Referrals to Mental Health Services

It is interesting to analyze studies on pattern of referrals to clinical psychology services.

This study from Malaysia, analyzed 2179 referrals between January and December 2015 from 6 general hospitals and 3 mental health institutions that provide clinical psychology services. Results showed male referrals (60.3%), female referrals (39.7%), and adults (48.2%). Children (48.8%) and adolescents (28.1%) were mainly referred for psychological assessment.[8]

Parental Help Seeking Patterns Prior to Referral to Outpatient Child And Adolescent Mental Health Services

In this cross-sectional observational study, parents of 250 children were interviewed about pathways to outpatient child and adolescent mental health services (CAMHS). Educational services were the first help-seeking contact for the majority (57.5%) but referrals to CAMHS were most frequently from health care services (56.4%), predominantly general practitioners.[9]

Indian Scenario

The COVID-19 pandemic has given insight into the gaps in the current approach to mental health care and the need to expand India's mental health ecosystem.

According to a Lancet study and Global Health Data Exchange, India accounts for nearly 15% of the global mental health burden and 1 in 7 Indians is estimated to suffer from mental health disorders.[10]

Based on a WHO study, India has nearly 0.29 psychiatrists and around 0.07 psychologists per 100,000 population, compared with a median of 0.3 to 0.5 in low-mid income countries and 9 to 11 in high-income countries.[11]

HISTORY
Historical Aspects for Adolescent Psychology

G Stanley Hall first proposed the term *sturm und drang* which related to the internal turmoil and upheaval during adolescence in his book—*Adolescence* in 1904.

In 1950s, Anna Freuds formulated her psychodynamic theory that believed the psychological disturbances associated with youth were biologically based and culturally universal while Erik Erikson focused on the dichotomy between identity formation and role fulfilment.[12]

Only in the 1980s, the less turbulent aspects of adolescence, such as peer relations and cultural influence, were addressed.

The first official organization dedicated to the study of Adolescent Psychology was the Society for Research on Adolescence in 1984. It discussed issues like understanding interactions between adolescents' various issues in their environments such as culture, society, and the nature versus nurture to get insight into their behaviors.[13]

If people successfully deal with the conflict, they emerge from the stage with psychological strengths that will serve them well for the rest of their lives.[14]

Child Psychologist David Elkind has built on the work of the child Psychologist Jean Piaget and focused on the cognitive, perceptual, and social aspects of healthy development. His research and writing have included the effects of stress and the importance of creative spontaneous play for healthy development and academic learning.[15]

In 1927, Jane MacFarlane founded the Institute of Human Development at the University of California. She launched the Berkeley Guidance Study which focused on the development of children in terms of their socioeconomic and family backgrounds.[16]

The Oakland Growth Study, initiated by Harold Jones and Herbert Stolz in 1931, aimed to study the physical, intellectual, and social development of children in the Oakland area. Longitudinal data were collected from 1932 to 1981 on the individuals that extended past adolescence into adulthood.[17]

The pioneering longitudinal studies of child development were launched in the 1920s and 1930s. These followed their young study members well past adolescence into the middle years and later life. Glen Elder in the 1960s proposed a life course perspective *of adolescent development* and formulated several descriptive principles of adolescent development.[18]

DISCUSSION

Adolescence has been defined as a period of storm and stress, and this is the time that young people develop their own independent identities and develop important competencies. They are very dependent on peer approval and acceptance, and this often pushes them into risk-taking behaviors to prove their mettle.

As an adult, one often finds it hard to figure out why adolescents take the risks they do. The reasons are twofold. On the one hand, they are doing it to impress their peers and gain acceptance in the group. The other is that the way they process information cognitively is fundamentally different from the patterns of cognition adults' show.

They may not calculate trade-offs between risk and reward the way adults might, in a linear, rational, logical, and verbal manner. Rather, they rely on the gist of what they know about the situation, and intuition to make the final call.

Many attribute this pattern of cognitive processing to the thinning of gray matter and pruning of synapses that occur at this developmental stage. However, it is also found that pruning is in fact essential for the young person to be able to develop sound and healthy decision making, which is also no doubt shaped by experience, contextual factors, and cultural values.[19]

Adolescent Identity

Many studies have been conducted on various aspects of adolescent Identity formation which gives good insight to decide interventions.[20]

Romantic Relationships

Romantic relationships constitute a new dimension in the adolescent's social life. Defined as developmental tasks, they have been associated with both positive and negative outcomes. This study analyzed data from a sample of 747 adolescents from Andalusia (Spain) between 13 and 17 years old (50.5% girls, mean age wave 1 = 14.55, SD = 0.84). The Structural Equation Modeling analysis showed romantic relationships as a predictor of psychological well-being, having a positive link with positive interpersonal relationships and with life development, and a negative link with autonomy and self-acceptance.[21]

Different Sexual Orientations - Lesbian, Gay, Bisexual, Transgender, and Questioning

The role of psychologists on issues of gender identity and gender expression is very important for adolescence. Adolescents will benefit from support from their educators in developing a professional, nonjudgmental attitude toward people who may have a different experience of gender identity and gender expression from their own.[22]

Perspectives from the Adolescents

When we think of psychological issues of adolescents it is also important to understand the perspective of the target group that is the AYA - adolescent and young adults themselves. This study concluded that generally, adolescents cared more about the psychosocial aspects of health than the physical dimensions. They also considered factors such as independence, communication, socioeconomic conditions, mental health, religion, and educational facilities synonymous with the concept of health.[23]

Intervention Areas in Adolescence

The key areas whereby medical and psychological intervention would be required can be divided into the broad categories of *disorder or deviance, distress, and development.*

Disorder or deviance: Horowitz has made an interesting distinction between these conditions, showing how extenuating circumstances can lead to disorder or deviance on the one hand, which can be diagnosed using a standard nosology.

These can be defined or described as internal psychological dysfunctions. However, a pediatrician can also identify conditions that are not internal psychological dysfunctions but instead are natural responses that nondisordered people make to stressful conditions.[24]

Distress and development.[25]

The conditions, which we may label as distress, are an important area of work for both the mental health professional as well as the adolescent pediatrician. Distress can occur due to chronic familial discord, body image issues arising out of social norms and stigmatization, broken relationships and so forth. A trained, sensitive pediatrician can pick up signs of these conditions and their impact on the physical and mental health of the young person.

Very often, in addition to the diagnostic skills or treatment of physical or mental disease, it is equally important to build on existing skills and resiliencies and empower the adolescent to deal with the stressors faced in life.

Positive psychology is the scientific study of the strengths that enable individuals and communities to thrive. The field is founded on the belief that people want to lead meaningful and fulfilling lives, and is thus concerned with *eudaimonia*, meaning "the good life" or flourishing.[26]

Whom to refer to[27]

The term psychologist clearly expresses the training background the person has in the field of Psychology, the minimal training being a Master's degree, with adequate supervised field experience; a Doctoral degree would be preferred. All psychologists are trained in the basics of psychometric assessment and psychotherapeutic intervention.

Clinical psychologists are specifically trained to work with persons with severe mental health conditions and typically work in a team with a psychiatrist or a neurologist, the latter if they specialize in neuropsychology. The psychometric assessments they are specially trained to use, therefore, align with these cases and would help to diagnose psychiatric (eg, psychosis, obsessive-compulsive disorder, and so forth) or neurologic conditions (eg, dementias, amnesic disorders, and so forth).

Psychotherapists preferentially choose intervention rather than focusing only on assessment and therefore take further specialized training in specific psychotherapeutic approaches.

The word Counselor has been overused and often loosely applies to persons who have backgrounds in psychology, social work, or even special education. If one goes to a counselor, it would be best to ask for their training background or certification before beginning intervention, to ensure that they have the qualifications one wishes for.

Integrated Behavioral Health

The collaborative training between the various stakeholders in the CAMH should be enhanced. Currently, the favored methods, to augment the training for practicing primary-care physicians, such as CME and short training programs with their specific goals, settings, and methodology are well documented.

Given the biopsychosocial nature of human development and functioning, the high rates of co-occurring biopsychosocial problems and the fact that individuals commonly seek help for mental health problems from their primary care providers, psychologists recognize the need to work collaboratively with professionals from other disciplines. The concept of mind-body medicine is emphasized in the ancient Indian medicine system Ayurveda.[28]

Clinical history taking and interviewing are one of the most powerful tools available to the child and adolescent mental health professionals to make a diagnosis and plan management. Other measures such as rating scales, diagnostic interviews, and laboratory investigations must be used in conjunction with the information obtained during history taking and interviewing. The clinician must be sensitive to the child's lived experience and culture as well as their developmental and cognitive capabilities. Confidentiality and the limits thereof must be discussed with the child and family. Documentation is a very important aspect of assessment and must be strictly maintained.

Team Approach to an Adolescent with Mental Health Issues

The roles of the pediatrician and psychologist in the area of adolescent medicine are complementary and supportive of one another. In a pediatric OPD, a team approach that includes a psychologist, a social worker, and perhaps even a nutritionist, can prove very useful.

History Taking and Physical Examination

The primary referral could be to the pediatrician, with the focus of complaints being on physical symptoms such as skin eruptions, weight gain or loss, menstrual problems, and so forth.[25]

However, on further exploration of psychosocial history by the pediatrician, the underlying psychological issues such as self-esteem issues, broken relationships or an upcoming long-term relationship commitment, poor body image, unhealthy lifestyle and poor eating habits, gender confusion, stress pertaining to examinations or interviews, competitive career pathways, and so forth may come into play and such cases will benefit by referral to a psychologist.

Psychological and Psychometric Assessment

The first step at this point is usually a thorough assessment, usually carried out by a psychologist. The following section outlines the use of various psychometric tools and rating scales by the psychologist to unveil underlying psychological issues.

Assessment of Personality

Projective tests

Psychology offers an armamentarium of projective techniques which can be used to evaluate the psychological condition of children and adolescents.[29] The concept underlying projective techniques is that, when faced with unstructured material, a respondent is likely to project their own inner impulses and urges onto the material, thereby revealing hidden motivations and anxieties, fears, and concerns. The natural advantage of projective techniques is that the person being assessed is not aware of what is likely to be evaluated and is thus quite natural and unaffected by tension or stress as they perform.

Examples of semi-structured projective techniques include the Thematic Apperception Test and the Children's Apperception Test.[30] For both, there are International as well as Indian versions available, to be used as applicable. The test consists of a set of cards that have some human figures drawn on them in the case of TAT and animal figures in the case of CAT. The animal figures once again as viewed with ease by younger children for whom this test is designed. Stories built by the respondent around these cards, and the pictures seen by them, allow the psychologist to assess the respondent as per scoring protocols made available by the test developers.

Other, more unstructured projective techniques include projective play, human figure drawing, sentence completion, and so forth.

Objective assessments

Personality can also be assessed using empirical, objective tests such as the Minnesota Multiphasic Personality Inventory (MMPI, MMPI 2, and MMPI 3), The Millon Clinical Multiaxial Inventory (MCMI I, II, III, and IV), and versions of these tools specially designed for adolescent populations, such as Millon Adolescent Clinical Inventory (MACI) and the Millon Adolescent Personality Inventory (MAPI).[31] These are internationally validated and normed tools and are used with equal comfort in India as well as in other countries.

Assessment of Intelligence

Another important area of assessment often needed in Child and Adolescent settings is the assessment of Intelligence. There are several tools available to the psychologist in this domain, ranging from tests that are internationally used, such as the Wechsler Intelligence Scale for Children (WISC, WISC III, and WISC IV) as well as local India tests such as the variants developed by Bhatia, Kamat, Mahendrika Bhatt, and Malin.[32,33] Several figural tests are also available for an intelligence assessment in case the child or adolescent has difficulty with verbal material, for example, the Raven's Colored, Standard, and Advanced Progressive Matrices, among others.

Surveys and Rating Scales

The pediatrician may also work together with the psychologist on the team, and use rating scales that proven reliability and validity and have been used earlier in the country and cultural setting whereby the pediatrician is working. A detailed review of rating scales and their interpretation can be reviewed.[34]

Interventions

Once a thorough evaluation has been completed, it is possible for the team, including the adolescent pediatrician and the psychologist, to conduct *individual or group interventions* to address the issue.

Individual counseling may use cognitive therapy, or client-centered approach as a base.

Supportive Role of Pediatricians/Adolescent Physicians in Psychological Issues in Adolescent

Though the role of the psychologist is so important in adolescent health, unfortunately such service may not be easily available at all centers and referral may not be easy. For this, it may often became necessary for adolescent pediatricians to get trained in delivering what we can call first aid counseling and play the important role in.

1. Helping to remove the stigma attached to going to a mental health professional and
2. Motivating clients to accept the referral to a psychologist when available

Psychosocial Interviewing of Adolescents by Adolescent Physicians

Adolescent pediatricians are trained to take a detailed psychosocial review of an adolescent in addition to the medical history and the physical examination. There are many specialized protocols:

1. American Medical Association (Guidelines for Adolescent Preventive Services, or GAPS[3]
2. American Academy of Pediatrics[35]
3. HEADSS

In India, most Adolescent Pediatricians are using the HEADSS while Interviewing teenagers.

- HEADSS was designed by Dr Henry Berman in1972 and modified by Eric Cohen in 1985. It has been successfully used in adolescent clinics across USA and many other countries.[36]
- *HEADSS* stands for - *H*ome environment, *E*ducation/*E*mployment, *A*ctivities -peer-related, *D*rugs, *D*iet, *S*exuality, *S*uicide/depression
- In 2004, HEADSS was further expanded to *version 2 HEEADSSS (or HE2 ADS3)*, whereby E for *E*ating, and S for *S*afety from injury and violence, was added.[36]
- The 2014 The HEEADSS 3.0 update includes 2 important additions:

(1) Media and (2) strength-based approach. An alternative acronym, SSHADESS, accounts for this strategy. *S*trengths, *S*chool, *H*ome, *A*ctivities, *D*rugs/substance abuse, *E*motion/depression, *S*exuality, *S*afety.[37]

Pediatricians are giving such guidance that can be called *preventive counseling* and *Anticipatory guidance* to the parents right from infancy in the well-baby clinic.

a. Handling of common behavioral issues such as temper tantrums, thumb sucking and so forth

b. Age-appropriate developmental aspects and behavior.
c. Guidance for the healthy lifestyle that promotes positive behavior—sleep, diet, exercise and so forth.

Preventive Counseling for Parents – Dealing with Adolescents

Use a strengths-based approach

- Approaches based on risk factors alone may induce feelings of shame and deter engagement.
- Identify strengths early, so that they can be "built on" when motivating to change or when encouraging ongoing success.
- Praise when it is warranted!
- Use reflective listening and pause. This allows the teenager time to confirm and expand on his or her thoughts.
- Create a comfortable, trusting, nonjudgmental setting that communicates respect.
- Share your concerns.[37] (**Table 1**)

The following *case scenario* shows how a combination of pediatric approaches to health and lifestyle management, psychological evaluation of overlaid mental health issues, and positive psychology/life skills-based approaches can be used to diagnose and course correct for a disorder, alleviate distress and guide a patient toward development.

Case Scenario - SSHADESS Approach of History taking[37]

Strengths - excels in academics.

School – has consistently conducted well at school.

Home - Her parents are going through a lot of conflicts which threatens to culminate in a divorce. They often vent their anger by scolding her over her relatively poorer grades and her body shape and weight.

Activities - She was good at sports and was taking part in extracurricular activities enthusiastically.

Drugs/substance abuse – No significant history.

Emotion/depression - she finds herself unable to concentrate on the studies. She feels she is unattractive and obese and has begun resorting to fad diets and intermittent fasting over long spells.

Sexuality - No significant history.

Safety - No significant history.

Team approach of pediatrician and psychologist

The pediatrician places Sonia on a healthy nutritive diet and exercise routine after proper counseling, and the psychologist on the team speaks to her over 4 to 5 sessions, showing her how focusing on her own wellbeing may not only render her happier, but perhaps yield additional gains in terms of better self-esteem which in turn will help her deal with her parents' anger, which she comes to understand and empathize with, over the counseling sessions. Counseling of parents is also conducted to improve the home atmosphere.

Screening Tools Used to Identify Referrals to Mental Health Professionals

Various screening tools we use are *CRAFFT Screening Test* is a short clinical assessment *tool* designed to *screen* for substance-related risks and problems in adolescents.[38]

Table 1
Role of Pediatrician in preventive counseling and anticipatory guidance

Items	Psychological Impact and Risky Teen Behavior	Preventive Counseling	Anticipatory Guidance
Issues related to puberty and body changes	Body image issues affecting self-esteem Eating disorders Anxiety, depression affecting other domains – academics, interpersonal relationships and so forth Guilt regarding masturbation	Life skill education Enhancing self-esteem and coping skills	To prevent reproductive tract infections
Sexuality Gender-related issues	Risky sexual behavior Anxiety confusion regarding sexual orientation/identity	Age-appropriate sexuality education	Safe sex and healthy intimacy
Romantic relationships	Inability to handle toxic/abusive relationship	Life skills to understand negotiating skills and learning the ability to say no when necessary	Age-appropriate education about the intimacy and prevention of teenage pregnancy
Tobacco alcohol substance abuse	Peer pressure to experiment leads to recreational use to dependence on addiction	Impact on the developing brain with teen use of tobacco, alcohol, impact on a fetus in teen pregnancy and understanding addiction to prevent experimentation	Parental guidance to discuss and also look for flag signs.
Internet addiction – social media, chat rooms, porn gaming and so forth	Not being happy or feeling lonely due to various psychological issues and turning to media for solace or under peer pressure	Scientific knowledge of all these issues including suppression of melatonin by a blue screen and adverse effects of sleep deprivation	Parental guidance to monitor media use and flag signs of internet addiction and being role models for healthy media use
Healthy lifestyle	Obesity and risk of NCDs due to unhealthy diet and lack of physical activity	Scientific knowledge and prevention	Parental guidance
Underage driving DUI - Driving under influence Lack of helmet and safety belts.	Legal issues that can affect career prospects.	Respecting rules and laws and consequences of flouting them	Parental guidance and monitoring for safe vehicles us

Source: table made by authors.

If one gets a history that is suggestive of depression, we use screening tools such as PHQ (Patient Health Questionnaire) Beck's depression inventory screening for suicide behaviors' such as Suicide Behaviors Questionnaire (SBQ-R)[39,40]

Collaboration Between Psychologist and Adolescent Pediatrician

Development

The role of the pediatrician in Development areas is amply clear and unambiguous. These are areas whereby the client clearly has no psychological problems, but some issues are preventing the full expression of potential. Let us use a Case example of Sports Psychology here.

Case scenario. A pediatrician may see a youngster who has shown excellence in sports and has the potential to reach State or National levels in sports competitions. However, it is clear that the client loses confidence at a key juncture or seems to lack the focus and mindset needed during important matches to win.

The pediatrician and psychologist may work together along with a trainer or coach and help develop strategies, self-messages, and cues for the young person to use at these junctures, whereby they are on their own and cannot turn to others for help.

Having learned these strategies and techniques and practiced them thoroughly, the player is now set to use them at short notice even when they are on the field of in the midst of a tournament.

Distress

The pediatrician's role may vary from mere sharing and self-disclosure to take away the stigma of counseling, to some problem solving and advice-giving whereby the client seems puzzled and cannot choose between various alternatives that present themselves.

Going deeper, the pediatrician may also gently explore pain points that exist either in the client's surround, such as parents who are conflicted and thus not empathic. Or the issues may exist with the client, such as poor self-esteem or indecisiveness and lack of confidence.

All of the above may fall within the domain of Distress, and can safely be handled by a pediatrician, sensitized fully to the notion that referral to a psychologist would be required if the matter seems to be moving into the domain of Disorder.

Disorder

This is the domain whereby there is a clear-cut presence of mild mental conditions such as anxiety, or severe conditions such as an imminent psychotic breakdown. In these instances, a trained psychologist needs to step in, and in the case of severe mental illness, a psychiatrist's help would also be recruited to medicate the client appropriately.

Child and Adolescent Depression

This is a particularly delicate and sensitive area. Cases involving depression, suicidality, or depressed and traumatized states arising out the abuse of a physical and sexual nature, mandate intervention by a psychiatrist at the earliest to protect the wellbeing and safety of the client. POCSO is an Act passed in India to protect clients exposed to Child Sexual Abuse and protocols are very stringent for the same [SB45].[41]

The table later in discussion addresses a very important area, which falls under the domain of consultation liaison, whereby the pediatrician and psychologist can work together to make a difference to the client. Not much work is happening in this area at present, but there is a high felt need for the same.

This is the area whereby the young person is suffering from purely physical complaints, which in turn affect their self-image, their self-esteem, and their adjustment to social settings. Some examples of such problems include.

 i. Body weight-related issues such as obesity or being underweight, which lead the client to believe that they are very unattractive and makes them step back from other life situations whereby they could easily succeed.
 ii. Skin-related complaints such as Vitiligo or Acne, which once again lead to poor self-image making clients shy away from public appearances.
 iii. PCOS, with associated complications of menstruation, weight gain, and skin problems.
 iv. Deficiencies due to nutritional imbalance which leads to associated problems that once again reflects in behavior and lifestyle.
 v. Chronic pain due to conditions such as autoimmune problems or sports injuries which lead the young person to be embittered and in a constant state of distress and negativity.
 vi. Chronic illness such as juvenile diabetes, epilepsy, early-onset arthritis, allergies, and so forth force the young person to retreat into their shell, and make them believe that they can never live a "normal" life of a youngster like their friends can enjoy.

It is important that a pediatrician–psychologist team creates modules to intervene in the above issues, beginning with a broad universal application whereby awareness about the conditions is built up in a community and following up with support groups, lectures, and webinars as well as audio–visual and reading material which can be used for self-help.

A detailed history taking following the earlier elaborated HEADSS protocol would be a precursor to this management process (**Tables 2** and **3**)

Importance of Nongovernmental Organizations Working for Awareness and Education on Mental Health Issues

In low- and middle-income countries (LMICs) like India, trained mental health professionals are low in number, when one keeps the overall ratio of the huge population to be served in mind. A large portion of this population is difficult to reach as they are in villages and smaller towns, and do not have access to large urban and metropolitan health centers. A purely biomedical and institutional-based approach can work in settings with lower and more accessible populations, whereas LMICs do not have the necessary infrastructure. Also, several important sociocultural factors come into play, which demands a more community-based approach. In India, the District Mental Health Programs and National Mental Health programs have accepted nongovernmental organization (NGO) partnerships as the means for primary care delivery.[10]

Role of Nongovernmental Organizations to Promote Awareness and Education About Mental Health Issues and Removing Stigma for Going to Mental Health Professionals

All 3 authors are actively working in AACCI – Association of Adolescent and Child Care in India for the last 15 years. *AACCI* works for the holistic health of children and adolescents through parents and teachers who are the main pillars of their well-being.

Its core group consists of doctors from various mental health professionals, educationists, parents, sports experts, and family lawyers (http://www.aacci.in/ and http://www.aaccitrainingprograms.com/).

Table 2
What can the pediatrician handle and when to refer

Issues to Be Handled	Role of Primary Physician/ Pediatrician	Referral to Psychologist	Referral to Psychiatrist
Chronic physical illness, for example, epilepsy, diabetes Or Chronic Pain	Pediatrician/physician would advise on the medical management of the condition	Psychologist and/Pediatrician/ Physician may handle the psychological sequelae of anger about the condition.	May not be required unless there is serious depression, and so forth
Chronic conditions that undermine self-image, for example, Obesity, Vitiligo, PCOS and so forth	Pediatrician/physician would advise on the medical management of the condition	Psychologist and/Pediatrician/ Physician may handle the psychological sequelae of the conditions for example, shame, feeling self-conscious about body, or facing body shaming.	May not be required unless there is serious depression.
Life threatening conditions such as Cancers.	Pediatrician may not be the primary treating physician, but families often prefer to follow-up with trusted pediatrician in spite of availing of specialist help.	Psychologist may help conduct support groups, offers supportive counseling.	May not be required.
Anxiety spectrum disorders, Panic, Phobias, OCD	To identify and explain to the patient about the symptomatology	Psychotherapy – CBT REBT will be required for specific phobias Generalized anxiety disorders PTSD and OCD	Severe cases will require the medication and identification and treatment of comorbidities
Depression and Suicide risk	To identify and explain to the patient about the symptomatology Primary counseling can be conducted for mild depression.	Moderate depression will need counseling and psychotherapy. Urgent psychiatric referral and admission in case of suicide risk.	Moderate to severe depression will require medications in addition to counseling

Personality disorders	To identify flag signs and explain them to parents. It must be kept in mind that PDs are not formally diagnosed till 18 y	For assessment with scales such as MCMI, MACI, and so forth. Psychotherapy for serious conditions such as borderline personality disorder.	Medication to address specific symptoms whereby possible; identification and treatment of comorbidities
Psychotic spectrum disorders	To identify flag signs and explain to parents. Motivation to referral to psychiatrist	Supportive counseling in addition to psychiatrist treatment, Psychosocial interventions. Rehabilitation and support groups.	Medication for the condition, identification, and treatment of comorbidities
Substance and Nonsubstance addictions	To identify flag signs and explain to parents. Motivation to Referral to psychiatrist	Supportive counseling in addition to psychiatrist treatment. Work with parents and support system, behavioral interventions.	Deaddiction treatment and identification and treatment of comorbidities
ADHD, Autism spectrum and neurodevelopmental disorders, LD, Intellectual Disability, and so forth	To identify flag signs and explain to parents. Motivation to Referral to psychologist and psychiatrist/ neurologist/educator.	Supportive counseling in addition to psychiatrist treatment. Work with parents and support system, behavioral interventions.	Deaddiction treatment and identification and treatment of comorbidities

Source: table made by authors.

Table 3
Approach to the management of and adolescent

Clinical Presentation	Steps in Management	Intervention Approach
Body image issues	Treatment of minor ailments	Medical intervention
	Ensure knowledge about normal pubertal changes	Psychoeducation
	Counseling to increase self-esteem	Client-centered approach
	Assessment of psychological and psychiatric problems	Referral to psychologist/ psychiatrist
Eating disorders: Anorexia Nervosa and Bulimia	Nutritional counseling and maintenance of healthy weight	Nutritionist, Physician plans meals
	Medical management of comorbidities	OPD monitoring Vitamin, mineral supplements Hospitalization if required
	Psychotherapy	Referral to psychologist for cognitive behavior therapy or acceptance and commitment therapy for body image issues Family and group therapy
	Suicide risk assessment and management	Psychiatric referral whereby needed. Teamwork to ensure risk management.
Internet addiction	Treatment of minor ailments such as poor diet	Medical intervention
	Counseling to explore reasons for addiction	Client-centered approach Family and group therapy
	Behavioral methods to manage addictive behavior	Psychologist referral
	Cognitive behavior therapy, rational emotive behavior therapy	Psychologist referral
Poor academic performance	Medical management	Pediatrician explores systemic illness, genetic disorders, visual, or hearing impairment
	Management of psychological comorbidities	Psychologist referral to assess low or borderline IQ, learning disabilities, attention deficit hyperactive disorder, conduct disorder, oppositional defiant disorder.

Source: table made by authors.

Group Surveys for Adolescent Mental Health

We have conducted many surveys in many schools across India using rating scales and focused group discussions to try to find out trends seen in the population to be addressed [SB47][42–45]

Group Interventions

We regularly conduct Group interventions such as interactive workshops, small group discussions, which use the Life Skills perspective as a base, using pre and postworkshop surveys to reassess postintervention to study impact.

Life skills Life skills have been defined by the World Health Organization (WHO) as "the abilities for adaptive and positive behavior that enable individuals to deal effectively with the demands and challenges of everyday life."[46] LSE programs can reduce risky adolescent sexual behavior and also reduce the incidence of HIV transmission and AIDS[47,48]

WHO Life skill education -LSE program trains adolescents in Life skill training .This empowers young peple to take positive actions to protext themsleves to promote health and positive social relationships.

CLINICS CARE POINTS

- Adolescents don't open up easily. Hence Rapport building rapport is crucial
- Adolescents may often come with physical symptoms that are the result of their mental turmoil
- Observe body language carefully as it may tell you more than what is being said verbally
- Important to take the help of psychological assessments whereby necessary
- Important to refer serious cases to mental health professionals
- Involvement of family is very important for getting good results
- Anticipatory guidance and preventive counseling can be conducted by the primary physician
- Psychologist should be involved in specific counseling and psychotherapy

DISCLOSURE

The authors certify that they do not have any commercial or financial conflicts of interest and any funding sources from anywhere for writing this article.

REFERENCES

1. Available at: https://www.azquotes.com/author/13382-William_Shakespeare/tag/youth Accessed November 01, 2022.
2. Adolescent Psychology. (n.d.). In Alleydog.com's online glossary. Available at: https://www.alleydog.com/glossary/definition-cit.php?term=Adolescent+Psychology. Accessed January 6, 2022.
3. Elster A. The American Medical Association Guidelines for Adolescent Preventive Services. Arch Pediatr Adolesc Med 1997;151(9):958–9.
4. Patel V, Fisher AJ, Hetrick S, et al. Mental Health of Young people a Global public health challenge. Lancet 2007;369(9569):1302–13.
5. Trent M. Why adolescent Medicine? JAMA Paediatrics 2020;174(11):1023–4.
6. Xiong J, Lipsitz O, Nasri F, et al. Since January 2020 Elsevier has created a COVID-19 resource centre with free information in English and Mandarin on the novel coronavirus COVID- 19. The COVID-19 resource centre is hosted on Elsevier Connect, the company' s public news and information. J Affect Disord 2020; 277(January):55–64.
7. WHO. Available at: https://www.who.int/activities/improving-the-mental-and-brain-health-of-children-and-adolescents. Accessed March 01, 2022.
8. Martadza M, Saedon UI, Darus N, et al. Patterns of referral to clinical psychology services in the Ministry of Health Malaysia. Malays J Med Sci 2019;26(6):111–9.

9. Anna SH, Gry KT, Emil F, et al. Help-seeking pathways prior to referral to outpatient child and adolescent mental health services Clinical child Psychatrary and psychology Volume: 26 issue: 2, page(s): 569-585. Available at: https://journals.sagepub.com/doi/abs/10.1177/1359104521994192#abstract. Accessed January 7, 2021.

10. Available at: https://www.businesstoday.in/opinion/columns/story/how-india-can-make-mental-healthcare-affordable-and-accessible-to-all-311224-2021-11-03 Assessed January 9, 2022.

11. Available at: https://www2.deloitte.com/in/en/pages/about-deloitte/articles/How-India-can-make-mental-healthcare-affordable-and-accessible-to-all.html. Accessed January 9, 2022.

12. a b c Lerner RM, Steinberg LD. Handbook of adolescent psychology. 2nd edition. Hoboken (NJ): John Wiley & Sons; 2004.

13. Petersen AC. The Early Adolescence Study: An Overview. J Early Adolescence 1984;4(2):103–6.

14. Widick C, Parker CA, Knefelkamp L. Erik Erikson and psychosocial development. New Dir Student Serv 1978;1978(4):1–17.

15. Doorey, Marie. "David Elkind." Psychology Encyclopaedia. 2012. Available at: http://psychology.jrank.org/pages/210/David-Elkind.html.

16. Macfarlane J. 95, Psychology Professor. The New York Times; 1989. Retrieved August 16, 2013.

17. "The Oakland Growth and Berkeley Guidance Studies of the Institute of Human Development at the University of California, Berkeley". University of North Carolina. Archived from the original on September 12, 2012. Retrieved October 4, 2012.

18. Elder G. The life course as developmental theory. Child Development 1998; 69(1):1–12.

19. Institute of Medicine (US) and National Research Council (US) Committee on the Science of Adolescence. The Science of Adolescent Risk-Taking: Workshop Report. Washington (DC): National Academies Press (US); 2011. 4, The Psychology of Adolescence. Available at: https://www.ncbi.nlm.nih.gov/books/NBK53420/. Accessed January 9, 2022.

20. Meeus W. The study of adolescent identity formation 2000–2010: A review of longitudinal research. J Res Adolescence 2011;21(1):75–94.

21. Gómez-López Mercedes, Viejo Carmen, Ortega-Ruiz Rosario Psychological Well-Being During Adolescence: Stability and Association with Romantic Relationships Frontiers in Psychology VOLUME=10: 2019PAGES=1772. Available at: https://www.frontiersin.org/article/10.3389/fpsyg.2019.01772   DOI=10.3389/fpsyg.2019.01772.

22. American Psychological Association - Guidelines for Psychological Practice with Transgender and Gender Nonconforming People. American Psychological Association 0003-066X/15/$12.00 Vol. 70, No. 9, 832– 864 https://doi.org/10.1037/a0039906.

23. Soroor P, Zeinab H. Adolescents' view of health concept and its risk factors: a literature review. Int J Adolesc Med Health 2014;26(3):351–9.

24. Horowitz AV. Distinguishing distress from disorder as psychological outcomes of stressful social arrangements. Health: An Interdisciplinary. J Social Study Health 2007;11(3):273–89.

25. Scott JG, Mihalopoulos C, Erskine HE, et al. Childhood Mental and Developmental Disorders. Dis Control Priorities 2016;145–61. https://doi.org/10.1596/978-1-4648-0426-7_ch8. Third Ed (Volume 4) Ment Neurol Subst Use Disord.

26. Kashdan T, McKnight PE, Goodman FR. Evolving positive psychology: A blueprint for advancing the study of purpose in life, psychological strengths, and resilience. J Positive Psychol 2021. https://doi.org/10.1080/17439760.2021.2016906.
27. Meadows G, Paul F, Dipclinpsych RM. Psychological medicine when to refer to a psychologist. Published online 2007.
28. Lele Dr RD – Ayurveda and modern medicine. Body and mind chapter 12: 267-280 Published by Bharatiya Vidya Bhavan, Mumbai Printed by R. Raman at Inland Printers Mumbai; 1986.
29. Piotrowski C. On the decline of projective techniques in professional psychology training. N Am J Psychol 2015;17(2):259–66.
30. Aronow E, Weiss KA, Rezinkoff M. A practical guide to the Thematic apperception test. Philadelphia: Brunner Routledge; 2001.
31. Strack S. Essentials of Millon inventories assessment. 2nd edition. New York: John Wiley and Sons; 2002.
32. Wechsler D. The Wechsler intelligence scale for Children. 4th edition. London: Pearson; 2003.
33. Kaufman AS, Lichtenberger E. Assessing adolescent and adult intelligence. 3rd edition. Hoboken (NJ): Wiley; 2006.
34. Bhave S, Sovani A. Chapter 20 adolescent medicine in Partha's investigations and interpretations in paediatrics and adolescent practice. New Delhi India: Jaypee Brothers Medical publishers; 2019. p. 272–8.
35. Hagan JR, Shaw JS, Duncan PM, editors. Bright futures: guidelines for health supervision of infants, children, and adolescents. 3rd edition. Elk Grove Village (IL): American Academy of Paediatrics; 2008.
36. Goldenring JM, Cohen E. Getting into adolescent heads. Contemp Pediatr 1988; 5(7):75–90.
37. Goldenring JM, Rosen DS. Getting into adolescent heads: an essential update. Contemp Pediatr 2004;21(1):64–90.
38. Knight JR, Shrier LA, Harris SK, et al. Validity of the CRAFFT Substance Abuse Screening Test Among Adolescent Clinic Patients. Arch Pediatradolesc Med 2002;156(6):607–14.
39. Beck AT, Steer RA, Brown G. Beck depression inventory–II. Psychol Assess 1996.
40. Osman A, Bagge CL, Guitierrez PM, et al. The Suicidal Behaviors Questionnaire Revised (SBQ-R): Validation with clinical and nonclinical samples. Assessment 2001;(5):443–54.
41. POCSO 2012 act. Available at: https://wcd.nic.in/sites/default/files/POCSO-ModelGuidelines.pdf. Accessed January 28, 2022.
42. Swati YB, Sovani A, Joshi S, et al. An Analysis of Communication Patterns. Asian J Paediatrics Pract 2011;15(Number 2).
43. Swati YB, Sovani A, Raghavan SV, et al. Examination Anxiety in Junior College Youth of Mumbai Who Participated in LSE Training Workshops. Asian J Paediatrics Pract 2011;15(Number 1):12–5.
44. Swati YB, Sovani A, Joshi S, et al. An Analysis of Anger Management in Participants of LSE Workshops from Junior Colleges in Mumbai. Asian J Paediatric Pract 2012;15(Number 3):12–7.
45. Joshi M, Mane S, Sovani A, et al. Internet usage trends in male and female college students. Bombay Psychol 2012;27(1 and 2):44–50.
46. World Health Organization (WHO) - Information Series on School Health, Document 9, Skills for Health – Skills-based health education including life skills: An

important component of a Child-Friendly/Health-Promoting School. Available at: http://www.who.int/school_youth_health/media/en/.

47. Perry CL, Grant M. A Cross-cultural pilot study on alcohol education and young people. World Health Statistics Quarterly – Rapport. Trimestriel de Statistiques Sanitaires Mondiales 1991;44:70–3. As cited in Hubley, 2000.

48. Magnani R, Macintyre K, Karim AM, et al. The impact of life skills education on adolescent sexual risk behaviours in KwaZulu-Natal, South Africa. J Adolesc Health 2005;36(4):289–304.

Role of Psychologists in Pediatric Congenital Heart Disease

Kanhai Amin[a], Keshav Patel, MD, MS[b],*

KEYWORDS

- Infant • Adolescent • Child • Mental health • Psychology • Cardiology

KEY POINTS

- Congenital heart disease (CHD) is a significant stressor for infants and their families into adulthood.
- Psychologists can aid the parents and child at all stages of CHD from pregnancy to the child's transition to adulthood.
- More research needs to be performed on the role and types of psychological intervention that may be beneficial in CHD.

BACKGROUND

Congenital heart disease (CHD) is the most common congenital disorder in liveborn infants and the most prevalent cause of infant death arising from birth defects.[1–3] The definition of CHD is not concrete as some definitions include the complete cardio-vascular system, whereas others specify the lesions. Here, along with most studies, we follow the definition proposed by Mitchell and colleagues[4] in 1971 articulating that CHD is a structural irregularity of the heart or the great vessels with the capacity to affect functionality.

Many children are born with heart defects and disorders. The incidence of CHD is estimated to be 6 to 11.1 per 1000 live births, but this may under-represent the true total as many miscarriages are a result of CHD.[5] The incidence of moderate-to-severe CHD is estimated to be approximately 6 of 1000 live births but this increases to 19 of 1000 live births when including potentially serious bicuspid aortic valves.[6] CHD is also prevalent in stillborns. In a study by Reinhold-Richter and colleagues

[a] Yale University, 261 Park St, New Haven, CT 06511, USA; [b] Department of Internal Medicine, University of Illinois at Chicago College of Medicine, University of Illinois at Chicago, 840 South Wood Street, Room 440, MC 718, Chicago, IL 60612-7323, USA
* Corresponding author.
E-mail address: kpate447@uic.edu
Twitter: @kpatelMD (K.P.)

Pediatr Clin N Am 69 (2022) 865–878
https://doi.org/10.1016/j.pcl.2022.05.002
0031-3955/22/© 2022 Elsevier Inc. All rights reserved.

analyzing the autopsies of 3071 stillborn and deceased children younger than 16 years of age between 1969 and 1983, CHD was found in 26.5% of the autopsies.[7] In another study by Hoffman and colleagues,[8] the incidence of CHD in stillborn fetuses was 7.9%. There has been a significant increase in prevalence over the last century. A meta-analysis of 114 papers indicates that the birth prevalence (<5 years) has increased from 0.6 of 1000 live births in 1930 to 9.1 of 1000 live births post 1995.[9]

Research and knowledge regarding the etiology of CHD is increasing and many risk factors are known, but most individual cases of CHD have an unknown cause.[10] Although this knowledge is beneficial to providers, the knowledge or lack thereof serves as a significant possible stressor and/or source of guilt for parents.[11] For example, chromosomal aneuploidies are the cause of approximately 8% to 10% of CHD cases. Examples of these chromosomal aneuploidies include Down syndrome, Turner syndrome, Patau syndrome, and DiGeorge syndrome among others.[10] Meanwhile, single-gene defects are attributed to 3% to 5% of CHD cases.[2] Various risk factors for CHD are also known. These include the definite risk factors: maternal rubella, pregestational diabetes, phenylketonuria, and exposure to retinoids or thalidomide. Other potential risk factors are maternal age greater than 40 years, paternal age greater than 35 years, maternal obesity, and maternal alcohol use.[2]

Early recognition of CHD greatly improves outcomes.[5] Prenatal diagnosis is instrumental regarding long-term neurocognitive function.[12] Prenatal screening includes fetal echocardiography if there is an abnormal screening ultrasound or a greater than 3% risk for CHD.[5,13] Between 1996 and 2013, the accuracy of prenatal detection of major CHD significantly increased from 4.5% to 71.0%.[14] Accurate detection aids in parental decisions regarding the termination of pregnancy. After birth, common presentations include chest pain, syncope, and irregular heart rhythm; these findings by pediatricians should result in a referral to a pediatric cardiologist.[5]

This early recognition has resulted in a decrease in CHD mortality. In a study by Oster and colleagues,[15] the one year survival rate of infants with CHD increased from 67.4% between 1979 and 1993 to 82.5% between 1994 and 2005. This trend has been seen in most of the developed world with Belgium and Sweden reporting that 90% to 95% of children born with CHD between 1972 and the early 1990s are surviving into adulthood.[16–18] However, the increased survival and improved diagnostic capabilities have greatly increased the financial costs of CHD as more patients are surviving and requiring medical interventions. More patients surviving CHD has also led to a greater number of babies requiring noncardiac surgery and hospitalization.[19,20] An analysis of the 2012 Kid's Inpatient Database found that hospital costs for children with CHD accounted for 23% of the global costs while only representing 4.4% of discharges.[20] The median cost was $51,302 for children who underwent cardiac surgery, $21,920 for children who underwent cardiac catheterization, $4,134 for children who underwent noncardiac surgery, and $23,062 for children who underwent medical treatment.[20] These costs continue after discharge. Data from the 2009 to 2010 National Survey of Children with Special Health Care Needs (NS-CSHCN) suggest that families of 89.1% of CSHCN with CHD experience at least one financial burden and 14.9% require mental health services because of their child's condition. Furthermore, when comparing families of CSHCN with and without CHD, families with a child with CHD had a greater financial burden.[21] When compared with the general population, children with CHD require 1.5 times the educational services, three times the prescriptions, five times the home health services, and eight times the special medical equipment.[21] Families with at least one financial burden were also found to be three times more likely to use mental health services.[21]

DISCUSSION
Infants

Infants with CHD undergo tremendous stress in the neonatal, cardiac, and/or pediatric intensive care units (NICU, CICU, and PICU, respectively). This is the result of the physical, clinical, and psychosocial environment. The early childhood adversity and toxic stress caused by these environments, especially repeated stress, has significant long-term effects on the child, including their neurodevelopment.[22,23] In the physical environment, infants are routinely subjected to loud sounds, bright lights, foul odors, and unrest.[11,24] Many of these result in infant awakenings during sleep.[25] Neonates in intensive care also undergo repeated invasive procedures during a time when it is developmentally unexpected.[26] Neonates, especially preterm neonates, are also more sensitive to pain than older infants, children, and adults.[27] Additional stressors in the clinical environment include mechanical ventilation, heelsticks, nasogastric tube insertion, intravenous catheter insertions, handling, suctioning, other life-sustaining procedures and interventions, pharmacologic therapy, and analgesia.[28–30] For this article, the psychosocial effects are emphasized, but the physical and clinical environments coincide with the psychosocial environment. Primarily, there is limited time for interaction with parents, thus decreasing infant–parent bonding. In addition, caregivers have diminished opportunity to provide developmentally important interactions. This may be linked to insecure attachment issues later in development.[11,31] Infants may also undergo delirium and opioid withdrawal.[32] Infants with CHD, especially critical CHD, are also overwhelmed by sensory and social stimulation.[33]

These infants face tremendous neurodevelopmental issues not only due to the physical, clinical, and psychosocial environments in the ICU but also as a result of their CHD.[11] These issues lead to further problems in adolescence and adulthood. Up to 70% of infants with CHD are at risk for neurodevelopmental impairments.[34–38] A study by Limperopoulos and colleagues found that neurobehavioral abnormalities were present in greater than 50% of newborns and 38% of infants before surgery. After surgery, status remained unchanged in most.[35] In infants, atrial oxygen saturation less than 85% was significantly associated with neurodevelopmental abnormalities.[35] This fits other studies indicating that abnormal neurobehavior is present before open heart surgery.[38,39] Surgical stresses and invasive diagnostic procedures may also contribute to brain injury, thus placing children with critical CHD at risk for neurobehavioral issues.[35,40] Other risk factors of neurodevelopmental issues include prematurity, cardiopulmonary resuscitation, seizures, strokes, and longer hospital stays.[11] Maternal stress during pregnancy may also contribute towards fetal programming, which has been shown to increase the risk for neurodevelopmental sequelae in other populations.[41] As a result, many survivors of CHD are at risk for behavioral, learning, cognitive, and motor impairments later in life.[33]

Psychologists play a minimal role in alleviating these issues faced by infants during this time; however, substantial research is coming out on how to diminish and mitigate these adverse effects.[28,42,43] Nevertheless, long-term effects are noticeable in adolescence and psychologists can play a significant role during this developmental period.

Adolescents

Owing to improved medical and surgical practices, there has been a significant improvement in survival rates, and CHD is now regarded as a chronic disease compared to a terminal one in many developed nations.[44] Adolescents face various stressors including additional surgeries, insurance coverage, and body image concerns.[45] Some studies indicate greater internalizing symptoms, whereas others show significantly more externalizing symptoms than controls.[46] A meta-analysis by Karsdorp and colleagues[47] found that only older children and adolescents with CHD displayed an increased risk of internalizing problems such as depressive and anxiety symptoms and externalizing behavior such as aggression and hyperactivity. The relationship with age is not clear; age may be a factor in the emotional conceptualization of CHD or natural puberty changes may play a role.[45] Many children with severe cyanotic defects post-surgery also deal with psychiatric disorders with one study noting a rate of 46%.[48] A systematic review by Latal and colleagues[46] found that maladjustment, the inability to function successfully and cope with difficulties in various domains and the inability to maintain effective relationships, ranges from 5% to 41% according to parental reports. In parental reports, individual characteristics such as postoperative developmental delay were also regularly related to psychological maladjusment.[46,49–51]

Research suggests that individuals with severe CHD or physical limitations as a result of their CHD have lower intelligence than their counterparts.[47,52,53] This may be a result of the increased care and severity of procedures required by those with more severe CHD. For example, research has shown that there is significant retardation of mental development in infants who were operated on with deep hypothermic cardiopulmonary bypass.[53] This difference in intelligence is noticeable during school-age years and poses different developmental requirements. A meta-analysis by Karsdorp and colleagues[47] found that patients with severe CHD experienced lower cognitive functioning than those with less severe CHD, especially in regards to performance intelligence. Karsdorp and colleagues suggest that children with severe CHD may benefit from therapy and interventions focused on perceptual organizational abilities, including visual and spatial abilities. Furthermore, the meta-analysis found that psychological interventions focused on reducing anxiety and depression may benefit adolescents and older children with CHD.[47]

The psychosocial needs of children and adolescents with CHD are not well understood. Regardless, there is growing consensus that surgical treatment should be accompanied by interventions concerning the psychological needs of adolescents and children.[54–56] Research by McMurray and colleagues[57] found five areas of emphasis: difficulty coping with one's own CHD, physical limitations, social exclusion, bullying and discrimination, and hope for improvement. Coping with the presence of disease includes sentiments of why me?, anger, fear, and regret, especially during instances where CHD serves as a limiting factor or subjects children to different experiences. Children also feel limited by impairment. This includes not being able to participate in the same activities such as sports and parties and limitations regarding future vocational goals. Many adolescents have reported that these limitations adversely affect their confidence.[57] Impairment is one of the more common ways adolescents define their difficulties especially when it comes to being limited by pace or stamina leading to partial or total social exclusion.[52,58] Many children and adolescents also face bullying. In McMurray and colleagues' study, all participants viewed themselves as normal and wanted others to do the same. However, this was not always the case as 32% reported being bullied. This bullying stemmed from physical differences such as lack of stamina, athletic inability, different coloration (blue-tinge), and short stature.[57] Bullying and lower self-esteem may be more prevalent in boys, potentially due to the greater emphasis on athleticism.[59] Reports indicate that up to 81% of those with cyanotic CHD may face teasing and bullying. Many also feared discrimination by future employers.[57] Regarding hopes and future improvement, many participants in McMurray's study hoped for alleviation of their physical impairment, never requiring surgery and medication again, educating others, and getting rid of their scars.[57]

A study by Horner and colleagues regarding adults with complex CHD found that their study was the first time many participants had talked about the social and personal consequences of their condition even though 52% were tearful and remembered disliking school. Many of these participants reported that they kept their pain and feelings private while acting as if everything was fine. For girls, this involved attempting to cover up their scars and cyanosis with makeup.[59]

School psychologists and outside psychologists play a crucial role in addressing bullying. This begins with recognition by teachers, nurses, and other school faculty.[60] For cardiac patients with anxiety and depression, cognitive behavioral therapy has proven to be one of the most effective interventions.[61] Cognitive behavioral therapy includes restructuring anxiety-provoking thoughts and learning relaxation techniques. A cognitive behavior therapy approach may also assist in counteracting unproductive thoughts arising from being unable to do similar activities as peers.[62]

Positive psychology is also useful towards psychocardiology as it improves the quality of life of not only the patient but also family members.[63] Positive psychology focuses on optimism and improving traits such as perseverance and courage while focusing on individual abilities instead of what is wrong and dysfunctional.[64,65] A Rogerian client-centered approach may also serve as a useful approach in assisting with the processing of surgical interventions.[62] Although there are many more methodologies psychologists may use not mentioned here, adolescents need individual care. Research regarding outcomes after receiving psychological care in children with CHD is lacking, but it seems that children may benefit from this care. Many children also do not fully understand their ailment even though they wish to do so. Thus, there may be benefits to research regarding when, how, and to what degree children and adolescents should be told of their disease by health professionals and parents.[57]

Parents

During pregnancy
Having a child with CHD is difficult for parents at all stages, from pregnancy to adulthood. Many studies have shown high levels of stress and distress for parents during diagnosis and hospitalization for CHD.[66,67] Many babies with severe and complex CHD are now diagnosed *in utero* at approximately 20 weeks gestation. Whether this diagnosis occurs during pregnancy or later, it creates feelings of tremendous guilt, fear, anger, sadness, and grief which can continue for many years. Earlier diagnostic capabilities also allow for parents and families to consider abortion.[68] CHD is also a cause of many spontaneous abortions.[6,69] In both of these instances, there is room for psychological intervention to address feelings of guilt and sadness.[70,71] Maternal anxiety during pregnancy is linked with many adverse perinatal outcomes including preterm birth, lower mean birth weight, smaller head circumference, and lower mental developmental scores at age 2.[72,73] Research regarding the effect of psychological intervention towards the parents during this time on the child is sparse. Regardless, parents will benefit from intervention.

After birth
After birth, the ICU environment is very stressful to families, especially mothers.[74] A recent systematic review by Woolf-King and colleagues found that 25% to 50% of parents reported clinically elevated symptoms of anxiety and/or depression, whereas 30% to 80% of parents reported severe psychological distress. Furthermore, 80% of parents at infant discharge had clinically significant symptoms of trauma, whereas up to 30% of parents had symptoms consistent with a diagnosis of post-traumatic stress disorder.[66] This may be the time of highest distress.[75] This is particularly true for

parents of children with more severe lesions.[76] Among other things, many parents fear that their child will die and threats to infant health are a known risk factor for psychological disturbance.[11,76] For many parents, the alteration of parental role is the most stressful aspect during this time.[75] Moreover, the bright lights, machinery, strange sounds, infant appearance, and general unfamiliarity may heighten parental distress.[75,77–79] Mothers of children with cyanotic CHD have significantly higher levels of depression than mothers with acyanotic children.[80] Other possible stressors include having to make hard, time-sensitive decisions, witnessing painful medical care, deterioration to personal physical health (poor nutrition, disrupted sleep, and fatigue), missing work, financial strain, and difficulty understanding medical information.[11] These stressors in combination with the ICU environment may heighten or result in the expression of previous mental illness; early childhood adversity such as physical, emotional, or sexual abuse; and other stressful events.[81,82]

High levels of parental distress, including anxiety and depression, during this time are predicted to interfere with the parent–infant attachment process; as a result, infant behavioral and intellectual development and mental health may be negatively impacted.[83–85] Parents with higher stress also report worse physical health, higher health service use, greater suicidal ideation, and worse parent and child quality of life.[11,86–89]

The severity and prevalence of distress among parents is often underestimated by providers.[90] However, there is still the opportunity to minimize psychological distress and improve bonding at this time. This includes individualized task-focused coping skills. A study analyzed the benefits of a Congenital Heart Disease Intervention Programme (CHIP), a relatively brief early psychosocial intervention. This program had the goals of assisting parents deal with the grief of not having a "normal" child through narrative therapy processes; promoting mother–infant interactions in feeding, care-taking, and social and sensory stimulation; and teaching mothers problem-solving strategies to counteract worries regarding having a child with CHD.[91] Problem-solving therapy includes active coping skills to decrease worry and distress to improve child development.[92] In a controlled trial, CHIP was shown to improve neurodevelopment, feeding practices, maternal anxiety, and worry. Another randomized trial found that early palliative care decreased maternal anxiety, improved positive reframing, and improved family relationships.[93] A trial by Giménez and Sánchez-Luza also analyzed the benefits of individualized support in the NICU delivered by a psychologist. They found that individualized intervention resulted in significantly less anxiety and depression after 15 days.[94] A systematic review by Kasparian and colleagues[11] analyzed these findings and determined that more high-quality trials are needed to establish better psychological care. There may be potential benefits from other therapies such as psychodynamic psychotherapies and cognitive-behavioral mindfulness.[11] Infants in the ICU with CHD are a unique population, and research specific to this population should be conducted.[75]

After discharge

The transition from the hospital to home also brings additional stresses and disruptions. There may still be uncertainty about the child's survival and this has been shown to increase parental stress.[95] An infant with CHD also requires additional levels of vigilance resulting in a physical and mental toll. In turn, the sleep deprivation and significant amount of work amplifies the parental stress, anxiety, and exhaustion.[96] After worries about survival, feeding problems are one of the greatest stressors for parents due to weight gain worries.[97] Dysphagia is a major contributor to this as it occurs in up to 20% of infants who have undergone open heart surgery.[98] Moreover, more than 50% of infants who have had open heart surgery are discharged with some sort of feeding device.[99] Parents face many fears and difficulties regarding these feeding devices, so more advanced training and practice may prove beneficial.[96] Additional psychological care during this time period may also assist in alleviating stress and anxiety. During routine medical care, medical professionals should ask about parental stress and family function while appropriately recommending and providing care.

There are few longitudinal studies analyzing the long-term mental health problems of parents of children with CHD. However, these longitudinal studies conflict regarding whether the parental symptoms decline over time or persist. For example, Menahem and colleagues[100] found that the emotional distress including anxiety at the time of surgery largely dissipated by 12 to 50 months following surgery. Meanwhile, Lawoko and Soaros[89] found in a 1-year follow-up that 7% to 22% of parents had persisting problems. In this study, mothers demonstrated higher levels of hopelessness and distress.[89]

A difference between mothers and fathers is a routine finding with mothers typically taking the burden of care and expressing higher rates of distress.[11,94] Fathers are also noticeably absent from the data with only one study in Kasparian and colleagues's[11] systematic review presenting paternal data. Treatment specific to fathers may improve engagement and efficacy; this includes language adaptation, action-orientated treatment styles, and self-disclosure.[101–103] However, none of these strategies have been tested on fathers of children with a critical illness.[11]

Transition to Adulthood

Many patients with CHD struggle during the transition from adolescence to adulthood and adult care. This stems from challenges regarding employment, health insurance, and not fully understanding their condition if left sheltered.[104–106] This can lead to depression.[107] Research has shown that adolescents more knowledgeable about their condition have an easier transition to adult care. In one study, adolescents with a higher level of understanding of their condition were significantly more likely to directly communicate with their provider and demonstrated a better understanding regarding the transtion to adult care.[108] This is similar to another study by Stewart and colleagues, which also found that transition readiness was better in patients more knowledgeable about their condition. Patient knowledge was also positively correlated with parental knowledge.[109] Providers should address any shortcomings in patient knowledge during the transition to adulthood.

SUMMARY

CHD is the most prevalent cause of infant death arising from birth defects.[1–3] CHD is extremely stressful to both pediatric patients and their caregivers, but this aspect is often overlooked. This article focuses on the role of psychologists in pediatric CHD.

Prolonged hospital and/or ICU stay can be taxing on the infant and caregiver. This stress can have negative long-term effects, including neurodevelopmental delays, on the child.[22,23] Important interaction time between caregivers and infants also becomes limited, leading to adverse effects. Maternal anxiety during pregnancy is associated with many poor perinatal outcomes, including preterm birth and lowerdevelopmental scores.[72,73] Intervention with a psychologist in the NICU decreases parental anxiety and depression.[94] There are many possible therapies, but there is a lack of research specific to psychological intervention for CHD.

Children and adolescents continue to face stressors related to CHD, including additional surgeries.[45] Beyond the medical stressors, children face difficulty coping with their CHD, their physical limitations, social exclusion, and bullying.[57] Outcomes after psychological care in children are lacking; however, most children will likely benefit from psychological intervention.

Many with CHD struggle during the transition from adolescence to adulthood. Adolescents who understand their condition are better suited for this transition.[108] However, many children do not understand their CHD even though they wish to do so. Psychologists may help children and adolescents both understand and cope with their condition.

CLINICS CARE POINTS

- The mental health effects on both children and parents arising from a child with congenital heart disease (CHD) are often overlooked
- Adverse maternal mental health during and after pregnancy can have long-term adverse effects on child development
- CHD continues to serve as a stressor for infants and their families into adulthood
- Adolescents with CHD often do not understand their condition, face bullying, and have psychological disturbances
- There is tremendous capacity for psychologists to improve parental and child mental health at various time points

DISCLOSURE

The authors have nothing to disclose.

REFERENCES

1. Jorgensen M, McPherson E, Zaleski C, et al. Stillbirth: the heart of the matter. Am J Med Genet A 2014;164A(3):691–9.
2. van der Bom T, Zomer AC, Zwinderman AH, et al. The changing epidemiology of congenital heart disease. Nat Rev Cardiol 2011;8(1):50–60.
3. Tennant PWG, Pearce MS, Bythell M, et al. 20-year survival of children born with congenital anomalies: a population-based study. Lancet 2010;375(9715): 649–56.
4. Mitchell SC, Korones SB, Berendes HW. Congenital Heart Disease in 56,109 Births Incidence and Natural History. Circulation 1971;43(3):323–32.
5. Garcia RU, Peddy SB. Heart Disease in Children. Prim Care 2018;45(1):143–54.
6. Hoffman JIE, Kaplan S. The incidence of congenital heart disease. J Am Coll Cardiol 2002;39(12):1890–900.
7. Reinhold-Richter L, Fischer A, Schneider-Obermeyer J. Congenital heart defects. Frequency at autopsy. Zentralbl Allg Pathol 1987;133(3):253–61.
8. Hoffman JI, Christianson R. Congenital heart disease in a cohort of 19,502 births with long-term follow-up. Am J Cardiol 1978;42(4):641–7.
9. van der Linde D, Konings EEM, Slager MA, et al. Birth prevalence of congenital heart disease worldwide: a systematic review and meta-analysis. J Am Coll Cardiol 2011;58(21):2241–7.
10. Nora JJ, Berg K, Nora AH. Cardiovascular diseases: genetics, epidemiology, and prevention. New York: Oxford University Press; 1991.
11. Kasparian NA, Kan JM, Sood E, et al. Mental health care for parents of babies with congenital heart disease during intensive care unit admission: Systematic review and statement of best practice. Early Hum Dev 2019;139:104837.

12. Kipps AK, Feuille C, Azakie A, et al. Prenatal diagnosis of hypoplastic left heart syndrome in current era. Am J Cardiol 2011;108(3):421–7.
13. Donofrio MT, Moon-Grady AJ, Hornberger LK, et al. Diagnosis and treatment of fetal cardiac disease: a scientific statement from the American Heart Association. Circulation 2014;129(21):2183–242.
14. Lytzen R, Vejlstrup N, Bjerre J, et al. The accuracy of prenatal diagnosis of major congenital heart disease is increasing. J Obstet Gynaecol 2020;40(3):308–15.
15. Oster ME, Lee KA, Honein MA, et al. Temporal trends in survival among infants with critical congenital heart defects. Pediatrics 2013;131(5):e1502–8.
16. Moons P, Bovijn L, Budts W, et al. Temporal trends in survival to adulthood among patients born with congenital heart disease from 1970 to 1992 in Belgium. Circulation 2010;122(22):2264–72.
17. Mandalenakis Z, Rosengren A, Skoglund K, et al. Survivorship in Children and Young Adults With Congenital Heart Disease in Sweden. JAMA Intern Med 2017;177(2):224–30.
18. GBD 2017 Congenital Heart Disease Collaborators. Global, regional, and national burden of congenital heart disease, 1990-2017: a systematic analysis for the Global Burden of Disease Study 2017. Lancet Child Adolesc Health 2020;4(3):185–200.
19. Massin MM, Astadicko I, Dessy H. Noncardiac comorbidities of congenital heart disease in children. Acta Paediatr 2007;96(5):753–5.
20. Faraoni D, Nasr VG, DiNardo JA. Overall Hospital Cost Estimates in Children with Congenital Heart Disease: Analysis of the 2012 Kid's Inpatient Database. Pediatr Cardiol 2016;37(1):37–43.
21. McClung N, Glidewell J, Farr SL. Financial burdens and mental health needs in families of children with congenital heart disease. Congenit Heart Dis 2018;13(4):554–62.
22. Shonkoff JP, Garner AS. Committee on Psychosocial Aspects of Child and Family Health, Committee on Early Childhood, Adoption, and Dependent Care, Section on Developmental and Behavioral Pediatrics. The lifelong effects of early childhood adversity and toxic stress. Pediatrics 2012;129(1):e232–46.
23. Grunau R. Early pain in preterm infants. A model of long-term effects. Clin Perinatol 2002;29(3):373–94, vii - viii.
24. Shoemark H, Harcourt E, Arnup SJ, et al. Characterising the ambient sound environment for infants in intensive care wards. J Paediatr Child Health 2016;52(4):436–40.
25. Daniels JM, Harrison TM. A case study of the environmental experience of a hospitalized newborn infant with complex congenital heart disease. J Cardiovasc Nurs 2016;31(5):390–8.
26. Anand KJS, Aranda JV, Berde CB, et al. Summary proceedings from the neonatal pain-control group. Pediatrics 2006;117(3 Pt 2):S9–22.
27. Anand KJ. Clinical importance of pain and stress in preterm neonates. Biol Neonate 1998;73(1):1–9.
28. Carbajal R, Rousset A, Danan C, et al. Epidemiology and treatment of painful procedures in neonates in intensive care units. JAMA 2008;300(1):60–70.
29. Newnham CA, Inder TE, Milgrom J. Measuring preterm cumulative stressors within the NICU: the Neonatal Infant Stressor Scale. Early Hum Dev 2009;85(9):549–55.
30. Weber A, Harrison TM. Reducing toxic stress in the neonatal intensive care unit to improve infant outcomes. Nurs Outlook 2019;67(2):169–89.

31. Gonya J, Nelin LD. Factors associated with maternal visitation and participation in skin-to-skin care in an all referral level IIIc NICU. Acta Paediatr 2013;102(2): e53–6.

32. Harris J, Ramelet A-S, van Dijk M, et al. Clinical recommendations for pain, sedation, withdrawal and delirium assessment in critically ill infants and children: an ESPNIC position statement for healthcare professionals. Intensive Care Med 2016;42(6):972–86.

33. Massaro AN, Glass P, Brown J, et al. Neurobehavioral abnormalities in newborns with congenital heart disease requiring open-heart surgery. J Pediatr 2011; 158(4):678–81.e2.

34. Mebius MJ, Kooi EMW, Bilardo CM, et al. Brain Injury and Neurodevelopmental Outcome in Congenital Heart Disease: A Systematic Review. Pediatrics 2017; 140(1). https://doi.org/10.1542/peds.2016-4055.

35. Limperopoulos C, Majnemer A, Shevell MI, et al. Neurodevelopmental status of newborns and infants with congenital heart defects before and after open heart surgery. J Pediatr 2000;137(5):638–45.

36. Miller SP, McQuillen PS, Vigneron DB, et al. Preoperative brain injury in newborns with transposition of the great arteries. Ann Thorac Surg 2004;77(5): 1698–706.

37. Tavani F, Zimmerman RA, Clancy RR, et al. Incidental intracranial hemorrhage after uncomplicated birth: MRI before and after neonatal heart surgery. Neuroradiology 2003;45(4):253–8.

38. Owen M, Shevell M, Donofrio M, et al. Brain volume and neurobehavior in newborns with complex congenital heart defects. J Pediatr 2014;164(5):1121–7.e1.

39. Owen M, Shevell M, Majnemer A, et al. Abnormal brain structure and function in newborns with complex congenital heart defects before open heart surgery: a review of the evidence. J Child Neurol 2011;26(6):743–55.

40. Bloom AA, Wright JA, Morris RD, et al. Additive impact of in-hospital cardiac arrest on the functioning of children with heart disease. Pediatrics 1997;99(3): 390–8.

41. Kim DR, Bale TL, Epperson CN. Prenatal programming of mental illness: current understanding of relationship and mechanisms. Curr Psychiatry Rep 2015; 17(2):5.

42. Weiner J, Sharma J, Lantos J, et al. How infants die in the neonatal intensive care unit: trends from 1999 through 2008. Arch Pediatr Adolesc Med 2011; 165(7):630–4.

43. Lipner HS, Huron RF. Developmental and Interprofessional Care of the Preterm Infant: Neonatal Intensive Care Unit Through High-Risk Infant Follow-up. Pediatr Clin North Am 2018;65(1):135–41.

44. Park JH, Park SW, Lee JY, et al. Survival rates of patients with congenital heart disease. Korean Soc Matern Child Health Conf 2003;2:81–2.

45. Jackson JL, Misiti B, Bridge JA, et al. Emotional functioning of adolescents and adults with congenital heart disease: a meta-analysis. Congenit Heart Dis 2015; 10(1):2–12.

46. Latal B, Helfricht S, Fischer JE, et al. Psychological adjustment and quality of life in children and adolescents following open-heart surgery for congenital heart disease: a systematic review. BMC Pediatr 2009;9:6.

47. Karsdorp PA, Everaerd W, Kindt M, et al. Psychological and cognitive functioning in children and adolescents with congenital heart disease: a meta-analysis. J Pediatr Psychol 2007;32(5):527–41.

48. Bjørnstad PG, Spurkland I, Lindberg HL. The impact of severe congenital heart disease on physical and psychosocial functioning in adolescents. Cardiol Young 1995;5(1):56–62.
49. Hövels-Gürich HH, Konrad K, Wiesner M, et al. Long term behavioural outcome after neonatal arterial switch operation for transposition of the great arteries. Arch Dis Child 2002;87(6):506–10.
50. Bellinger DC, Rappaport LA, Wypij D, et al. Patterns of developmental dysfunction after surgery during infancy to correct transposition of the great arteries. J Dev Behav Pediatr 1997;18(2):75–83.
51. Miatton M, De Wolf D, François K, et al. Behavior and self-perception in children with a surgically corrected congenital heart disease. J Dev Behav Pediatr 2007; 28(4):294–301.
52. Kramer HH, Awiszus D, Sterzel U, et al. Development of personality and intelligence in children with congenital heart disease. J Child Psychol Psychiatry 1989;30(2):299–308.
53. Sharma R, Choudhary SK, Mohan MR, et al. Neurological evaluation and intelligence testing in the child with operated congenital heart disease. Ann Thorac Surg 2000;70(2):575–81.
54. Casey FA, Sykes DH, Craig BG, et al. Behavioral adjustment of children with surgically palliated complex congenital heart disease. J Pediatr Psychol 1996; 21(3):335–52.
55. Gantt LT. Growing up heartsick: the experiences of young women with congenital heart disease. Health Care Women Int 1992;13(3):241–8.
56. Masi G, Brovedani P. Adolescents with congenital heart disease: psychopathological implications. Adolescence 1999;34(133):185–91.
57. McMurray R, Kendall L, Parsons JM, et al. A life less ordinary: growing up and coping with congenital heart disease. Coron Health Care 2001;5(1):51–7.
58. Wray J, Sensky T. How does the intervention of cardiac surgery affect the self-perception of children with congenital heart disease? Child Care Health Dev 1998;24(1):57–72.
59. Horner T, Liberthson R, Jellinek MS. Psychosocial profile of adults with complex congenital heart disease. Mayo Clin Proc 2000;75(1):31–6.
60. Hymel S, Swearer SM. Four decades of research on school bullying: An introduction. Am Psychol 2015;70(4):293–9.
61. Compare A, Germani E, Proietti R, et al. Clinical Psychology and Cardiovascular Disease: An Up-to-Date Clinical Practice Review for Assessment and Treatment of Anxiety and Depression. Clin Pract Epidemiol Ment Health 2011;7:148–56.
62. Compare A, Zarbo C, Bonaiti A. Psychocardiology and the Role of the Psychologist in Acquired and Congenital Heart Disease. In: Callus E, Quadri E, editors. Clinical psychology and congenital heart disease. Milan: Springer; 2015. p. 133–46.
63. Callus E, Quadri E, Chessa M. Elements of psychocardiology in the psychosocial handling of adults with congenital heart disease. Front Psychol 2010;1:34.
64. Alex Linley P, Joseph S, Harrington S, et al. Positive psychology: Past, present, and (possible) future. J Posit Psychol 2006;1(1):3–16.
65. Livneh, H., Martz, E. (2007). An Introduction to Coping Theory and Research. In: Martz, E., Livneh, H. (eds) Coping with Chronic Illness and Disability. Springer, Boston, MA. https://doi.org/10.1007/978-0-387-48670-3
66. Woolf-King SE, Anger A, Arnold EA, et al. Mental health among parents of children with critical congenital heart defects: A systematic review. J Am Heart Assoc 2017;6(2). https://doi.org/10.1161/JAHA.116.004862.

67. Franck LS, McQuillan A, Wray J, et al. Parent stress levels during children's hospital recovery after congenital heart surgery. Pediatr Cardiol 2010;31(7):961–8.

68. Menahem S, Grimwade J. Pregnancy termination following prenatal diagnosis of serious heart disease in the fetus. Early Hum Dev 2003;73(1–2):71–8.

69. Roos-Hesselink JW, Kerstjens-Frederikse WS, Meijboom FJ, et al. Inheritance of congenital heart disease. Neth Heart J 2005;13(3):88–91.

70. Séjourné N, Callahan S, Chabrol H. The utility of a psychological intervention for coping with spontaneous abortion. J Reprod Infant Psychol 2010;28(3):287–96.

71. Adler NE, David HP, Major BN, et al. Psychological responses after abortion. Science 1990;248(4951):41–4.

72. Grigoriadis S, Graves L, Peer M, et al. Maternal Anxiety During Pregnancy and the Association With Adverse Perinatal Outcomes: Systematic Review and Meta-Analysis. J Clin Psychiatry 2018;79(5). https://doi.org/10.4088/JCP.17r12011.

73. Brouwers EPM, van Baar AL, Pop VJM. Maternal anxiety during pregnancy and subsequent infant development. Infant Behav Dev 2001;24(1):95–106.

74. Pleck JH, Masciadrelli BP. Paternal Involvement by U.S. Residential Fathers: Levels, Sources, and Consequences. The role of the father in child development, 4th ed. 2004;4:222-271.

75. Diffin J, Spence K, Naranian T, et al. Stress and distress in parents of neonates admitted to the neonatal intensive care unit for cardiac surgery. Early Hum Dev 2016;103:101–7.

76. Brosig CL, Whitstone BN, Frommelt MA, et al. Psychological distress in parents of children with severe congenital heart disease: the impact of prenatal versus postnatal diagnosis. J Perinatol 2007;27(11):687–92.

77. Miles MS, Funk SG, Kasper MA. The neonatal intensive care unit environment: sources of stress for parents. AACN Clin Issues Crit Care Nurs 1991;2(2):346–54.

78. Barr P. A dyadic analysis of negative emotion personality predisposition effects with psychological distress in neonatal intensive care unit parents. Psychol Trauma 2012;4(4):347–55.

79. Franck LS, Cox S, Allen A, et al. Measuring neonatal intensive care unit-related parental stress. J Adv Nurs 2005;49(6):608–15.

80. Üzger A, Başpınar O, Bülbül F, et al. Evaluation of depression and anxiety in parents of children undergoing cardiac catheterization. Turk Kardiyol Dern Ars 2015;43(6):536–41.

81. Leigh B, Milgrom J. Risk factors for antenatal depression, postnatal depression and parenting stress. BMC Psychiatry 2008;8:24.

82. Lancaster CA, Gold KJ, Flynn HA, et al. Risk factors for depressive symptoms during pregnancy: a systematic review. Am J Obstet Gynecol 2010;202(1):5–14.

83. Feldman R, Granat A, Pariente C, et al. Maternal depression and anxiety across the postpartum year and infant social engagement, fear regulation, and stress reactivity. J Am Acad Child Adolesc Psychiatry 2009;48(9):919–27.

84. Gravener JA, Rogosch FA, Oshri A, et al. The relations among maternal depressive disorder, maternal expressed emotion, and toddler behavior problems and attachment. J Abnorm Child Psychol 2012;40(5):803–13.

85. Murray L, Arteche A, Fearon P, et al. Maternal postnatal depression and the development of depression in offspring up to 16 years of age. J Am Acad Child Adolesc Psychiatry 2011;50(5):460–70.

86. Pinelli J, Saigal S, Bill Wu Y-W, et al. Patterns of change in family functioning, resources, coping and parental depression in mothers and fathers of sick newborns over the first year of life. J Neonatal Nurs 2008;14(5):156–65.

87. Lawoko S. Factors influencing satisfaction and well-being among parents of congenital heart disease children: development of a conceptual model based on the literature review. Scand J Caring Sci 2007;21(1):106–17.

88. Werner H, Latal B, Valsangiacomo Buechel E, et al. The impact of an infant's severe congenital heart disease on the family: a prospective cohort study. Congenit Heart Dis 2014;9(3):203–10.

89. Lawoko S, Soares JJF. Distress and hopelessness among parents of children with congenital heart disease, parents of children with other diseases, and parents of healthy children. J Psychosom Res 2002;52(4):193–208.

90. Kasparian N, Barnett B, Sholler G, Winlaw D, Kirk E. When hearts and minds meet: A psychological perspective on fetal cardiac diagnosis. Infant Mental Health Journal 2011;31:103–4.

91. McCusker CG, Doherty NN, Molloy B, et al. A controlled trial of early interventions to promote maternal adjustment and development in infants born with severe congenital heart disease. Child Care Health Dev 2010;36(1):110–7.

92. D'Zurilla TJ, Nezu AM. Problem-solving therapy: a social competence approach to clinical intervention. New York: Springer Pub; 1999.

93. Hancock HS, Pituch K, Uzark K, et al. A randomised trial of early palliative care for maternal stress in infants prenatally diagnosed with single-ventricle heart disease. Cardiol Young 2018;28(4):561–70.

94. Cano Giménez E, Sánchez-Luna M. Providing parents with individualised support in a neonatal intensive care unit reduced stress, anxiety and depression. Acta Paediatr 2015;104(11):e476.

95. Tak YR, McCubbin M. Family stress, perceived social support and coping following the diagnosis of a child's congenital heart disease. J Adv Nurs 2002;39(2):190–8.

96. Hartman DM, Medoff-Cooper B. Transition to home after neonatal surgery for congenital heart disease. MCN Am J Matern Child Nurs 2012;37(2):95–100.

97. Davis D, Davis S, Cotman K, et al. Feeding difficulties and growth delay in children with hypoplastic left heart syndrome versus d-transposition of the great arteries. Pediatr Cardiol 2008;29(2):328–33.

98. Einarson KD, Arthur HM. Predictors of oral feeding difficulty in cardiac surgical infants. Pediatr Nurs 2003;29(4):315–9.

99. Medoff-Cooper B, Irving SY. Innovative strategies for feeding and nutrition in infants with congenitally malformed hearts. Cardiol Young 2009;19(Suppl 2):90–5.

100. Menahem S, Poulakis Z, Prior M. Children subjected to cardiac surgery for congenital heart disease. Part 2 – Parental emotional experiences. Interactive CardioVascular Thorac Surg 2008;7(4):605–8.

101. Seidler ZE, Rice SM, River J, et al. Men's mental health services: The case for a masculinities model. J Mens Stud 2018;26(1):92–104.

102. Seidler ZE, Dawes AJ, Rice SM, et al. The role of masculinity in men's help-seeking for depression: A systematic review. Clin Psychol Rev 2016;49:106–18.

103. Seidler ZE, Rice SM, Ogrodniczuk JS, et al. Engaging Men in Psychological Treatment: A Scoping Review. Am J Mens Health 2018;12(6):1882–900.

104. Reid GJ, Irvine MJ, McCrindle BW, et al. Prevalence and correlates of successful transfer from pediatric to adult health care among a cohort of young adults with complex congenital heart defects. Pediatrics 2004;113(3 Pt 1):e197–205.

105. Fekkes M, Kamphuis RP, Ottenkamp J, et al. Health-related quality of life in young adults with minor congenital heart disease. Psychol Health 2001;16(2): 239–50.
106. van Rijen EHM, Utens EMWJ, Roos-Hesselink JW, et al. Psychosocial functioning of the adult with congenital heart disease: a 20-33 years follow-up. Eur Heart J 2003;24(7):673–83.
107. Popelová J, Slavík Z, Skovránek J. Are cyanosed adults with congenital cardiac malformations depressed? Cardiol Young 2001;11(4):379–84.
108. Clarizia NA, Chahal N, Manlhiot C, et al. Transition to adult health care for adolescents and young adults with congenital heart disease: perspectives of the patient, parent and health care provider. Can J Cardiol 2009;25(9):e317–22.
109. Stewart KT, Chahal N, Kovacs AH, et al. Readiness for Transition to Adult Health Care for Young Adolescents with Congenital Heart Disease. Pediatr Cardiol 2017;38(4):778–86.

Role of Psychologists in Child Abuse Pediatrics

Olga Jablonka, PhD[a],*, Vincent J. Palusci, MD, MS[b]

KEYWORDS

- Forensic interview • Medical evaluation • Safety • Screening
- Trauma-informed care

KEY POINTS

- Abuse and neglect harm child in a number of ways with emotional and developmental trauma in addition to physical injury and death.
- The child psychologist has a vital role to play to address these harms in the outpatient medical evaluation of child physical and sexual abuse.
- Important functions are preparing the team before, assessing the child during, and assisting in communicating safety and treatment needs after the evaluation.

INTRODUCTION

In addition to being clinicians assessing and treating children with possible child abuse and neglect, child psychologists have important roles in the interdisciplinary medical evaluation of child maltreatment (CM). In the 60 years since the publication of Dr C. Henry Kempe's landmark article, "The Battered Child Syndrome,"[1] the subject of CM has become universal and not restricted to one community or to one type of medical provider. The goal of all professionals dedicated to this field is to optimize a child's physical and mental health and to ensure that child abuse, like many other adverse childhood experiences and social determinants of health, will be improved or eradicated.[2,3] Early work suggested that the role of child psychologists is twofold: assessment of the dynamics involved in the particular case and treatment.[4] This article describes the extent of the problem and the medical evaluation of CM, focusing on the outpatient interdisciplinary assessment of suspected child physical and sexual abuse.

General Epidemiology and Emotional Effects

Although each state in the United States defines CM in its child welfare and criminal statutes, broad definitions have been developed for the Child Abuse Prevention and

[a] Department of Child and Adolescent Psychiatry, NYU Grossman School of Medicine, 462 First Avenue, GC-65, New York, NY 10016, USA; [b] Department of Pediatrics, NYU Grossman School of Medicine, 462 First Avenue, GC-65, New York, NY 10016, USA
* Corresponding author.
E-mail address: Olga.Jablonka@nyulangone.org

Pediatr Clin N Am 69 (2022) 879–893
https://doi.org/10.1016/j.pcl.2022.05.003
0031-3955/22/© 2022 Elsevier Inc. All rights reserved.
pediatric.theclinics.com

Treatment Act and by the World Health Organization (**Box 1**).[5,6] Although child abuse overall pertains to the variety of acts committed or omitted by parents or caretakers for children, the quality of the parent–child relationship and nurturing is often left out of state laws. Sexual abuse, for example, has been defined as sexual contacts or exploitation of children by adults that cannot be consented to by the child and which violate social laws or taboos, but the emotional effects far outweigh the physical findings.[7] Similarly, all of the major types of CM carry their emotional and behavioral harms.

The victimization of children through maltreatment remains an all too common occurrence. In the United States, 1%–2% of children are confirmed victims of abuse or neglect each year, and young children and infants have the highest rates. More than

---

Box 1
World Health Organization Child Maltreatment definitions

Child abuse: Child abuse or maltreatment constitutes all forms of physical and/or emotional ill-treatment, sexual abuse, neglect or negligent treatment or commercial or other exploitation, resulting in actual or potential harm to the child's health, survival, development, or dignity in the context of a relationship of responsibility, trust, or power.

Physical abuse: Physical abuse of a child is that which results in actual or potential physical harm from an interaction or lack of an interaction, which is reasonably within the control of a parent or person in a position of responsibility, power, or trust. There may be a single or repeated incidents.

Emotional abuse: Emotional abuse includes the failure to provide a developmentally appropriate, supportive environment, including the availability of a primary attachment figure, so that the child can establish a stable and full range of emotional social competencies commensurate with her or his personal potentials and in the society in which the child dwells. There may also be acts toward the child that cause or have a high probability of causing harm to the child's health or physical, mental, spiritual, moral, or social development. These acts must be reasonably within the control of a patent or person in a position of responsibility, power, or trust. Acts include restriction of movement, patterns of belittling, denigrating, scapegoating, threatening, scaring, discriminating, ridiculing, or other nonphysical forms of hostile or rejecting treatment.

Neglect and negligent treatment: Neglect is the failure to provide for the development of the child in all spheres: health, education, emotional development, nutrition, shelter and safe living conditions, in the conditions, in the context of resources available to the family or caretakers and causes or has a high probability of causing harm to the child's health or physical, mental, spiritual, moral, or social development. This includes the failure to properly supervise and protect children from harm as much as is feasible.

Sexual abuse: Child sexual abuse is the involvement of a child in sexual activity that he or she does not fully comprehend or is unable to give informed consent to, or that violates the laws or social taboos of society. Child sexual abuse is evidenced by this activity between a child and an adult or another child who by age or development is in a relationship of responsibility, trust, or power, the activity being intended to gratify or satisfy the needs of the other person. This may include but is not limited to:
• The inducement or coercion of a child to engage in any unlawful activity
• The exploitative use of a child in prostitution or other unlawful sexual practices
• The exploitative use of children in pornographic performances and materials

Exploitation: Commercial or other exploitation of a child refers to the use of the child in work or other activities for the benefit of others. This includes, but is not limited to, child labor and child prostitution. These activities are to the detriment of the child's physical or mental health, education, or spiritual, moral or social-emotional development.

one-third (37.4%) of all US children will experience a child protective services (CPS) investigation by age 18 years.[8] Maltreated children suffer from a variety of behavior problems and mental disorders in addition to physical injuries.[9,10] The adverse childhood experiences study has noted the powerful relationship between adverse childhood experiences and several conditions of adulthood, including risk of suicide, alcoholism, depression, illicit drug use, and other lifestyle changes.[11,12] Although the exact pathways are still being explored, childhood abuse is thought to affect adult physical and mental health by putting people at risk for depression, trauma and stress-related disorders, difficulties in relationships, destructive behaviors, and negative beliefs and attitudes toward others.

The National Child Abuse and Neglect Data System (NCANDS) provides information about the US annual incidence of CM with aggregate and case-level data on child abuse reports received by state CPS agencies. National estimates of the overall numbers of victims (substantiated or indicated CPS reports) and victims identified with physical and sexual abuse show decline over the 25 years of nationally collected data in NCANDS (**Fig. 1**) following similar trends in other national crime statistics.[13] However, there are still more than 650,000 US children in 2019 who were found to be victims of maltreatment, and more than 175,000 of them were physically or sexually abused.[14]

Maltreated children present with significantly more internalizing and externalizing problems than non-maltreated children and have greater risk for developing comorbid medical and/or psychiatric conditions that may further derail normal development.[15–17] Clinical presentations may vary, regardless of the identified trauma. Common emotional symptoms include fear, sadness, anger, and/or extreme difficulties in emotion regulation.[18] Young children, who may have more difficulty verbalizing their feelings as compared with older children, may present with notable behavioral difficulties, such as oppositional and/or defiant behavior, aggression, separation anxiety, and/or sexualized behavior.[19] In addition, children may show behavioral avoidance, a hallmark symptom of post-traumatic stress disorder (PTSD).[18]

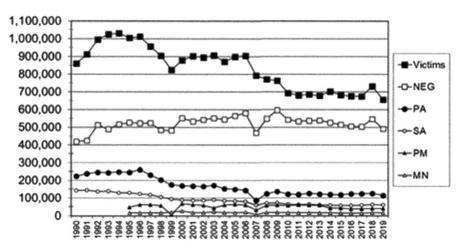

Fig. 1. US child maltreatment victims, NCANDS, 1990–2019. *Note.* Derived from United States Department of Health & Human Services (US DHHS) Child Maltreatment reports, 1990-2019 (12). MN, medical neglect; NEG, neglect; PA, physical abuse; PM, psychological maltreatment; SA, sexual abuse.

The diagnostic criteria for PTSD in the most recent Diagnostic and Statistical Manual of Mental Disorders (DSM-5)[20] identify four categories of post-traumatic stress symptoms: (1) intrusion symptoms, (2) avoidance symptoms, (3) negative alterations in thoughts and feelings that developed or worsened following the trauma, and (4) arousal and reactivity trauma-related alterations; many of which require language or highly attuned parent report. A thorough assessment of the child and their behavior is warranted following trauma exposure. Identifying mental health issues, and specifically PTSD, in maltreated children under the age of 6 is particularly difficult given their limited abilities to report on their psychological symptoms.[21–23] In addition, some research indicates that very young children may experience additional trauma symptoms that are not captured by the current DSM-5 criteria, such as constriction of play, regression to earlier functioning, aggression, separation anxiety, and development of new fears.[23]

More than two-thirds of children report experiencing a trauma before age 16 years.[24] Short-term distress following trauma exposure is common, and it is important to note that most of the children return to their prior levels of functioning. Current estimates suggest that 3% to 15% of girls and 1% to 6% of boys who are exposed to trauma will develop PTSD.[8] Factors that may increase risk for PTSD include female gender, previous trauma exposure or multiple traumas, prior psychiatric history and especially past history of anxiety, family adversity or parent psychopathology, and low social support.[10] When working with youth who have experienced a trauma, it is important to conduct a thorough evaluation of symptoms and history to better understand their clinical needs.

CM is given as a comorbid factor in a spectrum of adolescent problems, such as substance abuse, truancy, runaways, and psychiatric disorders.[25,26] According to findings from a longitudinal project examining the effects of maltreatment in adolescents, adolescents that experience CM were more likely to meet the clinical criteria for at least one mental health problems (eg, depression, anxiety, externalizing problems, PTSD, and psychological impairment) than their non-maltreated peers.[27,28]

MEDICAL EVALUATION
The Team Process

The interdisciplinary team uses multiple professional perspectives and expertise to identify and treat a number of harms that are related to one or more types of maltreatment. Thus, the diagnostic evaluation varies with the type of CM and the injuries of concern, be they physical or emotional.[29] An interdisciplinary team comprises professionals from various disciplines who work in collaboration to address multiple physical and psychological needs. Unlike a multidisciplinary team, it is not just a group of experts implementing separate treatments on a patient. The members of an interdisciplinary team work together to complement one another's expertise and to actively coordinate work toward shared treatment goals.[30]

Because of the complex nature of an optimal medical evaluation for CM, a number of team structures with additional professionals have been devised to add expertise and perspectives for the benefit of the child and to assist in the investigation for child protection.

Years before the publication of "Battered Child Syndrome," C. Henry Kempe originally formed a dedicated team of doctors, psychologists, nurses, and social workers to evaluate children with possible physical abuse.[1] At Los Angeles and Pittsburgh children's hospitals, these teams then spread throughout the country, beginning often with a physician–social worker team.[30] Teams have the potential to improve diagnosis and protection, and an early study noted that the teams' service recommendations and placement decisions were usually followed by CPS.[31] The Children's Hospital Association first offered guidelines for team structure and function in 2005, and teams have moved from the hospital to the community with the development of free-standing child advocacy centers (CACs) which can offer colocated investigators and streamlined evaluations can reduce trauma to the child.[32,33] There is reasonable evidence to support the idea that teams are effective in improving criminal justice and mental health responses compared with standard agency practices and that the team approach reduces bias.[34–36]

Referrals and evaluations can follow a number of pathways, from hospitals or emergency rooms, physicians, social workers, CPS caseworkers, or the legal system (**Fig. 2**). Differing from independent psychological evaluations, for which guidelines have been offered,[37] the child psychologist's role is not as an independent evaluator but is rather assisting the medical evaluation during three phases: information gathering, interviewing and physical assessment, and sharing opinions and recommendations. An assessment of the dynamics of child abuse necessitates a professional understanding of complicated interaction of social and personal factors, and the child psychologist's assessment can provide relevant information concerning whether to remove a child from the home, whether there is a danger to siblings, or whether the case would be amenable to treatment.[4]

Information gathering, a cornerstone of medical diagnosis that plays an important part in the diagnosis of CM, needs to begin before the actual evaluation as much as possible. It is the history, taken with the physical examination findings and imaging studies, that offers a sound basis for diagnosis and treatment recommendations for the child and family. Inquiring and recording the specific complaints and disclosures of maltreatment by the child and parent, if any, in their own words is vitally important to the ultimate protection of the child. Behavioral and emotional issues are equally important in this assessment. Certain nonspecific behaviors, developmental delays, and history of trauma should be recorded as part of the medical history; this history aids in assessing harm and planning for appropriate treatment.[7] The health history provides an opportunity to assess child and family resilience factors, social connectedness, parenting attitudes, and skills. The review of systems allows the medical provider to collect symptoms of trauma that may not have been identified in the chief

Before the Medical Visit	During the Medical Visit	After the Medical Visit
Referral	Team Huddle/Preparation[a]	Team Debriefing[a]
Information Gathering	Information Gathering[a]	Medical Diagnosis
Discipline-specific review[a]	Medical history	Psychological Assessments[a]
	Screening[a]	
Acuity Assessment[a]	Medical Preparation	Treatment[a]
Scheduling / Staffing	Interview[a]	Referrals[a]
	Physical Examination	Communicating Findings[a]
	Patient Support[a]	
	Safety Assessment[a]	

Fig. 2. The referral/evaluation/treatment process. [a]Potential role for child psychologist.

complaint but that can offer valuable insight into the current impact of trauma on the patient. Symptoms may be functional, neurodevelopmental, or related to immune function. It is important to obtain as much of this information as possible *before* proceeding with the evaluation. Collecting these data is often done best by members of the team with expertise in social work, psychology, and forensic interviewing.

After information gathering, the medical evaluation proceeds with physical assessment, testing, and clinical diagnosis, followed by treatment and referral. The medical clinician must be cognizant that multiple forms of maltreatment may coexist, understand the importance of certain risk factors, assist in choosing the appropriate location and timing of evaluation, the staff needed, and recognize that children being evaluated may have experienced significant trauma in their lives.

After the evaluation, the clinician integrates information from the referral source, history, examination, testing, and members of the interdisciplinary team to arrive at an assessment or diagnosis, often utilizing schema of diagnostic categories.[38–40] Documentation must be objective, with appropriate use of psychological screening, testing, and safety assessment as part of the comprehensive evaluation. This assessment of the child's physical and emotional health needs should be formulated with plans for any needed treatments and communicated to the caretakers or others responsible for the child so that appropriate services can be arranged.

Major Functions Before the Medical Evaluation

Child psychologists who work on interdisciplinary teams in medical settings spend a considerable amount of time teaching, whether formally, in the context of didactics and seminars, or informally, in the context of case discussions or clinical consultations.[41] Child psychologists can educate the medical team about mental health issues commonly seen in CM and provide a nuanced understanding of how symptoms and associated behavioral difficulties or functional impairment may develop over time. This is particularly true before the medical evaluation, when the interdisciplinary team is preparing for the evaluation by learning about the patient, their history, and the reason for the CM referral. In addition, child psychologists relay current research findings and discuss potential treatments with the team. Lastly, child psychologists have the unique opportunity to teach trainees, such as medical students, residents, and fellows, along with psychology externs and interns, about child abuse and its associated short-term and long-term mental health outcomes.[41]

As the mental health expert on the team, the child psychologist's primary role before the medical evaluation is to review relevant patient information and to synthesize this information to provide psychoeducation and support to the interdisciplinary team. By reviewing existing mental health records, neuropsychological testing reports, and individualized education plans, the child psychologist can have a better understanding of the patient, his strengths, and his limitations. The child psychologist can then integrate and relay these findings to the team to provide a greater contextualization of the child's presenting problems.[42] In addition, the child psychologist can suggest or recommend possible modifications that could facilitate the evaluation. Unfortunately, child psychologists are unable to access all relevant patient files at times and may need to use their clinical judgment in formulating case conceptualizations based on available data.

In preparing for the medical evaluation for the child presented in the first vignette (**Box 2**), there are several ways the child psychologist can gather information and help support the interdisciplinary team. First, the medical record may provide important information regarding the child and the specific symptoms associated with his ASD diagnosis (ie, language skills, cognitive delays, and behavioral issues). Data

---

Box 2
Physical abuse

A 9-year-old boy with patterned bruises and autism spectrum disorder has been referred by a local emergency room. The physician noted that the lesions appear to be "loop" or "cord marks," and the police have arrested his mother who reported hitting him with a belt to control his behavior. Limited medical information is available, but there is information that he sees a child psychiatrist, receives a number of medications for behavior control, and is in a classroom with additional personnel to provide services and close supervision. What additional information is needed to plan for his outpatient medical evaluation?

---

gathered from the emergency room may be limited to a specific snapshot in time, whereas notes from his psychiatrist may provide a closer look at the child's baseline functioning. Second, clinicians can outreach to existing providers, such as the treating psychiatrist, to gather collateral information that can aid the medical evaluation. For instance, what triggers the child's behavioral dysregulation? What strategies work well in soothing the child? If consultation and/or documentation are unavailable, child psychologists can relay the need to obtain these data from the caretakers who will be bringing the child in, such as the CPS caseworker who may have already gathered this collateral information. If no information is available, child psychologists can support team members in reviewing their general understanding and management of (**Box 3**) ASD.

Major Functions During the Medical Evaluation

Considering the high occurrence of mental health issues in maltreated youth, it is important to assess for clinically significant internalizing and externalizing symptoms, assist with acute patient decompensation, and refer to appropriate treatment.[3,4] Child psychologists can gather information regarding the child's emotional and behavioral functioning informally through the initial psychosocial assessment provided by the caregiver and/or CPS caseworker, or formally by administering standardized assessment measures. Ideally, screening instruments should be targeted, brief, and psychometrically sound. In addition, all measures should be reviewed before the child leaves the evaluation, as critical items related to non-suicidal self-injury, suicidal ideation, or homicidal ideation may be endorsed and will warrant further evaluation. Typically, a standard risk assessment with adequate safety planning will suffice.[43]

Although it is beyond the scope of this review to explore all available assessment measures, a number of screening tools are available that can be used as indicated (**Table 1**).[44,45] The child psychologist helps the medical team determine what routine screening is needed for mental health issues and whether a formal diagnostic tool is needed. In choosing a screening measure, it is important to consider various factors

---

Box 3
Sexual asault

A 15-year-old girl has been referred for an examination after she reported sexual assault by her boyfriend. She previously has resisted anogenital examination and the collection of sexually transmitted infection and forensic specimens and has a history of non-suicidal self-injury ("cutting") and suicidal ideation. Given her emotional reactions and the need for examination and testing, what steps can be taken during the medical evaluation to reduce further her trauma while identifying and treating her after the assault?

such as (1) age of the child, (2) availability of parent-report, (3) language preference, (4) length of measures, and (5) specific symptom cluster vs. general measure of pathology. It is important to remember that a screening tool is only helpful if it is used faithfully and results in timely clinical interventions and referrals if concerns are identified. In addition, if a patient is in imminent danger or acute crisis, an additional evaluation at a child psychiatric emergency room is recommended. Lastly, child psychologists are available to provide short-term patient support and parent education throughout the duration of the evaluation as well as promote elements of trauma-informed care (TIC).[46]

At times, children presenting for a medical evaluation may also be appropriate candidates for a forensic interview. "A forensic interview of a child is a developmentally-sensitive and legally sound method of gathering information regarding allegations of abuse and/or exposure to violence. This interview is conducted by a neutral professional utilizing research and practice-informed techniques as part of a larger investigative process" (p. 3)[60] Child psychologists are eligible to receive specialized training in forensic interviewing if they work in a CAC that conducts forensic interviews. However, it is important to note that the role of a forensic interviewer is significantly different from that of a treating clinician; therefore, in order to uphold ethical and legal standards, it is important to maintain boundaries around these relationships (ie, a child psychologist should not provide psychological treatment to the child they interviewed, nor should they interview existing therapy clients). Similarly, child psychologists may be asked to assist with medical preparation, which may include informing the child about what will happen during the medical examination, reviewing names of body parts, and providing skills coaching to mitigate any examination-related emotional distress. If the child psychologist is needed to be present during the physical examination, it is paramount to uphold professional and ethical standards and to refer out for treatment if needed.

To increase the chances of a successful medical evaluation with the adolescent presented in the second vignette (Box 3), it is important to consider TIC. "The basic definition of TIC is when every part of service is assessed and potentially modified to include a basic understanding of how trauma impacts the life of an individual seeking services" (p. 217)[61] Patient-centered communication and care is critical in TIC, and trauma survivors are encouraged to collaborate with their provider in their medical appointment. In this scenario, it is understandable that a patient with a sexual abuse history may have difficulty with a provider being in close proximity to the patient and needing to touch the patient's body. In an effort to increase subjective control and trust, the physician should provide the patient with options to mitigate anxiety, such as allowing a support person to be present during the physical examination and encouraging the patient to verbalize if they feel uncomfortable. "TIC creates a respectful and emotionally safe space in which to engage children, adolescents, and families around the discussion and management of these issues and to prevent retraumatization" (p. 8)[46]

Major Functions After the Medical Evaluation

On completion of the medical evaluation, the treatment team should meet to review the findings and formulate a plan. Child psychologists are present to support medical team members in these discussions and advocate for the child's mental health needs. Patients who endorse emotional and/or behavioral symptoms during the evaluation, and who are not already connected to mental health services, should be referred for appropriate care.[62] The child psychologist can assist with identifying referral options and longer term treatment planning. Lastly, child psychologists may collaborate

Table 1
Selected tools for mental health screening and diagnosis

Measure	Author	Construct Measured	Format (Report)	Age Group (in Years)	Time to Administer (in Minutes)	Language
Clinician administered PTSD scale for DSM-5-child/adolescent version	Pynoos, Weathers, Steinberg, Marx, Layne, Kaloupek, Schnurr, Keane, Blake, Newman, Nader, and Kriegler[47]	PTSD symptoms	Clinician	7+	45–60	English
Child PTSD symptom scale	Foa, Johnson, Feeny, and Treadwell[48,49]	PTSD symptoms	Child caregiver	8–18	15	English Spanish
Child trauma screen	Lang and Connell[50]	PTSD symptoms	Child	6–17	5–10	English
Eyberg child behavior inventory	Eyberg[51]	Externalizing symptoms	Caregiver	2–16	5	English Spanish
Generalized anxiety disorders and screener	Spitzer, Kroenke, Williams, and Loew[52,53]	Anxiety	Child	13+	1–2	English Spanish
Kiddie schedule for affective disorders and schizophrenia for school-age children	Kaufman and Schweder[54,55]	Comprehensive	Clinician	6–18	90	English
Patient health questionnaire—adolescents	Johnson, Harris, Spitzer, and Williams[56]	Depression	Child	11–17	< 3	English Spanish
Pediatric emotional distress scale	Saylor[57]	Traumatic stress internalizing symptoms	Caregiver	2–10	7	English Spanish
Revised children's anxiety and depression scale	Chorpita, Yim, Moffitt, Umemoto, and Francis[58,59]	Internalizing symptoms	Child caregiver	8–18	10–15	English Spanish

---

Box 4
Sexaul abuse

During her outpatient medical evaluation for sexual abuse, a 3-year-old girl was noted to have inappropriate sexualized behavior and other signs of emotional trauma. Her uncle has been removed from her home and any contact has been stopped pending further investigation by CPS and law enforcement. What plans will you make for services to address her behavioral and mental health needs?

---

with outside agencies, such as investigators and courts, by providing psychoeducation on the patient's mental health and helping to direct child welfare caseworkers to make referrals to appropriate providers and agencies.

The process of identifying the most appropriate mental health treatment for a patient and their family is rooted in evidence-based practice, which refers to the clinical decision-making process of considering and integrating clinical expertise, current research, and patient characteristics.[62] Child psychologists need to be aware of current evidence-based treatments, show competence and confidence in a given intervention model, and develop good clinical formulations of cases to determine goodness of fit with various available treatments.[62] In addition, clinicians need to be tuned in to patient characteristics, current risk and protective factors, prior traumas, family involvement, culturally influence beliefs and values, and existing access to services.[58] Child psychologists will factor in these variables when determining need for short-term crisis counseling versus long-term formal psychotherapy.

Child psychologists can directly provide a number of evidence-based therapies when indicated.[63–71] Although it is beyond the scope of this review to properly discuss all treatment options, we would like to highlight two treatments that the child psychologist would likely consider for the patient presented in **Box 4**. Trauma-focused cognitive behavioral therapy is an evidence-based treatment specifically designed for children and adolescents who have been impacted by trauma.[66] Treatment components include psychoeducation, parenting skills, relaxation, affective identification as well as modulation, cognitive processing, trauma narration and processing, in-vivo mastery of trauma reminders, conjoint parent child sessions, and safety planning. Backed by decades of research, it is a short-term, structured treatment model that significantly improves a range of trauma-related outcomes that would be appropriate for a child as young as 3-year old. Child–parent psychotherapy (CPP) is a long-term treatment intended for children aged 0–5 years who have experienced at least one traumatic event and their caregivers.[72] Rooted in attachment theory, the primary goal of CPP is to bolster the relationship between a child and their caregiver as a means to improving the child's emotional and behavioral functioning.[73] CPP was originally studied in mother–child dyads that had experienced domestic violence and would be particularly indicated if the child in **Box 4** had a prior history of exposure to domestic violence as well. A detailed assessment of the child's history, current symptoms, caregiver involvement, access to services, and patient preferences are all factored in the final treatment referral. In sum, the child psychologist is an invaluable resource in helping the team plan for services to meet the needs of children and families.

SUMMARY

This article has discussed the extent of the problem of CM and the role of child psychologists working with child abuse pediatricians, focusing on the outpatient evaluation of suspected physical and sexual abuse. The trauma of CM necessitates a comprehensive evaluation that includes obtaining medical and family history, behavioral and neurodevelopmental function, psychosocial information, and pertinent disclosures by the family and child regarding the immediate medical and safety concerns necessitating the evaluation. Although early work suggested that the role of child psychologists was to assess the dynamics involved in the particular case and provide treatment, we now know that the child psychologist is an integral member of the interdisciplinary team throughout the process, preparing for the evaluation (before the evaluation), preparing, interviewing, and screening/assessing the child (during) and assisting in determining immediate psychological safety and communicating the need for further treatment and follow-up (after). As Richard Krugman recently commented, our medical evaluations will be successful only "when there is an interprofessional, multidisciplinary approach to the problem at hand that includes the involvement of the children and families touched by the issue" (p. 536)[71] Integrating child psychologists into child abuse pediatric care offers the best approach to serve our children and families affected by child abuse and neglect.

CLINICS CARE POINTS

- Abuse and neglect harm child in a number of ways with emotional and developmental trauma in addition to physical injury and death.
- The child psychologist has a vital role to play to address these harms in the outpatient medical evaluation of child physical and sexual abuse.
- Important functions for the child psychologist are preparing the team before, assessing the child during, and assisting in communicating safety and treatment needs after the evaluation.
- There are a variety of screening tools and treatment models available.

DISCLOSURE

The authors have no commercial or financial conflicts of interest to disclose and have received no funding for the creation of this work.

REFERENCES

1. Kempe CH, Silverman FN, Steele BF, et al. Landmark article July 7, 1962: the battered-child syndrome. By C. Henry Kempe, FN. Silverman, BF. Steele, William Droegemueller, and Henry K. Silver. JAMA 1984;251(24):3288–94.
2. Shonkoff JP, Boyce WT, Levitt P, et al. Leveraging the biology of adversity and resilience to transform pediatric practice. Pediatrics 2021;147(2):e20193845.
3. Peterson MS, Urquiza AJ. The role of mental health professionals in the prevention and treatment of child abuse and neglect. U.S. Department of health and human services, administration for children and families, administration on children, youth and families, national center on child abuse and neglect. U.S. Government Printing Office; 1993. p. 722–441/80372.
4. Gerber GL. The role of the psychologist–Assessment and treatment of child abuse. Paper presented at: The Annual Convention of the American Psychological Association; August, 1978; Toronto, Ontario, Canada.
5. Child Welfare Information Gateway. About CAPTA: a legislative history. Washington, DC: U.S. Department of Health and Human Services, Children's Bureau; 2019.

6. Consultation on Child Abuse Prevention, World Health Organization. Violence and injury prevention team & global forum for health research. (1999). Report of the consultation on child abuse prevention, 29-31 March 1999, WHO, Geneva. World Health Organization. Available at: https://apps.who.int/iris/handle/10665/65900. Accessed January 28, 2022.

7. Jenny C, Crawford-Jakubiak JE. Committee on child abuse and neglect, american academy of pediatrics. The evaluation of children in the primary care setting when sexual abuse is suspected. Pediatrics 2013;132(2):e558–67.

8. Kim H, Wildeman C, Jonson-Reid M, et al. Lifetime prevalence of investigating child maltreatment among US children. Am J Public Health 2017;107:274–80.

9. Kaplan SJ, Sunday SR, Labruna V, et al. Psychiatric disorders of parents of physically abused adolescents. J Fam Viol 2009;24(5):273–81.

10. US Department of Veteran Affairs. PTSD in children and adolescents 2019. Available at: https://www.ptsd.va.gov/understand/common/common_children_teens.asp. Accessed May, 28, 2020.

11. Dube SR, Anda RF, Felitti VJ, et al. Childhood abuse, household dysfunction and the risk of attempted suicide throughout the lifespan: findings from the Adverse Childhood Experiences Study. JAMA 2001;286:3089–96.

12. Dube SR, Felitti VJ, Dong M, et al. The impact of adverse childhood experiences on health problems: Evidence from four birth cohorts dating back to 1900. Prev Med 2003;37(3):268–77.

13. Finkelhor D, Jones L, Shattuck A. Updated trends in child maltreatment, 2016. Durham, NH: University of New Hampshire Crimes Against Children Research Center; 2018. Available at: www.unh.edu/ccrc/pdf/Updated trends 2016.pdf.

14. U.S. Department. Of health and human services, administration on children, youth and families, children's bureau. Child maltreatment 2019: reports from the states to the National Child Abuse and Neglect Data System. Washington, DC: US Government Printing Office; 2020. Available at: https://www.acf.hhs.gov/cb/resource/child-maltreatment-2019.

15. Cohen JA, Berliner L, Mannarino A. Trauma focused CBT for children with co-occurring trauma and behavior problems. Child Abuse Negl 2010;34:215–24.

16. Humphreys KL, LeMoult J, Wear JG, et al. Child maltreatment and depression: A meta-analysis of studies using the Childhood Trauma Questionnaire. Child Abuse Negl 2020;102:104361.

17. Milot T, Éthier LS, St-Laurent D, et al. The role of trauma symptoms in the development of behavioral problems in maltreated preschoolers. Child Abuse Negl 2010;34:225–34.

18. Cohen JA, Mannarino AP, Deblinger E. Treating trauma and traumatic grief in children and adolescents. New York, NY: Guilford Publications; 2016.

19. Chu AT, Lieberman AF. Clinical implications of traumatic stress from birth to age five. Ann Rev Clin Psychol 2010;6:469–94.

20. American Psychiatric Association. Diagnostic and statistical manual of mental disorders. 5th edition. Arlington, VA: American Psychiatric Pub; 2013.

21. Levendosky AA, Bogat GA, Martinez-Torteya C. PTSD symptoms in young children exposed to intimate partner violence. Violence Against Women 2013;19:187–201.

22. Levendosky AA, Huth-Bocks AC, Semel MA, et al. Trauma symptoms in preschool-age children exposed to domestic violence. J Interpers Viol 2002;17:150–64.

23. Scheeringa MS, Zeanah CH, Myers L, et al. New findings on alternative criteria for PTSD in preschool children. J Am Acad Child Adolesc Psychiatry 2003;42: 561–70.
24. American Psychological Association. Children and trauma: Update for mental health professionals. 2008. Available at: https://www.apa.org/pi/families/resources/children-trauma-update. Accessed May 28, 2020.
25. Cohen JA, Mannarino AP, Zhitova AC, et al. Treating child abuse-related posttraumatic stress and comorbid substance abuse in adolescents. Child Abuse Negl 2003;27(12):1345–65.
26. Fergusson DM, Horwood LJ, Lynskey MT. Childhood sexual abuse, adolescent sexual behaviors and sexual revictimization. Child Abuse Negl 1997;21(8): 789–803. https://doi.org/10.1016/S0145-2134(97)00039-2.
27. Negriff S, Gordis EB, Susman EJ, et al. The young adolescent project: a longitudinal study of the effects of maltreatment on adolescent development. Dev Psychopathol 2020;32(4):1440–59.
28. Kearney CA, Wechsler A, Kaur H, et al. Posttraumatic stress disorder in maltreated youth: a review of contemporary research and thought. Clin Child Fam Psychol Rev 2010;13(1):46–76.
29. Hudson M, Kaplan R. Clinical response to child abuse. Pediatr Clin North Am 2006;53(1):27–39. https://doi.org/10.1016/j.pcl.2005.09.006.
30. Krugman S. Multidisciplinary teams. In: Krugman RD, Korbin J, editors. C. Henry Kempe: a 50 year legacy to the field of child abuse and neglect. Dordrecht, Germany: Springer Science; 2013. p. 71–7.
31. Hochstadt NJ, Harwicke NJ. How effective is the multidisciplinary approach? A follow-up study. Child Abuse Negl 1985;9(3):365–72. https://doi.org/10.1016/0145-2134(85)90034-1.
32. NACHRI (National Association of Children's Hospitals and Related Institutions). Defining the children's hospital role in child maltreatment. Alexandria VA: NACHRI; 2006.
33. Faller KC, Palusci VJ. Children's advocacy centers: Do they lead to positive case outcomes? Child Abuse Negl 2007;31(10):1021–9.
34. Asnes AG, Pavlovic L, Moller B, et al. Consultation for child physical abuse: Beyond the history and physical examination. Child Abuse Negl 2021;111: 104792.
35. Herbert JL, Bromfield L. Better Together? A review of evidence for multidisciplinary teams responding to physical and sexual child abuse. Trauma Violence Abuse 2019;20(2):214–28.
36. Palusci VJ, Botash AS. Race and bias in child maltreatment diagnosis and reporting. Pediatrics 2021;148(1). e2020049625.
37. American Psychological Association. Guidelines for psychological evaluations in child protection matters. Am Psychol 2013;68(1):20–31.
38. Adams JA, Kellogg ND, Farst KJ, et al. Updated guidelines for the medical assessment and care of children who may have been sexually abused. J Pediatr Adolesc Gynecol 2016;29(2):81–7.
39. Greiner MV, Palusci VJ, Keeshin BR, et al. A preliminary screening instrument for early detection of medical child abuse. Hosp Pediatr 2013;3(1):39–44.
40. Christian CW. Committee on child abuse and neglect, american academy of pediatrics. The evaluation of suspected child physical abuse. Pediatrics 2015; 135(5):e1337–54.
41. Wahass SH. The role of psychologists in health care delivery. J Fam Community Med 2005;12(2):63–70.

42. American Psychological Association. What do practicing psychologists do?. 2019. Available at: http://www.apa.org/topics/psychotherapy/about-psychologists. Accessed January 29, 2021.

43. Ngai M, Delaney K, Limandri B, et al. Youth suicide risk screening in an outpatient child abuse clinic. J Child Adolesc Psychiatr Nurs 2021. https://doi.org/10.1111/jcap.12335.

44. Stover CS, Berkowitz S. Assessing violence exposure and trauma symptoms in young children: A critical review of measures. J Trauma Stress 2005;18:707–17.

45. Strand VC, Sarmiento TL, Pasquale LE. Assessment and screening tools for trauma in children and adolescents: A review. Trauma Viol Abuse 2005;6:55–78.

46. Forkey H, Szilagyi M, Kelly ET, et al. Council on Foster Care, Adoption, and Kinship Care, Council on Community Pediatrics, Council on Child Abuse and Neglect, Committee on Psychosocial Aspects of Child and Family Health. Trauma-informed care. Pediatrics 2021;148(2). e2021052580.

47. Pynoos RS, Weathers FW, Steinberg AM, et al. Clinician-administered PTSD scale for DSM-5 - child/adolescent version 2015. National Center for PTSD.Available at: www.ptsd.va.gov.

48. Foa EB, Johnson KM, Feeny NC, et al. The Child PTSD Symptom Scale: a preliminary examination of its psychometric properties. J Clin Child Psychol 2001;30(3): 376–84.

49. Foa EB, Asnaani A, Zang Y, et al. Psychometrics of the Child PTSD Symptom Scale for DSM-5 for trauma-exposed children and adolescents. J Clin Child Adolesc Psychol 2018;47:38–46.

50. Lang JM, Connell CM. Development and validation of a brief trauma screening measure for children: The Child Trauma Screen. Psychol Trauma Theor Res Pract Pol 2017;9:390–8.

51. Eyberg S, Pincus D. Eyberg Child Behavior Inventory & Sutter-Eyberg Student Behavior Inventory-Revised: Professional Manual. Odessa (FL): Psychological Assessment Resources; 1999.

52. Spitzer RL, Kroenke K, Williams JB, et al. A brief measure for assessing generalized anxiety disorder: the GAD-7. Arch Intern Med 2006;166(10):1092–7.

53. Mossman SA, Luft MJ, Schroeder HK, et al. The generalized anxiety disorder 7-item (GAD-7) scale in adolescents with generalized anxiety disorder: Signal detection and validation. Ann Clin Psychiatry 2017;29(4):227.

54. Kaufman J, Birmaher B, Brent D, et al. Schedule for affective disorders and schizophrenia for school-age children-present and lifetime version (K-SADS-PL): Initial reliability and validity data. J Am Acad Child Adolesc Psychiatry 1997;36(7):980–8.

55. Kaufman J, Schweder AE. The Schedule for Affective Disorders and Schizophrenia for School-Age Children: Present and Lifetime version (K-SADS-PL). In: Hilsenroth MJ, Segal DL, editors. Comprehensive handbook of psychological assessment, vol. 2. Hoboken (NJ): John Wiley & Sons, Inc; 2004.

56. Johnson JG, Harris ES, Spitzer RL, et al. The Patient Health Questionnaire for Adolescents: validation of an instrument for the assessment of mental disorders among adolescent primary care patients. J Adolesc Health 2002;30:196–204.

57. Saylor CF, Swenson CC, Reynolds SS, et al. The pediatric emotional distress scale: a brief screening measure for young children exposed to traumatic events. J Clin Child Psychol 1999;28(1):70–81.

58. Chorpita BF, Yim L, Moffitt C, et al. Assessment of symptoms of DSM-IV anxiety and depression in children: A revised child anxiety and depression scale. Behav Res Ther 2000;38:835–55.

59. Chorpita BF, Moffitt CE, Gray J. Psychometric properties of the Revised Child Anxiety and Depression Scale in a clinical sample. Behav Res Ther 2005;43(3): 309–22.
60. Newlin C., Steele L.C., Chamberlin A., et al., US Department of Justice, Office of Justice Programs, Office of Juvenile Justice and Delinquency Prevention, Child Forensic Interviewing: Best Practices, 2015, 1-20. Available at: https://www.ojjdp.gov/pubs/248749.pdf. Accessed January 28, 2022.
61. Raja S, Hasnain M, Hoersch M, et al. Trauma informed care in medicine: Current knowledge and future research directions. Fam Community Health 2015;38(3): 216–26.
62. Greenbaum J, Celano M. Identification, mandated reporting requirements, and referral for mental health evaluation and treatment. In: Reece RM, Hanson RF, Sargent J, editors. Treatment of child abuse: common ground for mental health, medical, and legal practitioners. 2nd ed. Baltimore, MD: John Hopkins University Press; 2014. p. 3–28.
63. Sessa B. MDMA and PTSD treatment: "PTSD: From novel pathophysiology to innovative therapeutics". Neurosci Lett 2017;649:176–80.
64. Piacentini J, Bennett S, Compton SN, et al. 24-and 36-week outcomes for the Child/Adolescent Anxiety Multimodal Study (CAMS). J Am Acad Child Adolesc Psychiatry 2014;53(3):297–310.
65. Blaustein ME, Kinniburgh KM. Treating traumatic stress in children and adolescents: how to foster resilience through attachment, self-regulation, and competency. New York, NY: Guilford Publications; 2018.
66. Cohen JA, Mannarino AP. Trauma-focused cognitive behavioral therapy for traumatized children and families. Child Adol Psychiatr Clin 2015;24(3):557–70.
67. Saxe GN, Ellis BH, Brown AD. Trauma systems therapy for children and teens. New York, NY: Guilford Publications; 2015.
68. Chaffin M, Funderburk B, Bard D, et al. A combined motivation and parent-child interaction therapy package reduces child welfare recidivism in a randomized dismantling field trial. J Consult Clin Psychol 2011;79(1):84–95. https://doi.org/10.1037/a0021227.
69. McNeil CB, Hembree-Kigin TL. Parent-child interaction therapy. 2nd ed. New York, NY: Springer; 2010.
70. Timmer SG, Urquiza AJ, Zebell NM, et al. Parent-child interaction therapy: Application to maltreating parent-child dyads. Child Abuse Negl 2005;29:825–42.
71. Krugman RD. Medicine, mental health and child welfare: "Three different worlds that need to amalgamate". Fam Syst Health 2021;39(3):535–8. https://doi.org/10.1037/fsh0000647.
72. Lieberman AF, Ghosh Ippen C, Van Horn P. Don't hit my mommy: a manual for Child-Parent Psychotherapy with young children exposed to violence and other trauma. 2nd ed. Washington, DC: Zero to Three; 2015.
73. Lieberman AF, Ippen CG, Van Horn P. Child-parent psychotherapy: 6-month follow-up of a randomized controlled trial. J Am Acad Child Adolesc Psychiatry 2006;45(8):913–8.

Psychology and Developmental-Behavioral Pediatrics: Interprofessional Collaboration in Clinical Practice

Lauren Gardner, PhD[a],*, Jason Hangauer, PhD[a],
Toni Whitaker, MD[b], Ronald Espinal, MD[b]

KEYWORDS

- Interprofessional collaboration • Interdisciplinary • Psychology
- Developmental-behavioral pediatrics • Neurodevelopmental disabilities
- Autism spectrum disorder

KEY POINTS

- Neurodevelopmental disabilities (NDDs) are complex, and patients benefit from interdisciplinary collaboration to improve outcomes.
- Interprofessional collaboration between psychology and developmental-behavioral pediatrics (DBP) promotes diagnosis, treatment recommendations, and integrated care for patients and families.
- Collaboration between psychology and DBP is beneficial to patient care and health care professionals.

INTRODUCTION

Within the United States, research findings support that about one in six, or approximately 17%, of children aged 3 to 17 years have a diagnosed developmental disability.[1] Rates of diagnosis, particularly for attention-deficit/hyperactivity disorder, autism spectrum disorder (ASD), and intellectual disability, have continued to increase. Improved awareness, screening, and diagnosis by highly trained providers are likely part of the reason for increased rates of diagnosis. Data from the centers for disease control and prevention (CDC) Autism and Developmental Monitoring Network indicate that the percentage of children diagnosed with ASD varies widely across geographic areas ranging from 1.7% to 3.9%, but overall estimates that 1 in

a Johns Hopkins All Children's Hospital, 880 6th Street South, Suite 410, St. Petersburg, FL 33701, USA; b University of Tennessee Health Science Center, Center on Developmental Disabilities, 920 Madison, Suite 939, Memphis, TN 38160, USA
* Corresponding author.
E-mail address: lgardn18@jhmi.edu

Pediatr Clin N Am 69 (2022) 895–904
https://doi.org/10.1016/j.pcl.2022.05.004
0031-3955/22/© 2022 Elsevier Inc. All rights reserved.

44 (2.3%) 8 years old children have a diagnosis of ASD.[2] Medical providers, in particular pediatricians, are tasked with developmental monitoring and screening for concerns. Standardized screening for general developmental at 9, 18, and 30 months and for ASD at 18-month and 24-month well-child visits, with ongoing developmental surveillance, continues to be recommended in primary care.[3] Children who screen positive for possible neurodevelopmental disabilities (NDDs), including autism, should be referred for a comprehensive developmental evaluation, as a diagnosis by an experienced clinician is reliable by age 2 years.[4] Although general pediatricians can make an initial NDD diagnoses, many caregivers seek services from pediatric specialists to obtain diagnostic clarification through formal assessments of cognitive, language, and adaptive abilities, as well as sensory and other behavioral concerns.[3]

Referral to pediatric specialists who complete comprehensive diagnostic evaluations for NDDs may include specialists in developmental-behavioral pediatrics (DBP), psychology, neuropsychology, psychiatry, or neurology. Following evaluation and diagnosis, intervention and treatment for children diagnosed with NDDs also require specialists from a range of disciplines (eg, child psychiatry, psychology, DBP, speech–language pathology, and occupational therapy).[5] For both assessment and intervention, collaboration between health care providers is crucial in best practices in clinical care for patients with NDDs and to improve outcomes across care settings.

Interprofessional Collaboration in Clinical Practice

Interprofessional collaboration is defined as two or more professions working together to resolve complex issues of concern.[6] In working together collaboratively, professionals from differing areas of clinical practice can achieve more together working toward a shared goal than either could independently. Interprofessional collaborative practice is more than each health care provider working independently to provide service from their respective areas of expertise. Collaboration occurs when individuals have mutual respect for the other profession and act cooperatively for the benefit of a community of patients with a focus on improving outcomes.[6]

Previous research supports that both families and medical providers report high levels of satisfaction and improved pediatric patient care with the integration of psychology services.[7] Psychology and DBP are tasked with providing clinical care to a community of patients that present with NDDs. They represent two separate professions within pediatric healthcare who can work cooperatively to benefit a community of patients, assuring comprehensive services are provided for patients with NDDs and, in so doing, improving outcomes across settings. For instance, DBP and psychology can work together to answer complex questions related to differential diagnosis and appropriate treatment recommendations for pediatric patients with complex neurodevelopmental presentations. For the purposes of this article, emphasis will be on interprofessional collaboration between DBP and psychology within pediatric subspecialty clinical care for patients presenting with NDDs; however, interprofessional collaborative practice can occur between health care providers from various backgrounds who wish to provide a high-quality care to patients across settings.[8]

Taxonomy and Definition of Neurodevelopmental Disorders

NDDs encompass a wide range of neurologic and psychiatric conditions that are clinically and causally different in kind. (1) Key features of NDDs include disruption to brain development before puberty that results in the early onset of neurocognitive deficits that produce impairments of personal, social, academic, or occupational functioning and more commonly affect males. (2) Moreover, NDDs are highly heterogeneous in terms of their clinical characteristics, causes, treatment responses, and outcomes. There is no specific clinical or biological characteristic that clearly distinguishes this grouping from other neuropsychiatric disorders. The level of overlap in clinical symptoms between these disorders is high. This clinical heterogeneity in NDDs is reflected in extreme genetic heterogeneity, with a genetic diagnosis not possible for most cases. These disorders are defined by a phenotype that is not caused by one or two pathogenic variants in a single gene but by many genetic events with significant contribution from environmental factors. Nonetheless, rapid advances in molecular genetics allow NDDs to be increasingly defined by genetic variants, and all NDDs in the *Diagnostic and Statistical Manual of Mental Disorder, Fifth Edition*[9] (DSM-5) may include the specifier "associated with a known medical or genetic condition or environmental factor."

NDDs were introduced as an overarching disorder category in the DSM-5, replacing the chapter from DSM-IV, "Disorders usually diagnosed in infancy, childhood, or adolescence." The DSM-5 NDDs include intellectual disabilities, communication disorders, ASD, attention-deficit hyperactivity disorder, specific learning disorder, and motor disorders (including tic disorders). The validity of NDDs as a construct is supported by the high rates of comorbidity between various disorders within this diagnostic category.[9,10] From a clinical utility perspective, grouping these varied conditions as NDDs allows clinicians to find the categories that most accurately describe the patients they encounter as quickly, easily, and intuitively as possible and provide them with clinically useful information about treatment and management.[10] Distinct diagnostic categories also provide a means for clinicians to readily communicate about patients' difficulties with each other and with the patients themselves.[11]

Diagnosing Neurodevelopmental Disorders

Diagnosing NDDs is often not as straightforward as other medical diagnoses. Thus, medical professionals who specialize in NDDs are those with expertise in differential diagnosis of NDDs. Oftentimes, assessment and diagnosis of NDD may include significant overlap between DBP and psychology.[12] Both types of professionals can be properly trained to administer standardized assessment measures that reliably assess for NDDs; however, each professional brings unique contributions to this process. DBPs have extensive experience in the medical underpinnings that contribute to an NDD diagnosis. Integrating multiple sources of information, such as genetic testing, birth history, postdelivery complications, and current symptomology, requires a high level of expertise to synthesize all information. Psychologists present with expertise in conducting comprehensive diagnostic evaluations to assess for NDD using the diagnostic criteria presented in the DSM-5 and the provision of evidence-based interventions based on the unique needs of the patient and their family.

The "gold standard" for a diagnostic evaluation for NDDs, including ASD, involves the clinical judgment of a qualified interdisciplinary team, which includes using empirically-sound diagnostic instruments, clinical assessment, caregiver reports, and behavior observations.[13] Although a diagnosis made by an interdisciplinary team is ideal, this is not always feasible due to availability in a given location and extensive waitlists for such evaluations. Providers with expertise in ASD can also conduct evaluations independently. The core features of an evidence-based assessment for ASD in children and adolescents include caregiver reporting on interviews and questionnaires, autism-specific diagnostic tools and observation instruments, standardized assessment of intellectual/cognitive functioning, speech/language assessment, and adaptive behavior assessment.[14]

Both DBPs and psychologists are tasked with conducting diagnostic assessments and must recognize NDD signs and symptoms in early development. This requires a strong working knowledge of neurotypical development as well as the clinical aptitude to differentiate between NDDs. Although the behavioral symptoms of some NDDs, like autism, generally become apparent to experienced clinicians when children are between 1 and 2 years of age,[15] many children do not receive a diagnosis until almost two and a half years later, between the ages of 4 and 5 years.[16,17] Patients with NDDs provide a convergence point for increasing interdisciplinary collaboration between DBP and psychology. The following case examples provide an illustration of how these two disciplines can work collaboratively to provide integrated, high-quality patient care.

Case example I: A 30-month-old male patient with no significant medical history referred to a DBP by his primary care clinician (PCC) for assessment due to parental concerns of speech/language delays, behavioral difficulties, and picky eating habits. The PCC simultaneously referred the child to the state early developmental intervention program (Part C program of the Individuals with Disabilities Education Act, for children 0–3 years). The child has recently started once weekly speech–language therapy through the early intervention program.

The evaluation by the DBP at 35 months of age includes a detailed medical, developmental, and behavioral history for the child and family history with attention to developmental concerns. No vision or hearing concerns are reported, and a recent formal hearing screen was passed. No regression or plateau of skills is reported. General physical and neurologic examinations are appropriate for age. No dysmorphic physical features are noted. Developmental testing reveals delays in verbal and nonverbal communication as well as qualitative limits in socialization. Features of ASD are reported and observed, including some limitations in reciprocal social behavior and in initiating interaction, as well as some mildly repetitive behaviors. Because there is a mixed picture of possible features of ASD, the DBP seeks interprofessional collaboration by placing a referral to a Psychologist for a more formal assessment of ASD and additional data on developmental skills. In the interim, the DBP encourages the continuation of early developmental intervention services, but as language delays are mild to moderate, a recommendation is made to increase language therapy to twice weekly. DBP also provides anticipatory guidance for the transition to the public preschool program from the early intervention program in which the child is enrolled. A return appointment is set to ensure that appropriate interventions are provided and to discuss etiologic evaluation after the psychological assessment is complete.

The patient is scheduled for a comprehensive psychological evaluation that is completed at 40-month old. The psychologist uses a clinical interview, behavioral observations, and standardized testing measures to aid in their evaluation of the patient. This evaluation includes the use of accurate, reliable, and valid diagnostic instruments to assess for autism and other disorders that may be present, such as global developmental delay, language disorder, and other neurodevelopmental or behavioral disorders.

The psychologist administers several measures specific to autism, the results of which support social and communication deficits as well as restricted and repetitive patterns of behavior. The psychologist also administered standardized testing to appropriately assess cognitive development as well as a standardized assessment of adaptive functioning. Children with ASD demonstrate a pattern of adaptive skills that include deficits in socialization, moderate communication skills, and relative strengths and weaknesses in activities of daily living.[18] The assessment of adaptive functioning is important not only for diagnosing or ruling out intellectual disability but also in the determination of individualized educational and intervention planning for children with autism across the range of intellectual functioning. Standardized scores supported significant delays in cognitive development and adaptive skill acquisition.

In addition, the psychologist had the caregivers complete a broad-band behavior rating scale that measures children's behavioral difficulties, social-emotional concerns, and competency. Caregivers indicated elevated concerns on clinical scales assessing attention problems, withdrawal atypicality and adaptive scales assessing adaptability, functional communication, and social skills. Caregiver reporting and behavioral observations did not support the presence of significant disruptive behavior concerns.

Results of the psychological evaluation supported a diagnosis of autism. Information obtained from caregiver reports during the clinical interview, standardized rating scales, and behavioral observations indicated significant deficits in social communication and interaction, as well as in restricted, repetitive patterns of behaviors, interests, and activities. As such, the psychologist provides a diagnosis of ASD, requiring substantial support in both social communication and interaction and restricted and repetitive behaviors. Accompanying diagnoses included global developmental delay and language disorder. Treatment recommendations included the addition of comprehensive behavioral treatment for young children for at least 20 hours per week. These interventions are often described as applied behavior analysis (ABA) therapy or early intensive behavioral intervention. It was recommended that the family obtain a case manager through their insurance provider to assist with navigating services. The continuation of speech/language therapy services and follow-up with the DBP provider was also recommended. Following the completion of the psychological evaluation, the psychologist conferenced with the DBP provider to discuss the outcomes of the evaluation and treatment recommendations based on the patient's needs for individualized interventions targeting skill acquisition.

Case example II: The patient is a 7-year-old girl with a history of 18p partial monosomy syndrome confirmed through microarray analysis, alternating intermittent esotropia, apraxia, ASD, history of developmental delays, current academic performance, and behavioral difficulties. The patient presented to DBP due to increasing concerns for learning and behavioral difficulties. Given the patient has an NDD because of a genetic syndrome, she presented with multiple needs that were impacting her learning and behavioral regulation. This DBP practice routes new referrals for evaluation to an interdisciplinary team that includes a DBP and a child psychologist. The interprofessional approach allows each professional to evaluate different aspects of the patient's development that may impact functioning.[19] The family is scheduled for two visits. On the first day, the DBP and psychologist meet with the family to review child's previous medical records, academic support, and behavioral functioning with the family. The patient has a PCP that serves as her medical home coordinating the care of her multiple specialists. There are no recent illnesses or medical setbacks endorsed. Recent visits with neurology and ophthalmology are reviewed. Teacher Vanderbilt Assessment Rating Scales[20] reveal elevated concerns of hyperactivity and inattention with impairments noted in academics and classroom behavior.

Physical examination is remarkable for short stature with mild facial dysmorphism. The behavioral assessment determines that she developed mild self-injurious behavior and increased disruptive behavior once her mother returned to work after COVID-19 restrictions were eased. Developmental assessment reveals cognitive skills at a 4-year-old level. Though verbal, her speech is difficult to understand. The DBP shares concerns with the psychologist about possible co-occurring conditions, such as a mood disorder or attention-deficit/hyperactivity disorder (ADHD), before the patient's second upcoming visit.

During the second visit, the psychologist alone completes a comprehensive psychological evaluation examining behavioral and intellectual functioning using standardized assessment measures. The evaluation includes direct psychological testing and standardized rating scales completed by caregivers familiar with the patient (eg, parents, teachers). Results support the previous diagnosis of ASD and indicate intellectual functioning decreases significantly below age expectations as well as co-occurring adaptive skill deficits of similar severity. Standardized rating scales provide information about behavioral functioning across key areas of home and school. Significant inattentive, impulsive, and hyperactive behaviors seem to be impacting the patient's ability to function in the school setting, often resulting in disruptive behaviors and in difficulties accessing the curriculum due to deficits in intellectual functioning, as well as symptoms consistent with ADHD.

The DBP and psychologist meet to engage in interprofessional collaboration and review their findings to develop recommendations before providing feedback to the family. The review of the child's Individualized Education Program (IEP) reveals the need for a behavior intervention plan and intensified social skills and communication support. The team discusses and integrates their recommendations before the family meeting. The psychologist and DBP meet with the family together to explain the findings, discuss recommendations with the family, and answer their questions. The DBP recommends a trial of stimulant medication in response to medication data collected by school staff, whereas the psychologist provides educational recommendations related to IEP goals and a functional behavior assessment (FBA) to gain more clarity regarding the functions of various behaviors in the school setting. The psychologist engages in conjoint behavior consultation[21,22] with the school-based psychologist at the patient's school to further examine the response to medication and the recommendation for an FBA to be completed. The DBP and psychologist review assessment findings related to ASD and agree the current level of support is consistent with requiring substantial support and collaboratively agree to reinitiation of ABA therapy to target self-injurious behavior, increase task focus, and activities of daily living skills. Speech–language and occupational therapies are also indicated. The family is provided with comprehensive, customized recommendations with a plan to follow-up on progress in 1 month specific to medication response and 3 months for overall follow-up.

For both case examples, the interprofessional collaboration between DBP and psychology allows for a broader view of the patient's overall functioning and individualization of treatment recommendations supported by the standardized assessment of the patient's current ability level. Although broad developmental assessment found deficits in cognitive functioning, more detailed and intensive intellectual testing found significant cognitive/intellectual deficits, delayed adaptive skills, and informed co-occurring diagnoses that facilitate access to appropriate care based on the patient's unique needs. This information is then shared with their broader care team, including their family, school staff, and therapy providers, to best serve the needs of the patients and their families.

Benefits of Interprofessional Collaborative Practice for Neurodevelopmental Disability

Psychology and DBP working collaboratively in providing care to NDD patients results in an increased level of satisfaction reported by caregivers and physicians.[7,23]

Adjusting to cooperative care practices among DBP and psychology providers requires training for established and emerging professionals, including established DBP and psychologists as well as providers in-training (eg, medical residents and fellows, psychology interns, and postdoctoral fellows). Research supports that health care providers who engage in an interprofessional collaborative practice report increased job satisfaction, higher levels of perceived professional support, and reduced stress and chaos in the workplace.[24]

Different models of interprofessional collaboration and interdisciplinary practice exist across a variety of settings. Although various strategies for interdisciplinary collaboration between psychology and DBP may be useful, several considerations may impact the best fit in a specific practice circumstance. Engaging in interdisciplinary collaborative care requires proactive planning to assure successful implementation, including providers invested in collaborative practice, support from administration, and funding for ancillary care needs. Planful practices regarding billing and reimbursement, space, materials needed for assessment, scheduling coordination, and time for team collaboration are imperative to assure success. Scheduling coordination and team building are the biggest challenges.[25]

Building partnerships between multiple disciplines, including DBP and psychology, allows for more efficient use of resources while increasing access to comprehensive care provided to patients with NDDs. For example, the (S)Transdisciplinary Autism Assessment and Resources ([S]TAAR) model provides comprehensive diagnostic evaluations for young children using a transdisciplinary team. The use of this model has led to increased provider satisfaction among team members, reductions in wait-lists and time to diagnosis, and increased equitability in access to patient care.[26] Leadership Education in Neurodevelopmental and Related Disabilities (LENDs) provides interdisciplinary leadership training that is federally funded through Health Resources and Services Administration's Maternal Child Health Bureau. There are currently 60 LEND training programs serving nearly every state and many territories that provide interdisciplinary training to graduate-level trainees from diverse professional disciplines to advance the knowledge and skill of child health care professionals and improve health care delivery systems for children with NDDs.[27]

In addition to interprofessional collaborative practices, facilitating care across systems is important for NDD patients and their families. The American Academy of Pediatrics recognizes the importance of systems collaboration and recommends this type of collaboration to reduce costs and improve the detection, prevention, and management of health conditions affecting children.[28] By forging new partnerships among service providers, educational systems, and community members, evidence-based treatments and strategies can be adapted to be used more broadly in the school and community settings.

Barriers to Interprofessional Collaborative Practice for Neurodevelopmental Disability

The current DBP workforce struggles to meet current workforce demands, given a limited number of providers. A survey of the DBP workforce revealed significant barriers to providing DBP care, including a declining workforce, inadequate reimbursement, high demands for care coordination, lack of access to community services, and a need for more training to manage complex patients.[29] Interprofessional collaboration requires providers from at least two professions to work together toward solutions to patient health care needs. To decrease burnout and DBP providers feeling undervalued and overburdened, collaborative practice models provide an opportunity to expand the workforce and provide support to overburdened providers.[29]

ASD is a spectrum disorder, and, as such, it is associated with a broad range of symptoms that can affect individuals to varying degrees in severity, with the presentation of symptoms potentially changing over time.[4] Further, barriers that families face when seeking a diagnostic evaluation for ASD may include a lack of access to highly qualified professionals, increased levels of parental stress and anxiety, and financial barriers.[26] Unfortunately, interdisciplinary collaboration does not address barriers patients and families face related to access to care depending on public versus private insurance, school versus private services, and level of need for care.

Interprofessional collaboration should not be limited to only DBP and psychology, but this article provides a framework for collaboration between these two disciplines as a realistic starting point. Psychologists and DBPs working collaboratively with other health care providers with less specialized expertise in recognizing and diagnosing NDDs, including autism, could help to address issues related to age, gender, socioeconomic status, and racial/ethnic disparities in diagnosis.

SUMMARY

Assuring access to appropriate services, including identification of NDDs, requires collaboration between health care providers across settings. However, integrated and comprehensive care is negatively impacted by the lack of interprofessional collaboration between health care providers. The Interprofessional collaborative practice between psychologists and DBP represents two such health care providers who can readily work together to promote positive outcomes for individuals with NDDs.

Providing health care professionals with the opportunities to build skills and knowledge in interdisciplinary collaborative practice during their graduate training prepares emerging providers with the skills to effectively communicate and work together. Collaborative practice allows psychologists and DBPs the unique opportunity to learn from each other while reducing care silos and promoting integrated and high-quality services to autistic children and adolescents. Given the increased use of teleservices during the COVID-19 pandemic, collaborative practice between health care providers is more accessible than it has been in the past. As it is likely that telehealth will remain a staple of clinical care post-COVID-19, there is an increased opportunity for "face-to-face" collaboration between providers that may have previously been limited because of time constraints, access to video conference technology, or geographic location. As the incidence rates for NDD, particularly ASD, continue to increase, so does the need for integrated and comprehensive care for patients and their families.[30]

CLINICS CARE POINTS

- Interprofessional collaboration between psychology and developmental-behavioral pediatrics (DBP) is beneficial to patients and health care providers.
- Collaborative practices promote high-quality integrated services for patients with neurodevelopmental disabilities including autism.
- Psychology and DBP are two disciplines that, through collaborative practice, can provide interprofessional workforce support to overburdened providers.
- Established and emerging health care professionals need opportunities to build skills and knowledge in interdisciplinary collaborative practice to integrate this into professional practice effectively.

DISCLOSURE

The authors have nothing to disclose.

REFERENCES

1. Zablotsky B, Black LI, Maenner MJ, et al. Prevalence and trends of developmental disabilities among children in the United States: 2009–2017. Pediatrics 2019;144(4):e20190811.
2. Maenner MJ, Shaw KA, Bakian AV, et al. Prevalence and characteristics of autism spectrum disorder among children aged 8 years — autism and Developmental Disabilities Monitoring Network, 11 sites, United States, 2018. MMWR Surveill Summ 2021;70(11):1–16.
3. Hyman SL, Levy SE, Myers SM. Identification, evaluation, and management of children with autism spectrum disorder. Pediatrics 2020;145(1):e20193447.
4. Lord C, Risi S, DiLavore PS, et al. Autism from 2 to 9 years of age. Arch Gen Psychiatry 2006;63(6):694.
5. Thapar A, Cooper M, Rutter M. Neurodevelopmental disorders. Lancet Psychiatry 2017;4(4):339–46.
6. Green BN, Johnson CD. Interprofessional collaboration in research, education, and clinical practice: Working together for a better future. J Chiropractic Education 2015;29(1):1–10.
7. Ward WL, Smith A, Munns C, et al. The process of integrating psychology into medical clinics: pediatric psychology as an example. Clin Child Psychol Psychiatry 2020;26(2):323–41.
8. Gardner L, Campbell JC, Gilchrest C, et al. Identification of autism spectrum disorder and interprofessional collaboration between school and clinical settings. Psychol Schools 2022;(59):1308–18.
9. American Psychiatric Association. Diagnostic and statistical manual of mental disorders. 5th edition. Arlington, VA: American Psychiatric Association; 2013.
10. Doernberg E, Hollander E. Neurodevelopmental disorders (ASD and ADHD): DSM-5, ICD-10, and ICD-11. CNS Spectrums 2016;21(04):295–9.
11. Reed GM, Roberts MC, Keeley J, et al. Mental health professionals' natural taxonomies of mental disorders: implications for the clinical utility of the ICD-11 and the DSM-5. J Clin Psychol 2013;69(12):1191–212.
12. Desikan RS, Barkovich AJ. Hazards of neurological nomenclature. JAMA Neurol 2017;74(10):1165.
13. Ritzema AM, Sladeczek IE, Ghosh S, et al. Improving outcomes for children with developmental disabilities through enhanced communication and collaboration between school psychologists and physicians. Can J Sch Psychol 2014;29(4): 317–37.
14. Gardner L, Erkfritz-Gay K, Campbell J, et al. Purposes of assessment. In: Handbook of assessment and diagnosis of autism spectrum disorder. Cham: Springer; 2016. p. 27–43.
15. Ozonoff S, Goodlin-Jones BL, Solomon M. Evidence-based assessment of Autism Spectrum Disorders in children and adolescents. J Clin Child Adolesc Psychol 2005;34(3):523–40.
16. Kozlowski AM, Matson JL, Horovitz M, et al. Parents' first concerns of their child's development in toddlers with autism spectrum disorders. Developmental Neurorehabil 2011;14(2):72–8.
17. Maenner MJ, Shaw KA, Baio J, et al. Prevalence of autism spectrum disorder among children aged 8 years — autism and Developmental Disabilities

Monitoring Network, 11 sites, United States, 2016. MMWR Surveill Summ 2020; 69(4):1–12.

18. Carter AS, Volkmar FR, Sparrow SS, et al. J Autism Dev Disord 1998;28(4): 287–302.

19. Liu XL, Zahrt DM, Simms MD. An interprofessional team approach to the differential diagnosis of children with language disorders. Pediatr Clin North Am 2018; 65(1):73–90.

20. Clinical practice guideline: Treatment of the school-aged child with attention-deficit/hyperactivity disorder. Pediatrics 2001;108(4):1033–44.

21. Garbacz SA, Beattie T, Novotnak T, et al. Examining the efficacy of conjoint behavioral consultation for middle school students with externalizing behavior problems. Behav Disord 2020;46(1):3–17.

22. Sheridan SM, Eagle JW, Cowan RJ, et al. The effects of conjoint behavioral consultation results of a 4-year investigation. J Sch Psychol 2001;39(5):361–85.

23. Burt JD, Garbacz SA, Kupzyk KA, et al. Examining the utility of behavioral health integration in well-child visits: Implications for rural settings. Families, Syst Health 2014;32(1):20–30.

24. Fisher MD, Weyant D, Sterrett S, et al. Perceptions of interprofessional collaborative practice and patient/family satisfaction. J Interprof Educ Pract 2017;8: 95–102.

25. Barber JA, Frantsve LM, Capelli S, et al. Implementation and evaluation of an Integrated Care Program in a VA Medical Center. Psychol Serv 2011;8(4):282–93.

26. Brinster MI, Brukilacchio BH, Fikki-Urbanovsky A, et al. Improving efficiency and equity in early autism evaluations: the (s)taar model. J Autism Dev Disord 2022; 12:1–10.

27. About lend. AUCD. Available at: https://www.aucd.org//template/page.cfm? id=473. Accessed January 31, 2022.

28. Abdul Razzak H, Ghader N, Qureshi AA, et al. Clinical practice guidelines for the evaluation and diagnosis of attention-deficit/hyperactivity disorder in children and adolescents. Sultan Qaboos Univ Med J [SQUMJ] 2021;21(1):e12–21.

29. Bridgemohan C, Bauer NS, Nielsen BA, et al. A workforce survey on developmental-behavioral pediatrics. Pediatrics 2018;141(3):e20172164.

30. Matson JL, Goldin RL. Diagnosing young children with autism. Int J Dev Neurosci 2014;39(1):44–8.

Role of Psychologists in Pediatric Endocrinology

Marissa A. Feldman, PhD[a],*, Heather L. Yardley, PhD[b], Ayse Bulan, MD[c],
Manmohan K. Kamboj, MD[c]

KEYWORDS

- Pediatric • Psychologist • Psychosocial • Behavioral health • Endocrinology
- Diabetes • Obesity

KEY POINTS

- Psychologists' role in managing diabetes, obesity, and metabolic syndrome is diverse, including screening, in-clinic intervention, inpatient care, and outpatient psychological services.
- Best practice guidelines recognize the critical influence of psychosocial aspects in the physical and emotional functioning of youth with diabetes and obesity.
- Identification of psychosocial risk and resilience facilitates adherence and improved health and quality of life outcomes through psychological interventions.
- There is growing cost analysis research to support psychological interventions.

INTRODUCTION

The prevalence of pediatric diabetes (types 1 and 2) and obesity is rising.[1,2] Given the physical and emotional demands of diabetes and obesity management, there is a growing recognition of the need for multidisciplinary or interdisciplinary care. With expertise in managing the developmental, behavioral, and social needs of these patients, psychologists are being increasingly incorporated as essential team members.[3] This article provides context for the benefits of integrated psychological care by reviewing the diagnosis and management of diabetes, obesity, and metabolic syndrome. We then aim to outline the role of psychologists in the screening and treatment of youth with these chronic health conditions as research shows that a collaborative

The authors have nothing to disclose.
[a] Department of Psychology, Johns Hopkins All Children's Hospital, Saint Petersburg, 880 Sixth Street South, Suite 460, Saint Petersburg, FL 33701, USA; [b] Department of Pediatric Psychology and Neuropsychology, Nationwide Children's Hospital, 700 Children's Drive, Columbus, OH 43205, USA; [c] Section of Endocrinology, Department of Pediatrics, Nationwide Children's Hospital, 700 Children's Drive, Columbus, OH 43205, USA
* Corresponding author.
E-mail address: mfeldm25@jhmi.edu

treatment approach maximizes health and psychosocial outcomes for patients seen within pediatric endocrinology clinics.

DIABETES MELLITUS

Diabetes mellitus is a metabolic condition characterized by chronic hyperglycemia because of impaired insulin secretion and/or inadequate tissue response to insulin.[4–6] Hyperglycemia leads to characteristic symptoms of diabetes such as polyuria, polydipsia, nocturia, enuresis, and weight loss. Diagnostic criteria are based on hemoglobin A1c (HbA1c), blood glucose, and presence of symptoms. There are different sets of diagnostic criteria for diagnosing diabetes (**Table 1**).[4–6] Diabetes is classified into two categories: type 1 diabetes (T1D) and type 2 diabetes (T2D). T1D is characterized by severe insulin deficiency and dependence on exogenous insulin. T2D results from a combination of insulin resistance and inadequate compensatory insulin secretion. Patients with T2D may require insulin if an adequate response is not achieved with oral medications or initial presentation with high HbA1c and/or ketosis.[7] Features that differentiate T1D and T2D are listed in **Table 2**[6]; however, overlap in presentation or lack of clarity in differentiating between the two types may occur.

T1D is the most common form of diabetes in children and adolescents, with an annual incidence of 20 to 25 cases per 100,000 children.[8] T2D has increased substantially among children with obesity and children in high-risk ethnic populations, such as Africans, Latinos, Native American Indians, and other susceptible ethnic groups.[9] This increase represents an urgent public health challenge to patients' survival and quality of life. Patients with diabetes may face acute conditions such as hypoglycemia, ketoacidosis, and hyperglycemic hyperosmolar state necessitating emergency care or admission. Furthermore, studies show increased mortality and morbidity including cardiovascular disease (CVD), retinopathy, neuropathy, and nephropathy secondary to poor long-term glycemic control.[10] Optimal treatment is crucial to reduce the risk of life-threatening complications.[11]

Successful management of T1D involves blood glucose monitoring and insulin therapy. Patients need multiple blood glucose checks daily. Continuous glucose monitoring devices have improved monitoring, eliminating 4 to 10 finger sticks daily, and

Table 1	
Diagnostic criteria for diabetes mellitus	
Measurement	**Diagnostic Values**
Plasma glucose	Fasting plasma glucose $\geq$126 mg/dL OR 2-h plasma glucose $\geq$200 mg/dL during oral glucose tolerance test OR Random plasma glucose $\geq$200 mg/dL in a patient with classical symptoms of hyperglycemia such as polyuria, polydipsia, and weight loss OR
HbA1c	HbA1c $\geq$ 6.5%. The test should be performed in a laboratory using a method that is NGSP certified and standardized to the DCCT assay.[a]

Abbreviation: DCCT, Diabetes Control and Complications Trial.

[a] In the absence of unequivocal hyperglycemia, diagnosis requires two abnormal test results from the same or in two separate test samples.

Adapted from American Diabetes Association guidelines-2022. Draznin, B., et al., *2. Classification and Diagnosis of Diabetes: Standards of Medical Care in Diabetes-2022.* Diabetes Care, 2022. **45**(Supplement_1): p. S17-s38.

Table 2
Common clinical characteristics of T1D versus T2D

Characteristics	Type 1	Type 2
Age at presentation	>6–12 mo	Pubertal or later
Clinical presentation	Acute, rapid	Usually, gradual deterioration
Ketosis at presentation	Common	Not
Autoimmunity	Yes	No
Obesity	Same as in general population	More common
Acanthosis nigricans	Usually not seen	Usually seen
Genetics	Polygenetic	Polygenetic
Prevalence of all diabetes mellitus in children and adolescents	90% or more	Less common

Adapted from ISPAD guidelines-2018. Davis, E.J., et al., *ISPAD Clinical Practice Consensus Guidelines 2018: Definition, epidemiology, and classification of diabetes in children and adolescents.* Pediatr Diabetes, 2018. **19 Suppl 27**(Suppl 27): p. 7-19.

reducing frequent hypoglycemia. Insulin therapy may be provided by multiple daily injections,[12] insulin pumps, or closed-loop insulin delivery systems. Therapeutic option depends on individual patient/family preferences, age, diabetes duration, literacy, lifestyle, and insurance coverage.[13] Treatment of T2D may involve oral therapy or involve insulin therapy based on presentation and severity. Although technology improves diabetes care and glycemic control, management remains challenging for patients and families, and the impact of psychosocial factors influencing diabetes care is well recognized.[3]

Psychosocial Aspects of Diabetes Management

The management of diabetes, and multiple factors involved to facilitate positive health outcomes, makes it clear that a biopsychosocial approach and interdisciplinary team are essential. Youth with diabetes are at increased risk for emotional and psychosocial problems,[14] which have been associated with nonadherence, including fewer blood glucose checks and suboptimal glycemic control, even 1 year later.[15–17] Family conflict, low parental monitoring, and diffusion of responsibility have been associated with decreased adherence and poor outcomes,[15,18,19] as having sociodemographic variables, such as family density, socioeconomic status (SES), and minority status.[18]

Most youth do not meet the guidelines for HbA1c set forth by the American Diabetes Association (ADA).[20] Owing to the challenges youth and families face living with diabetes, clinical guidelines recommend psychological care for these patients. The International Society for Pediatric and Adolescent Diabetes (ISPAD) states, "psychosocial factors are the most important influences affecting the care and management of diabetes."[3] Given this, psychologists find themselves perfectly positioned to serve the psychosocial needs of youth with diabetes and are increasingly a member of the team.

Screening of Psychosocial Factors Associated with Diabetes

The ADA and ISPAD recommend routine psychosocial assessment across a variety of individuals (eg, quality of life, depressive and anxiety symptoms, and diabetes-specific distress), and social/family factors (eg, family conflict and communication).[3,21] Psychosocial screening may reduce health disparities, facilitate access to services, reduce unnecessary referrals and costs, promote resilience in at-risk youth,[21–23] and help identify intervention targets. Psychologists have been integral in developing and implementing screening protocols because of their training in child development, family systems, and psychosocial aspects of chronic health conditions.

There are different approaches to psychosocial screening that can be used, including clinical interviews and/or validated screening tools. There are evidence-based guidelines to enhance clinical care and improve psychosocial and health-related outcomes.[24] Screening should involve self-report and parent-proxy measures, beginning at diagnosis and occurring more often than annually.[25] Sequential screening carries several benefits (eg, reduction of false positives, unnecessary costs/referrals)[26] and has been used within diabetes clinics.[27]

Consistent with best practice, psychologists should be available during the clinic to conduct screening and assessments and to support the interdisciplinary team in recognizing and managing psychological concerns.[28] Psychologists can identify and appreciate psychosocial factors that may complicate care and lead to poorer outcomes. However, only 58.1% of ISPAD listserve members identified a psychologist as a member of the team on-site and in-clinic,[29] and less than half of US programs have integrated psychology.[30] When psychologists are not integrated, missed visits for mental health are higher than those for medical providers,[31] and less than a quarter of youth referred to psychological services successfully follow-up.[32]

Behavioral and Psychological Interventions for Pediatric Diabetes

Given the impact of psychosocial functioning on the management of diabetes, psychologists have an integral role in treatment. Psychologists can play a role in three areas: inpatient hospitalization, endocrinology clinic visits, and outpatient behavioral health.

Inpatient Behavioral Health Care: Psychology consultation for hospitalized youth with T1D is either for new-onset adjustment or chronic nonadherence. In newly diagnosed youth, treatment focuses on coping and adjustment to the diagnosis and hospital. Psychologists work with the child and family to help them understand the diagnosis and process some of the initial negative feelings. This may be the first time a child or family has interacted with a psychologist and thus it is important to define the psychologist's roles working with these families. Psychologists may refer for outpatient follow-up based on screening measures to address other factors. Finally, the family will make significant changes to their daily lives and may need time to discuss implementation and sharing information with others. Psychologists can aid in balancing concrete and emotional support during this transition to home.

For youth who are chronically nonadherent, the goal is to identify and reduce barriers preventing regimen adherence with the patient and family. Providers rely on cognitive-behavioral therapy (CBT) to increase adherence and coping.[33] Cognitively, the goal is to reduce distortions around adherence (ie, one mistake ruins everything) and encourage more neutral or positive thoughts (ie, I can do it). Behaviorally, the goal is to increase adherence to medication and lifestyle changes. These strategies, when part of a multicomponent treatment plan, have been shown to increase effectiveness and adherence.[34–37]

Clinic-Based Interventions: Studies show that collaborative or comanaged care for youth with T1D is effective.[38,39] The medical team guides treatment but receives more robust information regarding individual patient needs and helps keeping the patient accountable. During collaborative visits, psychologists can provide brief psychological interventions and facilitate communication between medical providers, patients, and caregivers. Psychologists work with families on improving management through setting appropriate expectations, providing incentives/discipline, identifying and increasing support, and reducing barriers. Motivational interviewing (MI) is a key intervention for diabetes adherence that uses communication skills to encourage change behaviors while addressing barriers.[40] In youth with diabetes, MI is used to increase adherence and facilitate communication about an individual's obstacles.

Outpatient Behavioral Health and Psychological Interventions: When youth with diabetes need longer intervention, they are referred for outpatient psychotherapy. Treatment goals are similar to those addressed in clinic or while inpatient but also include addressing traditional mental health concerns complicated by the diabetes diagnosis. For example, individuals with T1D are at higher risk for depression and anxiety.[41] Depression manifests with decreased motivation to care for activities of daily living (ADLs) and can exacerbate nonadherence. Using CBT, psychologists work on improving maladaptive thought patterns regarding self-efficacy, motivation for self-care, and help the individual engage in regimen tasks. Caregivers will learn behavioral strategies to encourage and support the youth living with diabetes. Finally, addressing any social support concerns including reconnecting to peer groups and other activities is key in reducing depressive symptoms.

Regarding anxiety, youth may experience specific phobias (eg, needle phobia) and/or health anxiety. Using CBT, goals include addressing the underlying cognitive distortions and approaching feared behaviors. Unlike other phobias, some diabetes-related fear is rational. Therefore, the goal is managing anxiety so the individual can care for their diabetes without being concerned that they are going to do permanent damage to their health or body. Exposures to physiologic symptoms and situations have to be managed with the help of a medical provider.

OBESITY AND METABOLIC SYNDROME

Obesity is an important public health problem,[42] as 35.4% of US children and adolescents (aged 2–19 years) are overweight or obese.[42] High prevalence rates of obesity and increased incidence of medical problems lead to the financial burden on the health systems. The Centers for Disease Control and Prevention (CDC) defines overweight as body mass index (BMI) between 85th and 95th percentile for age and sex, and obesity as BMI $\geq$95th percentile.[10,43–45] Obesity is associated with increased morbidity and mortality. Chronic inflammation noted in adipocytes may lead to insulin resistance and ultimately T2D.[46,47] This may also lead to vascular endothelial dysfunction, an abnormal lipid profile, and hypertension, promoting the development of atherosclerotic CVD.[47] The co-occurrence of these risk factors for both T2D and CVD is often referred to as metabolic syndrome characterized by abdominal obesity, hyperglycemia, dyslipidemia, and hypertension. Furthermore, obesity is associated with polycystic ovarian syndrome, nonalcoholic fatty liver disease, cholelithiasis, idiopathic intracranial hypertension, obstructive sleep apnea, orthopedic diseases, and psychosocial problems.[10] Recognition and prevention of obesity early in childhood is key to preventing complications. It is recommended that all children older than 2 years have BMI measurements calculated and plotted on age-appropriate growth charts annually to ensure early recognition and timely counseling and treatment.[48] Prevention and treatment of overweight and obesity in youth focuses on behavioral modifications, including decreasing energy intake and increasing energy expenditure.[44] Pharmacotherapy and weight loss surgery may be recommended in severe obesity and/or associated complications after intensive assessment and management by a comprehensive multidisciplinary weight management team.[49] Obesity in youth is associated with immediate and long-term medical and psychological problems.[50]

Psychosocial Factors Associated with Pediatric Obesity and Metabolic Syndrome

Childhood overweight and obesity have a deleterious impact on youth's psychosocial functioning. Youth who are overweight experience decreased quality of life and more distress, including anxiety and depression, weight-related teasing/bullying, and self-esteem issues as compared with healthy-weight peers.[51–53] In adolescents with severe versus moderate obesity, the incidence of depression and anxiety increases exponentially.[54] Although maternal psychopathology accounts for a large variance in child internalizing and social problems for overweight and obese youth, both maternal and child psychological problems predict treatment success.[55,56] These findings suggest the importance of detecting the presence of psychosocial issues, youth at-risk for negative psychosocial outcomes, and family factors that may influence functioning.

Screening of Psychosocial Factors Related to Pediatric Obesity and Metabolic Syndrome

The Pediatric Endocrine Society recommends psychosocial assessment as part of the standard of care given the impact of psychosocial variables on the development and maintenance of lifestyle behaviors[57] Screening psychological risk and comorbidities (eg, anxiety, depression, eating disorders), as well as family functioning (eg, child-rearing regarding diet and exercise, communication),[58] is critical. In addition, recommendations prescribe psychological evaluation for any patient pursuing bariatric surgery.[58] Although there is recognition of the importance of screening for social vulnerabilities and comorbid psychosocial problems that may impact the treatment of youth who are overweight or obese,[59] there have been no explicit recommendations regarding the initiation, frequency, or measurement of these psychosocial factors. In addition, for metabolic syndrome there are no recommendations regarding psychosocial screening, which may be due to the lack of consistency in the diagnostic criteria for pediatric metabolic syndrome.[60,61] One might suspect screening to be similar to the above recommendations for youth with overweight and obesity, but without expert consensus and explicit call for psychologists to be integrally involved with the screening, prevention, and treatment of pediatric obesity and metabolic syndrome, psychologists may have to make a case for integration into clinics. They may, however, be able to inform practice guidelines through research efforts and dissemination of clinical practice experiences as exemplars.

Behavioral and Psychological Interventions

Treatment of youth who are overweight or obese is similar but not identical to that of youth with T1D. For example, many youth with overweight or obesity are not seen inpatient by psychologists but are seen in outpatient weight management clinics and for outpatient treatment.

Clinic-Based Interventions: Research has shown several factors important to achieving good outcomes when working with youth who are overweight or obese: nutritional education, increasing exercise/physical activity, and utilization of cognitive and behavioral interventions to address behavior change.[62] Thus, psychologists are uniquely positioned to help support and provide these interventions in concert with medical professionals. During clinic visits, parents are more involved and thus can be engaged in treatment, which is linked to better outcomes for youth.[63,64]

Outpatient Behavioral Health and Psychological Intervention: As noted, youth with chronic health conditions may be referred for outpatient therapy to address other comorbid concerns. When youth who are overweight are referred for outpatient therapy, working on health behavior change using MI and addressing body-related dysmorphia are key. MI can be used alone but is recommended as one part of a multifactorial approach.[65] In addition, CBT may be used to help with monitoring intake, cognitive distortions, and stimulus control. It is important to be mindful that abstinence cannot be part of treatment of overweight and obesity and thus bringing behaviors to normal limits is more realistic and may involve behavior change for the whole family and not just the patient.

A CASE FOR INTEGRATING PSYCHOLOGISTS WITHIN PEDIATRIC ENDOCRINOLOGY

Integration of psychological services into diabetes management can improve health outcomes and decrease health care expenditures. Research has examined the cost-effectiveness of integrated psychological services in diabetes clinic visits by examining the impact on medical and psychosocial outcomes and found significant improvements in patient's HbA1c following psychological consultation, suggesting overall benefit given the potential for long-term cost savings of improved HbA1c.[66,67] Real-world limitations can make the integration of psychological services challenging (eg, space and reimbursement). However, integrated models have shown revenue generation or at minimum "break-even" outcome suggesting that embedding psychological providers is financially feasible.[68] Psychologists may bill direct patient care (eg, current procedural terminology (CPT) 90791, 90832, 96156, 96158), as well as the screening of behavioral, developmental, and psychosocial factors (eg, CPT 96127, 96110, 96161) that may affect diabetes management. Provider perspectives on routine psychosocial screening and experiences working with embedded psychologists suggest support for integrating behavioral health into routine care.[69]

Findings support cost-effectiveness in the behavioral health care of youth presenting with obesity. As many of the comorbidities of obesity are reversible with intervention, researchers have been exploring evidence-based behavioral and family-based interventions. There are emerging data suggesting the cost-effectiveness of interventions delivered by psychologists in the management of pediatric obesity;[70,71] however, there continue to be barriers to billing and reimbursement of psychological services, and ongoing research and advocacy is necessary.[72]

SUMMARY

The role of the psychologists working with youth and families with endocrine disorders is diverse and varied. Given best practice guidelines established by professional societies dedicated to the care of pediatric diabetes, embedding a psychologist is imperative to address the growing and evolving psychosocial needs of pediatric patients and families. Although there are several models of collaborative care ranging from minimal integration for the psychologist (eg, support/consultative) to a full interdisciplinary team member, overall psychologists are being recognized as important partners in the care of patients with diabetes, obesity, and metabolic syndrome.

CLINICS CARE POINTS

- Psychologists should be considered integral members of the multidisciplinary treatment team in the management of endocrine disorders, specifically diabetes, obesity, and metabolic syndrome.

- Best practice guidelines recommend routine psychosocial screening for all youth with diabetes at diagnosis and regularly during standard clinical care; screening recommendations in pediatric obesity are emerging.
- Psychologists can develop screening protocols, assess psychosocial functioning during clinic visits, and provide interventions to optimize health outcomes.
- For additional support, referrals to psychologists for evidence-based treatment can help improve adherence and comorbid psychological concerns (eg, anxiety and depression).
- Although CPT codes can be used for patient care (eg, screening, assessment, and treatment), greater advocacy and research is necessary to maximize reimbursement of integrated behavioral health care.

REFERENCES

1. Lawrence JM, Divers J, Isom S, et al. Trends in prevalence of type 1 and type 2 diabetes in children and adolescents in the US, 2001-2017. JAMA 2021;326(8): 717–27.
2. World Health Organization. Obesity and overweight. 2017.
3. Delamater AM, de Wit M, McDarby V, et al. ISPAD clinical practice consensus guidelines 2018: Psychological care of children and adolescents with type 1 diabetes. Pediatr Diabetes 2018;19:237–49.
4. Cameron FJ, Garvey K, Hood KK, Acerini CL, Codner E. ISPAD clinical practice consensus guidelines 2018: Diabetes in adolescence. Pediatr Diabetes 2018; 19(Suppl 27):161–250.
5. Draznin B, Aroda VR, Bakris G, et al. 2. classification and diagnosis of diabetes: Standards of medical care in diabetes-2022. Diabetes Care 2022; 45(Supplement_1):S17–38.
6. Mayer-Davis EJ, Kahkoska AR, Jefferies C, et al. ISPAD clinical practice consensus guidelines 2018: definition, epidemiology, and classification of diabetes in children and adolescents. Pediatr Diabetes 2018;19(Suppl 27):7.
7. Danne T, Phillip M, Buckingham BA, et al. ISPAD clinical practice consensus guidelines 2018: Insulin treatment in children and adolescents with diabetes. Pediatr Diabetes 2018;19:115–35.
8. Divers J, Mayer-Davis EJ, Lawrence JM, et al. Trends in incidence of type 1 and type 2 diabetes among youths—selected counties and indian reservations, united states, 2002-2015. Morb Mortal Weekly Rep 2020;69(6):161.
9. Bacha F, Gungor N, Lee S, et al. Progressive deterioration of β-cell function in obese youth with type 2 diabetes. Pediatr Diabetes 2013;14(2):106–11.
10. American Diabetes Association. 4. comprehensive medical evaluation and assessment of comorbidities: Standards of medical care in Diabetes—2020. Diabetes Care 2020;43(Supplement 1):S37–47.
11. Draznin B, Aroda VR, Bakris G, et al. 6. glycemic targets: Standards of medical care in diabetes-2022. Diabetes Care 2022;45(Supplement_1):S83–96.
12. Pihoker C, Forsander G, Fantahun B, et al. ISPAD clinical practice consensus guidelines 2018: the delivery of ambulatory diabetes care to children and adolescents with diabetes. Pediatr Diabetes 2018;19:84–104.
13. Sherr JL, Tauschmann M, Battelino T, et al. ISPAD clinical practice consensus guidelines 2018: diabetes technologies. Pediatr Diabetes 2018;19:302–25.
14. Reynolds KA, Helgeson VS. Children with diabetes compared to peers: Depressed? distressed? A meta-analytic review. Ann Behav Med 2011;42(1): 29–41.

15. Brodar KE, Davis EM, Lynn C, et al. Comprehensive psychosocial screening in a pediatric diabetes clinic. Pediatr Diabetes 2021;22(4):656–66.
16. Hilliard ME, Herzer M, Dolan LM, et al. Psychological screening in adolescents with type 1 diabetes predicts outcomes one year later. Diabetes Res Clin Pract 2011;94(1):39–44.
17. Hood KK, Beavers DP, Yi-Frazier J, et al. Psychosocial burden and glycemic control during the first 6 years of diabetes: Results from the SEARCH for diabetes in youth study. J Adolesc Health 2014;55(4):498–504.
18. Caccavale LJ, Weaver P, Chen R, et al. Family density and SES related to diabetes management and glycemic control in adolescents with type 1 diabetes. J Pediatr Psychol 2015;40(5):500–8.
19. Helgeson VS, Reynolds KA, Siminerio L, et al. Parent and adolescent distribution of responsibility for diabetes self-care: Links to health outcomes. J Pediatr Psychol 2008;33(5):497–508.
20. Wood JR, Miller KM, Maahs DM, et al. Most youth with type 1 diabetes in the T1D exchange clinic registry do not meet american diabetes association or international society for pediatric and adolescent diabetes clinical guidelines. Diabetes Care 2013;36(7):2035–7.
21. American Diabetes Association. 13. children and adolescents: Standards of medical care in diabetes—2019. Diabetes Care 2019;42(Supplement 1): S148–64.
22. Anderson LM, Papadakis JL, Vesco AT, et al. Patient-reported and parent proxy-reported outcomes in pediatric medical specialty clinical settings: A systematic review of implementation. J Pediatr Psychol 2020;45(3):247–65.
23. Wallace AS, Wang D, Shin J, et al. Screening and diagnosis of prediabetes and diabetes in US children and adolescents. Pediatrics 2020;146(3).
24. Young-Hyman D, De Groot M, Hill-Briggs F, et al. Psychosocial care for people with diabetes: A position statement of the american diabetes association. Diabetes Care 2016;39(12):2126–40.
25. Barry-Menkhaus SA, Stoner AM, MacGregor KL, et al. Special considerations in the systematic psychosocial screening of youth with type 1 diabetes. J Pediatr Psychol 2020;45(3):299–310.
26. Lavigne JV, Feldman M, Meyers KM. Screening for mental health problems: Addressing the base rate fallacy for a sustainable screening program in integrated primary care. J Pediatr Psychol 2016;41(10):1081–90.
27. Marker AM, Patton SR, McDonough RJ, et al. Implementing clinic-wide depression screening for pediatric diabetes: An initiative to improve healthcare processes. Pediatr Diabetes 2019;20(7):964–73.
28. Delamater AM. Psychological care of children and adolescents with diabetes. Pediatr Diabetes 2009;10(12):175–84.
29. De Wit M, Pulgaron ER, Pattino-Fernandez AM, et al. Psychological support for children with diabetes: Are the guidelines being met? J Clin Psychol Med Settings 2014;21(2):190–9.
30. Guttmann-Bauman I, Thornton P, Adhikari S, et al. Pediatric endocrine society survey of diabetes practices in the united states: What is the current state? Pediatr Diabetes 2018;19(5):859–65.
31. Markowitz JT, Volkening LK, Laffel LM. Care utilization in a pediatric diabetes clinic: Cancellations, parental attendance, and mental health appointments. J Pediatr 2014;164(6):1384–9.

32. Vassilopoulos A, Valenzuela JM, Tsikis J, et al. Pediatric diabetes patients infrequently access outpatient psychology services following screening and referral: Implications for practice. Child Health Care 2020;49(2):202–17.

33. Lemanek KL, Yardley H. Noncompliance and nonadherence. Handbook of cognitive behavioral therapy for pediatric medical conditions. Switzerland: Springer Nature; 2019. p. 407–16.

34. Kahana S, Drotar D, Frazier T. Meta-analysis of psychological interventions to promote adherence to treatment in pediatric chronic health conditions. J Pediatr Psychol 2008;33(6):590–611.

35. Dean AJ, Walters J, Hall A. A systematic review of interventions to enhance medication adherence in children and adolescents with chronic illness. Arch Dis Child 2010;95(9):717–23.

36. DiMatteo MR. The role of effective communication with children and their families in fostering adherence to pediatric regimens. Patient Educ Couns 2004;55(3):339–44.

37. Gould E, Mitty E. Medication adherence is a partnership, medication compliance is not. Geriatr Nurs 2010;31(4):290–8.

38. Bodenheimer T, Wagner EH, Grumbach K. Improving primary care for patients with chronic illness. JAMA 2002;288(14):1775–9.

39. Ginnard OZ, Alonso GT, Corathers SD, et al. Quality improvement in diabetes care: a review of initiatives and outcomes in the T1D exchange quality improvement collaborative. Clin Diabetes 2021;39(3):256–63.

40. Alvarado-Martel D, Boronat M, Alberiche-Ruano MdP, et al. Motivational interviewing and self-care in type 1 diabetes: a randomized controlled clinical trial study protocol. Front Endocrinol 2020;11:948.

41. Buchberger B, Huppertz H, Krabbe L, et al. Symptoms of depression and anxiety in youth with type 1 diabetes: a systematic review and meta-analysis. Psychoneuroendocrinology 2016;70:70–84.

42. Ogden CL, Fryar CD, Martin CB, et al. Trends in obesity prevalence by race and hispanic origin—1999-2000 to 2017-2018. JAMA 2020;324(12):1208–10.

43. Deurenberg P, Weststrate JA, Seidell JC. Body mass index as a measure of body fatness: age-and sex-specific prediction formulas. Br J Nutr 1991;65(2):105–14.

44. Chung YL, Rhie Y. Severe obesity in children and adolescents: metabolic effects, assessment, and treatment. J Obes Metab Syndr 2021;30(4):326.

45. Skinner AC, Skelton JA. Prevalence and trends in obesity and severe obesity among children in the united states, 1999-2012. JAMA Pediatr 2014;168(6):561–6.

46. Saltiel AR, Olefsky JM. Inflammatory mechanisms linking obesity and metabolic disease. J Clin Invest 2017;127(1):1–4.

47. Gállego-Suárez C, Bulan A, Hirschfeld E, et al. Enhanced myeloid leukocytes in obese children and adolescents at risk for metabolic impairment. Front Endocrinol 2020;11:327.

48. Krebs NF, Himes JH, Jacobson D, et al. Assessment of child and adolescent overweight and obesity. Pediatrics 2007;120(Supplement_4):S193–228.

49. Masarwa R, Brunetti VC, Aloe S, et al. Efficacy and safety of metformin for obesity: A systematic review. Pediatrics 2021;147(3).

50. Ruiz LD, Zuelch ML, Dimitratos SM, et al. Adolescent obesity: diet quality, psychosocial health, and cardiometabolic risk factors. Nutrients 2020;12(1):43.

51. Eisenberg ME, Neumark-Sztainer D, Story M. Associations of weight-based teasing and emotional well-being among adolescents. Arch Pediatr Adolesc Med 2003;157(8):733–8.

52. Nascimento MMR, Melo TR, Pinto RMC, et al. Parents' perception of health-related quality of life in children and adolescents with excess weight. J Pediatr 2016;92:65–72.

53. Rankin J, Matthews L, Cobley S, et al. Psychological consequences of childhood obesity: psychiatric comorbidity and prevention. Adolesc Health Med Ther 2016; 7:125.

54. Fox CK, Gross AC, Rudser KD, et al. Depression, anxiety, and severity of obesity in adolescents: Is emotional eating the link? Clin Pediatr 2016;55(12):1120–5.

55. Epstein LH, Wisniewski L, Weng R. Child and parent psychological problems influence child weight control. Obes Res 1994;2(6):509–15.

56. Myers MD, Raynor HA, Epstein LH. Predictors of child psychological changes during family-based treatment for obesity. Arch Pediatr Adolesc Med 1998; 152(9):855–61.

57. August GP, Caprio S, Fennoy I, et al. Prevention and treatment of pediatric obesity: an endocrine society clinical practice guideline based on expert opinion. J Clin Endocrinol Metab 2008;93(12):4576–99.

58. Styne DM, Arslanian SA, Connor EL, et al. Pediatric obesity—assessment, treatment, and prevention: an endocrine society clinical practice guideline. J Clin Endocrinol Metab 2017;102(3):709–57.

59. Sagar R, Gupta T. Psychological aspects of obesity in children and adolescents. Indian J Pediatr 2018;85(7):554–9.

60. Al-Hamad D, Raman V. Metabolic syndrome in children and adolescents. Translational Pediatr 2017;6(4):397.

61. Magge SN, Goodman E, Armstrong SC, et al. The metabolic syndrome in children and adolescents: Shifting the focus to cardiometabolic risk factor clustering. Pediatrics 2017;140(2).

62. Herrera EA, Johnston CA, Steele RG. A comparison of cognitive and behavioral treatments for pediatric obesity. Child Health Care 2004;33(2):151–67.

63. McLean N, Griffin S, Toney K, et al. Family involvement in weight control, weight maintenance and weight-loss interventions: A systematic review of randomised trials. Int J Obes 2003;27(9):987–1005.

64. Young KM, Northern JJ, Lister KM, et al. A meta-analysis of family-behavioral weight-loss treatments for children. Clin Psychol Rev 2007;27(2):240–9.

65. Suire KB, Kavookjian J, Wadsworth DD. Motivational interviewing for overweight children: A systematic review. Pediatrics 2020;146(5).

66. Gelfand K, Geffken G, Lewin A, et al. An initial evaluation of the design of pediatric psychology consultation service with children with diabetes. J Child Health Care 2004;8(2):113–23.

67. Caccavale LJ, Bernstein R, Yarbro JL, et al. Impact and cost-effectiveness of integrated psychology services in a pediatric endocrinology clinic. J Clin Psychol Med Settings 2020;27(3):615–21.

68. Yarbro JL, Mehlenbeck R. Financial analysis of behavioral health services in a pediatric endocrinology clinic. J Pediatr Psychol 2016;41(8):879–87.

69. Brodar KE, Leite RO, Marchetti D, et al. Psychological screening and consultation in a pediatric diabetes clinic: Medical providers' perspectives. Clin Pract Pediatr Psychol 2021;10(2):164–79.

70. Borner KB, Canter KS, Lee RH, et al. Making the business case for coverage of family-based behavioral group interventions for pediatric obesity. J Pediatr Psychol 2016;41(8):867–78.

71. Goldfield GS, Epstein LH, Kilanowski CK, et al. Cost-effectiveness of group and mixed family-based treatment for childhood obesity. Int J Obes 2001;25(12): 1843–9.
72. Gray JS, Filigno SS, Santos M, et al. The status of billing and reimbursement in pediatric obesity treatment programs. J Behav Health Serv Res 2013;40(3): 378–85.

A Hypothetical Case Example Illustrating the Importance of a Multidisciplinary Approach to Treating Chronic/Functional Abdominal Pain in Pediatric Patients

Orhan Atay, MD[a],*, Jennie David, PhD[b], Ami Mehta, MD[c]

KEYWORDS

- Irritable bowel syndrome • Functional abdominal pain
- Pediatric pain and palliative care • Pediatric gastroenterology • Pediatric psychology

KEY POINTS

- Functional abdominal pain is a complex condition that is treated by multidisciplinary care.
- Patients and families understanding the pathophysiology of functional abdominal pain is critical to support adherence to multidisciplinary recommendations.
- Providers benefit from multidisciplinary collaboration to support patients and their families with functional abdominal pain.

INTRODUCTION

In this co-authored article by a pediatric gastroenterologist, a pediatric pain and palliative care specialist, and a pediatric gastrointestinal (GI) psychologist, we present a hypothetical case of a pediatric patient who will undergo evaluation and treatment by each of these specialists. We outline, in detail, the patient's journey through the health care system and demonstrate how a collaborative effort among multidisciplinary specialists is the ideal approach to care for individuals such as this hypothetical patient.

---

[a] Neurogastroenterology Motility Program, Division of Pediatric Gastroenterology, Children's Hospital of The King's Daughters, Eastern Virginia Medical School, 601 Children's Lane, Norfolk, VA 23507, USA; [b] Pediatric Psychology and Neuropsychology, Department of Pediatrics, Nationwide Children's Hospital, The Ohio State University College of Medicine, 700 Children's Drive, Columbus, OH 43205, USA; [c] Pediatric Pain and Palliative Care, Children's Hospital of The King's Daughters, 601 Children's Lane, Norfolk, VA 23507, USA
* Corresponding author.
E-mail address: Orhan.Atay@CHKD.ORG

Pediatr Clin N Am 69 (2022) 917–927
https://doi.org/10.1016/j.pcl.2022.06.005
0031-3955/22/© 2022 Elsevier Inc. All rights reserved.

pediatric.theclinics.com

We present a hypothetical case involving a 15-year-old African American girl, "Jane," with a history of chronic, intermittent periumbilical abdominal pain for the past few years, now with worsening pain over the past 3 months. Her additional symptoms included intermittent nausea and irregular bowel movements, alternating between constipation and diarrhea. She is a high-achieving student athlete (plays soccer) with a history of anxiety. She was previously enrolled in therapy for anxiety but has not attended therapy over a year and has reported that therapy did not help in the past. School absenteeism has become a concern and she is no longer able to regularly participate in competitive sports because of missing school and leaving school early due to her symptoms. Aside from her current GI issues, she is otherwise healthy with no significant family medical history. Jane lives with her mother, father, grandmother, and twin sister, Julie. Jane is in the 10th grade.

Multidisciplinary Assessment and Treatment/Intervention

Pediatric gastroenterology
Jane was initially evaluated by her pediatrician. Several tests were performed but did not yield an etiology of her symptoms. Given the persistent abdominal pain and ongoing family concern, she was referred to a pediatric gastroenterologist for further evaluation and treatment.

Jane was accompanied by her parents at the time of her clinical visit. On initial impression, Jane seemed to have withdrawn with a noticeable flat affect. Her parents were noted to be very invested in identifying the cause of Jane's symptoms and were observed to talk for the majority of the visit about Jane's health. The family shared GI-related concerns of their close friends and was wondering whether Jane had Crohn's disease or celiac disease.

A thorough history was obtained, mostly through Jane's parents. There was acknowledgment of Jane's history of anxiety disorder and the pressure she was facing both in academics and through her athletic involvement at her school. In addition to Jane reporting that previous therapy focused on anxiety was not helpful, parents also reported that they did not think previous therapy had helped.

Jane was prescribed an antispasmodic and antiemetic by her pediatrician, which was helpful in reducing but not fully alleviating her abdominal pain and nausea. Of note, family reported that Jane generally only reports GI symptoms on school mornings and Jane tends to not report GI symptoms on weekends. The family also reported that over the past 3 years, symptoms have always improved to some extent over the summer.

Her bowel movements were described as variable in frequency and consistency. Jane was shown the Bristol stool chart and reported seeing a variety of stool consistencies from Bristol types 1–7 (**Fig. 1**). No history of rectal bleeding was reported.

Her history was negative for unexplainable fever, weight loss, oral aphthous ulcers, arthralgia, or unusual rash. Her family history was negative for inflammatory bowel disease, celiac disease, or polyposis syndrome.

Laboratory test results were reviewed that included a complete blood count, comprehensive metabolic panel, sedimentation rate, and C-reactive protein, all of which were unremarkable.

During examination, Jane remained quiet and reserved. Her abdominal examination showed a significant generalized tenderness without worrisome signs of rebound or guarding. No organomegaly was identified; however, a palpable mass was appreciated involving the left lower quadrant (LLQ).

A Patient Health Questionnaire was performed for depression. No suicidal ideation was identified at that time. These results were discussed during the visit and Jane's

Bristol Stool Chart

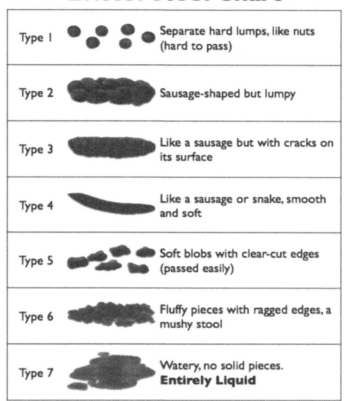

Type 1		Separate hard lumps, like nuts (hard to pass)
Type 2		Sausage-shaped but lumpy
Type 3		Like a sausage but with cracks on its surface
Type 4		Like a sausage or snake, smooth and soft
Type 5		Soft blobs with clear-cut edges (passed easily)
Type 6		Fluffy pieces with ragged edges, a mushy stool
Type 7		Watery, no solid pieces. **Entirely Liquid**

Fig. 1. Stool form scale as a useful guide to intestinal transit time.[21] (*From* Lewis, S.J. and K.W. Heaton, Stool form scale as a useful guide to intestinal transit time. Scandinavian journal of gastroenterology, 1997. 32(9): p. 920-924.)

parents voiced their concern and desire to reenroll Jane for therapy, with hesitation of finding the "right" therapist.

An abdominal x-ray, complete and pelvic ultrasound, and additional laboratory tests were ordered including a celiac disease panel, amylase, lipase, fecal calprotectin, hemoccult, and *Helicobacter pylori* stool antigen. Aside from stool retention noted on her x-ray, especially involving the rectosigmoid (which would explain the palpable LLQ mass) the remainder of Jane's test results were unremarkable. Jane was prescribed a stool softener for her constipation and was diagnosed with irritable bowel syndrome (IBS) with mixed presentation.

Despite reassurance and addressing her constipation, Jane's abdominal pain persisted, and she was subsequently referred to a pediatric pain and palliative care specialist for IBS refractory to conventional therapy.

Pediatric pain and palliative care specialist
Jane presented to the pain management clinic accompanied by her mother. She was quiet but appropriate during triage, and when asked questions by the triage nurse, her

mother would often jump in and answer for her. Directing questions specifically to Jane helped this tendency slightly.

During her visit with the physician, her pain was the specific focus of the conversation. Jane expressed that she was not exactly sure when her pain began, but thinks that maybe it started in the beginning of middle school, though there was no identifiable trigger or illness that precipitated this prolonged pain presentation. In her words, "I just noticed the pain was there 1 day."

Jane was able to articulate descriptions about her pain, including reporting that it was "stabbing and throbbing" in nature, and when asked where it was located, she gestured to her whole abdomen. She shared that she had a consistently present level of pain at baseline, usually 2 to 3 of 10, at which she could function. She expressed that she was never really pain free, though sometimes she would feel fleetingly pain free, first thing in the morning. Once she woke up and thought about her day and upcoming school assignments, her pain returned.

Jane expressed that pain was worse on school days, and when she was at school, though it was present at all times to some degree, but often a lower level of pain than when she was at home. She reported that pain flares were precipitated by stressful events at school, high levels of activity, and sometimes just randomly happened. Usually, her flares would jump as high as 7 to 8 of 10. She reported that sometimes Tylenol or ibuprofen would help, and sometimes the antispasmodics, but often they did not help at all, leading to notable feelings of frustration. Jane reported that she just stopped telling her parents all the time that she was having pain, as they would want to discuss the pain, offer medications, or would start talking again about what might be wrong with Jane to cause this pain.

Jane shared that pain was really starting to interfere with school, as she has had such bad pain on some days that she could not go at all. She was struggling with getting to school regularly, and often would get in late if pain flares were an issue. Generally, if she was able to get to school on any given day, she would be able to stay throughout the day, but getting there in the mornings was often a challenge. She reported that she was late at least 1 to 2 days a week, missed ~1 day per week, and would miss 2 to 4 days each month.

We spent some time discussing chronic pain and the pathophysiology behind this, including sensitization of nerve pathways to interpret all incoming stimuli as pain, rather than what they really are (stretch, pressure, and digestion). Jane understood the fact that being in pain for a long time can beget a chronic pain problem. Her mother took some time to understand the fact that though Jane has chronic abdominal pain, there is nothing "big, bad, or scary" happening in her abdomen. Jane and her mother began to understand that pain does not have to be due to the pathology at the target organ (the GI system, in this case), but can be due to misfiring in the pain pathways that carry information to the brain.

In addition, we spent some time discussing that the gut/brain connection is strong, and the GI system is full of nerves. The numerous nerve endings that allow the brain to interpret, from just one twinge, if one is sick, or nauseated, or hungry, or needs to have a bowel movement, or is having menstrual cramps, can misfire and send "incorrect" signals to the brain. Just as anxiety or cognitive stress can manifest with GI symptoms such as urgency to stool or void, those same pathways can lead to chronic sensation of GI discomfort, even in the absence of pathology. Jane did acknowledge that she noticed a connection, where her pain does seem worse when she has significant stressors, such as a test at school or something else she is nervous about.

We discussed that the best approach to pain management is a three-fold approach:

1. We treat the nerve dysfunction with a medication such as amitriptyline or gabapentin,[1] to help retrain nerves that not all stimulus is pain, and some can be normal gut sensations. This requires a real understanding and willingness to commit to a medication and to the concept that there is no gut pathology that is being missed.
2. We treat functionality, by assessing ability to attend school, participate in sports/extracurricular activities, and interactions with family. If there is a significant decline in functionality, which often happens as chronic pain leads to poor functioning that leads to deconditioning, we will send a patient to physical therapy to work toward achieving functional goals. If school attendance is an issue, we work with family to create a 504 plan to help support the patient in getting to school every day and staying in school when possible. Increasing and maintaining functioning was described as a critical component to managing Jane's chronic pain.
3. We treat the mental health and psychosocial components of living with chronic pain. The isolation, frustration, fear, and stress that come with a chronic pain diagnosis are a huge emotional burden, especially for a teenager. In addition to that the sensation of "feeling different than one's peers" and frequent statements from others (including teachers), of "you look fine, you can't really be in that much pain," can be a huge stressor, and even a cause for depression and anxiety. On the heels of that, explaining the gut-brain connection supports the fact that anxiety and depression can worsen abdominal pain (though it is important to point out that anxiety and depression do not "cause" the abdominal pain, ie, it is not "all in your head") and the role of evidence-based interventions like cognitive behavioral therapy (CBT) and biofeedback in management of chronic pain. This leads us to have frank conversations about mental health as a part of each clinical visit, and if warranted, prompts a referral to a pain psychologist or mental health therapist (depending on available resources).

Though Jane was initially hesitant, when she understood that the goal of this multidisciplinary approach is to really help improve her pain and functioning, she was willing to consider trying this approach. She did worry about her ability to comply with a daily medication such as amitriptyline. She and her parents were interested in the 504 plan, but Jane did report that she did not feel a need to do physical training, as she is still able to play soccer most of the time. She has also expressed her concern that a referral to therapy services implied that her "pain is made up, or all in my head." She was able to be dissuaded from this concept, and was grudgingly willing to see a pediatric psychologist to discuss the intersection of chronic pain and psychological stress.

Pediatric gastrointestinal/pain psychologist
Jane was accompanied by her father when she was presented to pediatric psychology to see the pediatric GI psychologist. Jane greeted clinician appropriately and easily engaged in discussion about the sports jersey she was wearing as Jane, her father, and GI psychologist walked back to the clinic.

Family was receptive to overview of confidentiality and plan to spend time together (Jane, her father, and psychologist) and also to spend time individually between Jane and psychologist during the visit. Jane and her father described a longstanding history of pain and reported normative frustration in Jane's ongoing symptoms and expressed worries that there may be an etiology to Jane's pain that had been missed. When gently prompted by clinician, family shared concerns about how Jane's pain may be perceived and addressed differently as a young person of color and worries that her pain may not be taken seriously. The family also shared tensions in their larger family system as Jane's grandparents have been encouraging family to pursue other interventions (eg, religious prayer) to improve Jane's pain; family reported that they wanted to continue with medical treatment and described hesitation about the role of psychology in pain and if seeing psychology implied that Jane was "making up" her pain. As Jane's symptoms have worsened in recent months, her father reported that parents and grandmother ask Jane often about her pain and ask her to rate it on a 0 to 10 scale. Jane reported that she tried the medications that her doctors have given her, but reported that she does not think they really help and it is very hard for her to swallow pills; when asked to estimate how often she takes her daily medicine as prescribed, Jane reported she takes her medicine as prescribed 2 to 3 days per week.

Jane's father reported that Jane had first begun therapy for anxiety when she was 8 years old after the family had been in a car accident and Jane subsequently refused to get in cars. Her father reported that therapy was effective in helping Jane get into cars, and as therapy continued Jane began to share other worries, such as about school, getting along with her twin sister Julie, and worries that she would not make the soccer team. Jane reported that she did not like her therapist and described feeling uncomfortable talking about her feelings with a stranger and felt different than the therapist, who was a middle-aged Caucasian woman. Jane also reported that the therapist once made a comment that the therapist was "color blind" in relation to race and Jane reported that this was frustrating for her and made her feel uncomfortable. Jane and her father reported that they discontinued therapy after 8 months when there were no noticeable changes with therapy and the initial care concern was resolved. The family did not report the type of therapy that Jane had done with her therapist, though reported that terms like "cognitive behavioral therapy" were not familiar and reported that Jane would see the therapist by herself without parents presence and her parents were not asked to implement any skills in the home settings. Jane reported not learning any skills or strategies during this time and reported that terms like "diaphragmatic breathing" were not familiar. The family reported some variability in Jane's mood and continued to report no safety or suicidal ideation (SI) concerns. Her father reported noticing that Jane is more likely to seem sad or irritable when she is more tired and days when she is in more pain, which Jane agreed with.

When the clinician asked the family about their understanding of the IBS diagnosis, the family reported knowing that this has been the diagnostic label though reported without understanding what this is and could not explain it. The family also reported that Jane's GI and pain doctor had strongly recommended GI psychology, though described uncertainty about why a psychologist is important for ongoing GI symptoms and pain. The family shared overall goals for Jane's care, including reducing pain and GI symptoms and helping Jane get to school every day. Jane reported wanting to not experience pain every day and not feel different than her sister and friends. The family reported that Jane has to wake up early on school days (6 am) and will often sleep until 11 am on weekends if she does not have soccer practice or a game. Jane reported that pain impacts sleep onset and she is often lying in bed awake for 1h before she falls asleep by her report. She reported feeling fatigued in the mornings and sometimes having a hard time staying awake during class. Jane reported napping after school on the days she does not have practice. At present, Jane and her father reported that Jane misses approximately one day of school per week and this is often a Monday. Consistent with previous reporting to her pediatric pain physician, Jane reported that she still is late approximately 1 to 2 days per week. Her father also shared that school will send Jane home if she experiences high pain that day and this may happen two to four times per month.

The clinician and Jane also spent time alone during the visit, and Jane was receptive to a re-review of confidentiality when her father was out of the room. When asked about other things she would like to share privately, Jane reported some recent stress with her sister as they both have a crush on the same person at school. Jane reported that sometimes she feels babied by her family when they ask about how she is feeling and described wanting to just be herself and go back to normal. Jane reported noticing at times that when she is really stressed or excited, like before an important soccer game or an examination, that her nausea and GI symptoms feel intense. Jane described some hopelessness about her pain and reported worries that she would not be able to continue playing soccer though wants to play soccer in college. Jane reported that she generally does not like to take medicine and thinks she should be able to handle it on her own and described feeling frustrated when the medicine did not work like she had wanted and reported not wanting to keep taking it.

The clinician invited Jane's father back into the room and thanked her family for their willingness to share Jane's story. The clinician proceeded to provide appropriate psychoeducation to Jane and her father about IBS and pain, including discussion of the autonomic and enteric nervous systems and the pathophysiology of pain. The family was receptive to use of metaphors about how stress and mood can be volume dials to turn up or down the pain experience. The clinician also provided psychoeducation on GI and pain psychology and how these interventions can reduce the pain experience and improve functioning through evidence-based care and consistent implementation of skills. The family seemed receptive to use of metaphorical language in discussing pain and GI psychology interventions, such as how distractions are like a creaky house (pain) and can make the creaky house (pain) feel quieter when there is a distraction and the difference between hurt and harm.[2] The family reported that although they had heard the same diagnosis and general information from Jane's doctors, they reported feeling like they understood Jane's IBS more after the explanation. The clinician provided psychoeducation on relaxation skills like diaphragmatic breathing, progressive muscle relaxation, and guided imagery, and discussed how these skills activate the parasympathetic autonomic nervous system (ANS) and work to reduce the pain experience. The psychologist and Jane practiced the skills together in the visit with some coaching to reduce thoracic breathing and promote diaphragmatic breathing. The family was receptive to discussion about how these skills, like soccer, take ongoing practice and consistent implementation to work. The clinician discussed how these skills are metaphorically like sunscreen at the beach in that they work effectively when used before or as soon as pain occurs (putting on sunscreen before or when you get to the beach) versus when pain is at its peak (putting on sunscreen when you are leaving the beach). The clinician also spent time discussing CBT and acceptance and commitment therapy (ACT) approaches to pain and GI symptoms, and how cognitions can negatively impact feelings about pain and pain behaviors, and shared hypothetical examples to illustrate this connection. The clinician shared the goal of CBT and ACT in Jane's care, such as how cognitive restructuring (eg, from "This pain will never end" to "I am working on my pain getting quieter") can support adaptive, flexible, and realistic thoughts about pain that can reduce the pain experience.

The family and clinician also spent time discussing the role of sleep in modulating the pain experience and how this is an important target in psychological care; family agreed to spend more time at the next visit discussing this. Jane's father was receptive to psychoeducation and recommendations related to how parents and family members can support reducing the pain experience, including not asking about pain and directing Jane to a skill if she reports being in pain. The family agreed to sign a release of information for psychologist to talk with the school to provide psychoeducation and encourage Jane to remain at school on days when she has pain with any acute medical symptoms (eg, high fever), and also to explore a 504 plan put in place to support Jane getting to and staying at school with her pain.

Lastly, the family was receptive to normalization and validation with reflective listening and empathetic statements as relevant throughout the visit. The psychologist and family also began to discuss the intersection of race and gender with health and pain and Jane seemed excited to be able to bring this part of her life experiences into GI psychology in supporting her pain experiences. Family reported feeling more positive about psychology at the end of the visit and expressed their understanding on why GI psychology is important to Jane's care. The family agreed to schedule biweekly psychology visits with the expectation of having home tasks after sessions to implement skills in her daily life.

DISCUSSION

The prevalence of IBS has raised over the past 20 years, with notable impacts on the physical, academic, and psychosocial functioning of pediatric patients, impact on the family system, and a burden on the health care system caring for these patients.[3] As a functional GI disorder, pediatric patients with IBS are thought to benefit from a multidisciplinary approach to target the biopsychosocial factors of this condition and support pediatric patients doing what they want to and have to in life (eg, school, sports).

The criteria for chronic abdominal pain consist of three or more episodes of pain occurring over three consecutive months.[4] Chronic abdominal pain is estimated to affect close to 12% of children and approximately 20% of teenagers.[5,6] Most of chronic abdominal pain is noted to be functional in nature.

Up to 50% of referrals to a gastroenterologist are due to IBS, a potentially debilitating GI condition that accounts for a 1.35 billion dollar loss in annual productivity in the United States alone.[7]

The Rome IV diagnostic criteria are used to assist in the diagnosis of IBS (**Box 1**). There are three subtypes of IBS that include constipation predominant (IBS-C), diarrhea predominant (IBS-D), and a mixed or alternating stool pattern (IBS-M).

Discussing the physiology of IBS can be challenging to patients unfamiliar with this condition. The terminology visceral hypersensitivity and brain–gut axis can be helpful visual. Patients with IBS have thought to have a low pain threshold due to increased sensitivity of pain receptors involving the digestive tract. These receptors detect distention from gas and/or stool along with chemoreceptors responsible for detecting pressure and pH change.[8,9]

Studies have shown that there is likely a strong genetic inheritance of IBS within a family.[10] In addition, anxiety and mood disorders are common comorbid conditions. Environmental stressors can play a strong role in exacerbating symptoms. Inquiring

---

Box 1
Rome IV diagnostic criteria for irritable bowel syndrome[6]

Must include all of the following:
1. Abdominal pain at least 4 days per month associated with one or more of the following:
   a. Related to defecation
   b. A change in frequency of stool
   c. A change in form (appearance) of stool
2. In children with constipation, the pain does not resolve with resolution of the constipation (children in whom the pain resolves have functional constipation, not irritable bowel syndrome)
3. After appropriate evaluation, the symptoms cannot be fully explained by another medical condition.

Criteria fulfilled for at least 2 month before diagnosis.

about stressors at home and/or school is an important part of the clinical history. Patients and their family should be encouraged to enroll is mental health counseling, especially if a strong psychosocial stressor is identified.[11]

Patients with IBS-C may benefit from anorectal manometry (ARM) with biofeedback. The concept of ARM involves the use of a specialized catheter that senses pressure change. This catheter is gently inserted into the rectum where a small balloon attached to the catheter is inflated. The catheter is connected to a computer where the patient can observe muscle contractions involving the anal sphincter muscle and rectum. Anorectal dyssynergia is a condition, commonly found in the patients who are unable to generate Valsalva pressure along with a paradoxic increase in anal sphincter pressure when asked to bear down. This condition can lead to a functional outlet obstruction and subsequent incomplete evacuation of stool. In addition, rectal sensory threshold is determined using balloon inflation within the rectum. Patients with IBS generally have a low sensory threshold and the quality of the sensation is generally described as pain rather than fecal urgency.[12] Also heart rate variability biofeedback has been identified as a promising intervention for pediatric patients with IBS and functional abdominal pain.[13] Heart rate variability biofeedback teaches autogenic relaxation to activate the parasympathetic ANS and reduce the pain experience.

Treatment of IBS-C should be focused on management of their underlying constipation in addition to their pain. Stool softeners should be prescribed and stimulant laxatives should be used cautiously as this may exacerbate their pain.

Lubiprostone is an approved medication for IBS-C and exerts its effect on the chloride channels of the intestinal epithelial cells. Lubiprostone acts by promoting fluid secretion into the lumen of the intestinal tract that leads to increased stool frequency and improvement of tenesmus.[14] Pediatric studies regarding the use of lubiprostone in this age group have not always yielded positive results.[15] The safety profile; however, has been equal to that of adults.

IBS-D can be equally as challenging to treat as IBS-C. Intestinal dysbiosis has been implicated as a cause of IBS-D and a probiotic therapy has been shown to be helpful.[16] In addition, antimicrobial therapy with rifaximin has been promising in the treatment of IBS-D with most of the patients reporting an extended duration of symptom relief after completing their therapeutic course.[17] As needed antispasmodic treatment (dicyclomine, hyoscyamine) are also effective in treating IBS. These medications have a relaxing effect on the smooth muscle lining of the digestive tract.[18]

In patients with refractory IBS, tricyclic antidepressants, and selective serotonin reuptake inhibitors may be beneficial in managing their symptoms.[19] These medications alter the visceral afferent nervous system that promotes an analgesic effect.

It has been increasingly acknowledged within the health care system that opioids prescribed for chronic pain should be used with caution given the substantial negative impact it can have on our patients, including the high risk of addiction. Narcotic bowel syndrome has been described in patients with IBS who are prescribed opioids to manage their longstanding abdominal pain. This condition leads to worsening of their abdominal pain along with higher likelihood of developing opioid addiction. Once a chronic pain syndrome has been diagnosed, patients will require a combination of treatment from a psychotherapist along with a pain management specialist to optimize a biopsychosocial approach to IBS and chronic pain.[20]

SUMMARY

This hypothetical case presentation seeks to demonstrate the unique and intersecting roles of multidisciplinary providers in treating IBS and chronic pain in pediatric patients, including medical evaluation, discussion of pathophysiology of pain, and critical roles of functioning and psychosocial care. The authors also hope that this hypothetical case presentation displays common clinical considerations in this population to support and optimize care, such as patient and family understanding and buy-in, assessing and supporting pill swallowing and adherence as needed, and interventions with parents/families to reduce attention and discussion on pain. The authors also hope that this work may serve as a resource to providers to provide insights into how multidisciplinary care can be delivered and to strengthen the validity and importance of the role other specialties (eg, pain/GI psychology) in the management of IBS and chronic pain.

CLINICS CARE POINTS

- Extensive laboratory testing for abdominal pain may include a complete blood count, comprehensive metabolic panel, erythrocyte sedimentation rate, C-reactive protein, amylase, lipase, celiac disease serology, fecal calprotectin, hemoccult, and *H pylori* stool antigen test.
- Addressing functional abdominal pain, identifying triggers, and teaching coping mechanisms are an important part of treatment.
- It is imperative to approach functional abdominal pain in a comprehensive manner with pharmacologic treatment, physical, and psychotherapy.
- Psychosocial stressors as well as underlying mental health issues are common influencing factors in functional abdominal pain and should be addressed as part of an overall treatment strategy.
- Understanding and addressing family system components (eg, dysfunction, family communication style) is a necessary approach for treating patients with functional abdominal pain.

DISCLOSURE

The authors have no financial or commercial conflicts of interest to disclose.

REFERENCES

1. Chao G-q, Zhang S. A meta-analysis of the therapeutic effects of amitriptyline for treating irritable bowel syndrome. Intern Med 2013;52(4):419–24.
2. Coakley R, Schechter N. Chronic pain is like... The clinical use of analogy and metaphor in the treatment of chronic pain in children. Pediatr Pain Lett 2013; 15(1):1–8.
3. Devanarayana NM, Rajindrajith S. Irritable bowel syndrome in children: current knowledge, challenges and opportunities. World J Gastroenterol 2018;24(21): 2211.
4. Apley J. The child with recurrent abdominal pain. Pediatr Clin North Am 1967; 14(1):63–72.
5. Ramchandani PG, et al. The epidemiology of recurrent abdominal pain from 2 to 6 years of age: results of a large, population-based study. Pediatrics 2005;116(1): 46–50.
6. Hyams JS, et al. Abdominal pain and irritable bowel syndrome in adolescents: a community-based study. J Pediatr 1996;129(2):220–6.

7. Saito YA, Schoenfeld P, Locke GR III. The epidemiology of irritable bowel syndrome in North America: a systematic review. Am J Gastroenterol 2002;97(8): 1910–5.
8. Kanazawa M, Hongo M, Fukudo S. Visceral hypersensitivity in irritable bowel syndrome. J Gastroenterol Hepatol 2011;26:119–21.
9. Saha L. Irritable bowel syndrome: pathogenesis, diagnosis, treatment, and evidence-based medicine. World J Gastroenterol 2014;20(22):6759.
10. Saito Y, et al. Irritable bowel syndrome aggregates strongly in families: a family-based case-control study. Neurogastroenterol Motil 2008;20(7):790–7.
11. Fadgyas-Stanculete M, et al. The relationship between irritable bowel syndrome and psychiatric disorders: from molecular changes to clinical manifestations. J Mol Psychiatry 2014;2(1):1–7.
12. Prior A, Maxton D, Whorwell P. Anorectal manometry in irritable bowel syndrome: differences between diarrhoea and constipation predominant subjects. Gut 1990; 31(4):458–62.
13. Stern MJ, Guiles RA, Gevirtz R. HRV biofeedback for pediatric irritable bowel syndrome and functional abdominal pain: a clinical replication series. Appl Psychophysiology Biofeedback 2014;39(3):287–91.
14. Lacy BE, Chey WD. Lubiprostone: chronic constipation and irritable bowel syndrome with constipation. Expert Opin Pharmacother 2009;10(1):143–52.
15. Benninga MA, et al. Lubiprostone for pediatric functional constipation: randomized, controlled, double-blind study with long-term extension. Clin Gastroenterol Hepatol 2021;20(3):602–10.e5.
16. Didari T, et al. Effectiveness of probiotics in irritable bowel syndrome: Updated systematic review with meta-analysis. World J Gastroenterol WJG 2015;21(10): 3072.
17. Pimentel M, et al. Rifaximin therapy for patients with irritable bowel syndrome without constipation. N Engl J Med 2011;364(1):22–32.
18. Annaházi A, et al. Role of antispasmodics in the treatment of irritable bowel syndrome. World J Gastroenterol WJG 2014;20(20):6031.
19. Tack J, et al. A controlled crossover study of the selective serotonin reuptake inhibitor citalopram in irritable bowel syndrome. Gut 2006;55(8):1095–103.
20. Grunkemeier DM, et al. The narcotic bowel syndrome: clinical features, pathophysiology, and management. Clin Gastroenterol Hepatol 2007;5(10):1126–39.
21. Lewis SJ, Heaton KW. Stool form scale as a useful guide to intestinal transit time. Scand J Gastroenterol 1997;32(9):920–4.

The Role of Psychologists in Pediatric Hospital Medicine

Brittany N. Barber Garcia, PhD[a,b,*], Amy Pugh, PsyD[a,b], Christina Limke, PsyD[a,b], Nicholas Beam, MD[b,c]

KEYWORDS

- Pediatric psychology • Consultation-liaison • Hospital medicine • CL psychology

KEY POINTS

- Psychologists who function in children's hospital medical settings, referred to as pediatric consultation-liaison (CL) psychologists, perform numerous roles including consulting to patients, caregivers, and medical staff, and supporting system-wide and community-wide initiatives to promote the mental and behavioral health of youth.
- Pediatric CL psychologists commonly evaluate and treat patients who are hospitalized with somatic/functional symptoms, trauma, eating disorder, acute/chronic pain, and difficulty adjusting to new diagnosis with a variety of evidence-based assessment and intervention strategies.
- Physicians should request pediatric CL psychology involvement with patients in the hospital early in the admission to ease patient and family acceptance of the services and to facilitate addressing behavioral health challenges that can impact medical care.

ROLE OF PSYCHOLOGISTS IN PEDIATRIC HOSPITAL MEDICINE

Psychologists working in pediatric hospital medicine settings are commonly referred to as pediatric consultation-liaison (CL) psychologists. This article describes the development of CL psychology, current models of practice, how CL psychologists serve as consultants to children and caregivers (including evaluation and management of pediatric inpatients), how CL psychologists engage with physician colleagues, and ways in which CL psychologists offer advocacy and prevention strategies to hospital systems and the communities they serve. This article concludes with clinical pearls for the pediatric physician regarding how to engage pediatric CL psychologists for their patients.

[a] Spectrum Health Helen DeVos Children's Hospital, Pediatric Behavioral Medicine, 35 Michigan Street Northeast Suite 5301 MC 261, Grand Rapids, MI 49503, USA; [b] College of Human Medicine, Michigan State University, 15 Michigan Street Northeast, Grand Rapids, MI 49503, USA; [c] Spectrum Health, Office of Graduate Medical Education, 100 Michigan Street Northeast, Grand Rapids, MI 49503, USA
* Corresponding author. Spectrum Health Helen DeVos Children's Hospital, Pediatric Behavioral Medicine, 35 Michigan Street Northeast Suite 5301 MC 261, Grand Rapids, MI 49503.
E-mail address: brittany.barbergarcia@helendevoschildrens.org
Twitter: @drbbarbergarcia (B.N.B.G.)

Pediatr Clin N Am 69 (2022) 929–940
https://doi.org/10.1016/j.pcl.2022.05.006
0031-3955/22/© 2022 Elsevier Inc. All rights reserved.

pediatric.theclinics.com

Introduction: What Is a Consultation-Liaison Psychologist

History of consultation-liaison psychology

When pediatric psychology was first established in the 1960s, pediatric psychologists were described by Wright as "... any psychologist who finds himself dealing primarily with children in a medical setting which is nonpsychiatric in nature."[1] By the mid-1970s, psychologists working in pediatric hospital settings began testing strategies for hospitalized children[2] and used clinical and scientific expertise to translate developmental research into individualized clinical interventions that benefited pediatric hospitalized patients.[3]

Pediatric CL psychologists have a long-established history of evaluating the needs of medically hospitalized youth in their role as "consultants," including (1) evaluating behavioral health challenges associated with medical diseases and hospitalization, (2) providing psychoeducation to parents and medical colleagues, and (3) delivering brief, solution-focused treatments to youth. In addition to these primary assessment and intervention roles, pediatric CL psychology has evolved to include additional "liaison" duties, such as (4) liaising with hospital, school, and community partners to assist with transitions for hospitalized youth, (5) developing and implementing quality improvement programs in the hospital, and (6) providing advocacy to impact policy and practice relating to pediatric patients and their families.[4]

Current training for consultation-liaison psychologists

As the role of pediatric CL psychologists has evolved over the past 50 years, education and development of CL psychologists have become simultaneously broader and deeper in scope as well.[5] The first training recommendations for pediatric psychologists were developed in the 1980s[6] and identified that training should include broad coursework in developmental and clinical child psychology, specialized clinical experiences in pediatrics and health psychology and a postdoctoral experience specific to pediatric psychology. By 2014, the competencies for pediatric psychology practice were revised to include six competency clusters (i.e., science, professionalism, interpersonal skills, application, teaching and supervision, and systems functioning) and 10 cross-cutting knowledge competencies (e.g., clinical child and developmental psychology, child health and illness, understanding familial, cultural, and socioeconomic factors influence on health and health disparities, how systems and policies impact health outcomes, and so forth).[5,7–9] Pediatric psychology trainees are expected to develop competencies through didactic coursework, research, and clinical experiences in preparation for their doctoral degrees.[10] Further, a one or two-year postdoctoral fellowship is often necessary to develop independence in specific skills, systems functioning, and professional competencies.[5] On achieving licensure, some pediatric CL psychologists may go on to pursue board certification through the American Board of Clinical Child and Adolescent Psychology, of which pediatric psychologists make up approximately half of those certified.[5]

Studies indicate that CL psychologists may benefit from being trained in a practice elements approach to treatment for medically hospitalized youth.[11] In this approach, psychologists are trained in specific techniques that are shared among various evidence-based interventions instead of relying on one standardized protocol to treat one presenting disorder, which is often unlikely to be accomplished during a hospital admission given variability in patient length of stay, medical needs, and presence of co-occurring disorders. Using a practice elements approach allows CL psychologists to treat co-occurring psychiatric conditions (e.g., depression, adjustment to illness) simultaneously and tailor treatments to unique patient presentations.[11]

Models of consultation-liaison psychology practice

Theory-driven approaches to pediatric CL psychology have focused on identifying the systems in which children function and may require support, the level of support needed, and what question or problem needs to be addressed to help the child return to their usual level of functioning. As such, current pediatric CL practice rests on two foundational theories: the bioecological systems theory of Bronfenbrenner[12] and the pediatric psychosocial preventative health model of Kazak.[13] These two theories help explain that CL psychologists provide services across various systems in which children function, which include the individual (child), microsystem (family, school), mesosytem (level of interaction within microsystem), exosystem (neighbors, social services, legal system), macrosystem (cultural/societal attitudes), and chronosystem (time). According to Kazak, intervention approaches then vary depending on the level of need. The universal need level is when the family is adapting adequately and needs more general support, such as psychoeducation. The targeted level involves preventative measures for at-risk families with the larger system which the child is involved (e.g., school). The clinical/treatment level is needed when symptoms are causing a greater level of interference with functioning and require direct intervention.

Carter and colleagues[4,14] have developed and refined over time a model of CL psychology that depends on the Bronfenbrenner and Kazak theories and is commonly referred to as the "Six Cs of CL."[4] The six Cs are derived from the six areas/roles in which CL psychologists typically function: crisis, coping, compliance/adherence, communication, collaboration, and changing systems. Each of the "Cs" coincides with a unique level of intervention. The communication, collaboration, and changing systems functions relate to CL psychologists intervening on universal themes of distress and resiliency. The coping and compliance functions are generally the focus of more targeted consultation questions related to acute distress or risk factors. Finally, the crisis-oriented referral questions involve direct psychological intervention to address persistent or escalating symptoms and stabilize the patient so that medical care can proceed. Therefore, the role of the pediatric CL psychologist can vary depending on a child or family's current level of symptomatology and distress, existing support, goals, and the system in which the child is functioning.

Discussion: The Multiple Roles of the Pediatric Consultation-Liaison Psychologist

The consultation-liaison psychologist as a clinical consultant: providing evaluation, treatment, and more

Involving a CL psychologist in the care of a hospitalized child adds significant value in their care.[15] Psychological consultation may provide diagnostic insight, aid in pain and anxiety management, improve compliance with care, minimize caregiver stress, and guide treatment. Some hospitals are including a psychologist in the multidisciplinary team introduced to patients on admission. Including or consulting a psychologist early in a patient's care can help minimize stigma and resistance. Each hospital has a different process on *how* to consult a CL psychologist; however, all hospitalist teams are encouraged to clearly state the question they need answered by the consulting CL psychologist and any relevant background. The American Psychological Association specifically highlights the importance of effective and timely communication between health care providers and the CL psychologist, as communication is one of the most important variables in successful collaboration.[16]

Once consulted, the CL psychologist will interview the patient and caregivers. This interview includes time to build rapport, explain the psychologist's role, and normalize the child's experience all while considering a patient's chronological age and developmental level. The CL psychologist will review medical records, develop behavioral observations, and confer with ancillary personnel as needed (e.g., outpatient therapist, school counselor). Once the initial assessment is complete, the CL psychologist will discuss findings and recommendations with the family and the referring team and document the assessment in the patient's medical record. CL psychologists provide brief, tailored, solution-focused interventions for multiple different presenting concerns at bedside, determine appropriate care needed after discharge, and identify any additional services in and out of the hospital that may be helpful in managing symptoms.

Somatic/functional disorders. Somatic symptoms and related disorders (SSRDs) are one of the most common consultation targets for pediatric CL psychologists. In general, SSRDs are physical symptoms in the absence of a medical cause or identifiable disease, or when an organic cause for the physical symptoms is present, somatic symptoms are more frequent, severe, or chronic than what would be expected for the diagnosis.[17] Patients have related distress and functional impairment because of their symptoms. Children with SSRDs present with both physical and psychological symptoms and most often seek care in a medical facility. Somatic symptoms include a variety of complaints from gastrointestinal issues such as abdominal pain and neurologic changes such as weakness and gait abnormalities to cardiac difficulties such as syncope. The field has moved to use the term "Functional Disorder" to discuss somatic complains that result from body system dysfunction rather than organic disease, as this term is more palatable to patients and families and easier to understand.[18,19]

The role of the psychologist with these patients is to first identify possible psychological factors contributing to physical symptoms. Studies have shown that youth with SSRD exhibit elevated emotional responses to stress and implement fewer adaptive coping strategies compared to healthy peers.[20] Patient and families must be educated on the nature of the symptoms as functional. To do so appropriately, the medical team must answer the family's medical questions and provide reassurance that the presenting concerns are real, but not a medical emergency.[18] The medical team and the psychologist must work together to present a united message about the diagnosis to help improve acceptance and adherence to treatment plan. Some recommendations about this messaging include the following: clearly state there is no organic disease, empathize with patient's symptoms and distress,[21] provide a positive diagnosis (e.g., functional disorder), support the mind–body connection,[22] normalize functional symptoms, and talk about treatments that work including cognitive behavioral therapy, physical therapy, and medication options.[18]

Eating and feeding disorders. Another patient population commonly assessed by CL psychologists are those with eating and feeding concerns. Patients may present with typical anorexia nervosa and/or bulimia nervosa symptoms; however, some may present with restrictive eating related to food and sensory sensitivities or food aversion (and may meet criteria for a newer eating disorder classification, avoidant/restrictive food intake disorder). When a patient with eating and feeding concerns is admitted into the hospital, there is often severe nutritional deficiency, significant weight loss, and concern for refeeding syndrome.

The medical team and the psychologist must work closely together to manage patients with disordered eating and/or feeding habits. A patient must be assessed medically for possible diagnoses that can drive weight loss such as cancer malignancies and gastrointestinal disease[23] and monitored for refeeding syndrome. A dietician is also part of the team to guide meal planning and nutrition. The CL psychologist assesses for psychiatric issues and behavioral concerns that may contribute to a patient's poor nutritional intake.[24] These may include learned feeding avoidance due to aversive conditioning (e.g., choking event, vomiting episodes following eating, abdominal pain), inappropriate mealtime interactions, maladaptive environmental contingencies on behavioral refusals, and familial and cultural expectations for feeding.[25]

Another role of the psychologist is evaluating patient and family insight and understanding of the disorder as this can influence readiness for and adherence to treatment.[26] Often families are unaware of the pervasiveness of the patient's eating and feeding difficulties and may be naïve to the appropriate level of treatment needed for healthy and long-lasting recovery. The CL psychologist provides psychoeducation on eating/feeding disorder severity, prognosis, and realistic expectations of empirically supported treatment. Within a medical hospital, the goal of initial care is to get the patient medically stable until they can be transferred to the appropriate level of care (e.g., residential, inpatient, partial hospitalization, or intensive outpatient). Educating the family on this process is a necessity. There are often high levels of caregiver and patient distress when first treating eating and feeding concerns, thus the CL psychologist must respond to, and help the medical team navigate, these affective changes and effectively enlist the patient and family's agreement with the treatment model.[23]

Pain. In the hospital, pediatric patients may present with procedural, acute, or chronic pain. Psychologists are often asked to consult on patients who are in pain, especially when pain is not congruent with a recognized disease process. Assessment of the biopsychosocial factors influencing the child's pain experience is critical to developing an appropriate treatment plan.[27] A child's history with pain including their pain tolerance, prior acute and chronic pain episodes, and previously helpful pain mitigation strategies is important variables in the CL psychologist's assessment of the present pain experience. Preexisting psychiatric conditions, especially anxiety or trauma, may have significant influence in a patient's current perception of pain. Assessment of pain also should include frequent child self-report whenever possible[28] or standardized behavioral observations.[27] Special consideration needs to be taken for young children and children with developmental or intellectual disabilities, as they are at a greater risk of experiencing pain due to communication challenges.[29] A number of tools (e.g., behavioral observation, caregiver report, proxy measures) and assistive technologies have been studied to help ensure all youth receive appropriate pain assessment and management.[30]

When helping a child cope with acute pain, or pain related to a procedure in the hospital, several intervention strategies are commonly used by the CL psychologist. Exposure-based therapy is recommended for children with needle phobia, which ideally should be done before any scheduled procedures.[31] The CL psychologist also helps manage environmental factors such as determining which caregivers are present, the number of people in the room, including engaging a Certified Child Life Specialist who can provide training for the procedure, which has been shown to help reduce distress and pain[32] and offering distraction options and activities. CL psychologists also provide psychoeducation to coach caregivers in working with their child to help manage acute pain (e.g., encouraging positive statements about patient's coping vs. problem-focused statements).[27]

Children can also be admitted to the hospital for acute exacerbations of chronic pain experiences. A patient's psychological functioning and coping style can impact the chronic pain experience. In addition, greater functional impairment due to pain has been associated with pain-related anxiety and pain catastrophizing (e.g., believing the worst about the pain, feeling unable to cope with pain).[33,34] Further, there is a bidirectional relationship between parent/family functioning and child adjustment to chronic pain[35] such that higher levels of parent distress and family dysfunction are related to more pain-related disability in children.[36] Therefore, the CL psychologist must help to identify and manage these psychological factors to reduce distress and promote coping. Common strategies used include bedside teaching of relaxation skills, promotion of daily functioning using behavioral reinforcement schedules, and teaching basic cognitive coping skills.[37] Hospitalized patients with chronic pain may also benefit from a multidisciplinary team approach with nurses, physicians, psychologists, psychiatrists, and physical/occupational therapists.

Traumatic stress. Acute trauma within the hospital is another common concern that leads to a psychology consultation motor vehicle accident, burn injury, or other traumatic injury, and CL psychologists are often called to help with these patients. In addition to children who are admitted for reasons of traumatic injury, children who spend time in the pediatric intensive care unit are at risk for developing medical trauma as the result of their complex care including new diagnoses, exacerbations of existing medical conditions, high-risk treatments, extended isolation, exposure to multiple and ever-changing providers and specialists, and removal from typical coping environments (e.g., home, school, friends).[38] Initial psychological experience after a trauma can include exhaustion, confusion, sadness, anxiety, agitation, numbness, dissociation, confusion, physical arousal, and blunted affect; however, there is significant variability in children's and parent's responses to pediatric illness and injury.[39]

In the case of a child who has recently experienced a trauma or has undergone a traumatic hospitalization, it is helpful for a trusted and familiar medical provider to introduce the psychologist and their role on the team.[38] Because patients experience different reactions to trauma, "early and ongoing screening for pediatric medical traumatic stress are needed to determine the appropriate level of psychological support."[40] Adding other service lines including Child Life, School Liaisons, and Music Therapy may be helpful in supporting a child with difficult care in the moment (e.g., burn dressing changes)[41] as well as with their long-term care and return to functioning. Caregivers and loved ones may also experience traumatic stress because of the child's hospitalization, because caregiver mental health is closely related to pediatric patient recovery, it is an important role of the CL psychologist to address parental anxiety, depression, and acute stress.[42]

Complex neonatal course and caregiver mental health. Parental factors can also affect infant development, which is why increasingly pediatric CL psychologists are being consulted in hospital's neonatal intensive care units (NICUs). NICU parents exhibit elevated rates of emotional distress and are at greater risk for developing a diagnosable mental disorder during the first year postpartum as compared with parents of newborns who do not need NICU treatment.[43] NICU consultation, different from other hospital-based care, focuses on the parent or caregiver rather than the child, and the goal is to identify maladaptive coping or "elevated clinical presentations that may require more targeted intervention."[44] Involving a CL psychologist as a part of the multidisciplinary team is recommended when there is concern about a caregiver's mental health, coping challenges impacting parental bonding with infant, or extensive or complex parental mental health history. The CL psychologist can address parental mental health, promote adjustment, and improve interactions between parents and staff.

Coping with new chronic illness diagnosis. Another common reason for referral in pediatric CL psychology is to assist with adjustment to a new medical diagnosis or assist with coping with a complicated chronic medical condition (e.g., cancer, diabetes mellitus).[45] Physicians request this type of consultation when they have impression that the child and/or family are having difficulty processing the implications of a serious illness and would benefit from assistance learning specific coping skills for the psychological impact of the diagnosis. The role of the CL psychologist is to assist with adaptive adjustment by helping the family identify and express feelings about the diagnosis, normalize the adjustment experience, and provide psychoeducation about coping skills to help the child and family handle their "new normal." The CL psychologist also communicates to the medical team how they can mitigate furthering the child's psychological distress in the face of an already traumatic situation. Finally, the CL psychologist offers recommendations as to how to foster adaptive functioning after discharge (e.g., outpatient psychotherapy, school accommodations).

Adherence. Finally, a pediatric CL psychologist can be particularly helpful when a child and family are struggling to implement their medical regimen. This includes situations where a lack of adherence caused the current hospitalization (e.g., Diabetic ketoacidosis (DKA) for a child with diabetes) and where poor adherence prevents the child from reaching medical milestones necessary for discharge (e.g., not limiting fluid intake so diagnostic tests can be performed).

In these instances, the role of the psychologist is primarily focused on three main objectives: (1) assess psychological barriers to adherence; (2) problem-solve these barriers with the patient to improve adherence; and (3) communicate the adherence plan to the medical team to implement changes. The areas of focus for barriers to adherence typically include individual factors (e.g., motivation), family factors (e.g., parental management), community factors (e.g., peer support), and disease and regimen factors (e.g., complexity of treatment).[46,47] Once the CL psychologist identifies the specific barriers, they work with the child and family to create solutions that can be realistically implemented. Finally, the CL psychologist communicates the solutions generated to the medical team, so they can follow-up on these strategies as they continue to manage the medical condition. Further, if the psychologist makes the diagnosis of a comorbid psychological disorder, they provide recommendations for treatment to reduce symptomology both while the patient is admitted and after discharge.

The consultation-liaison psychologist as consultant: engaging with physicians and other medical staff

One of the keys to successful engagement of pediatric CL psychology is integration into the multidisciplinary medical team. This approach recommended for any environment in which psychologists are a part of health care delivery.[16] In any multidisciplinary team, establishing joint goals is a key to ensuring successful intervention. For medical providers, clearly establishing these goals with the CL psychologist and ensuring communication is critically important to the most effective management of patients. As is discussed above, the collaboration process ideally begins when a patient is admitted, but if not, it begins with the initial consultation request to the psychologist. Involving CL psychologists early in the diagnostic process can lead to improved patient acceptance of the involvement of the psychologists. This bidirectional communication should occur throughout the inpatient stay, allowing the CL psychologist to weigh in and contribute to decision for further evaluation and management as it serves the needs of the patient and their management. This would ideally through frequent, in-the-moment verbal communication, written treatment plans, and family-centered rounds.

The consultation-liaison psychologist as change agent: system and community advocacy

In addition to their roles as consultant and liaison within the evaluation and treatment of individual patients, the CL psychologist also engages on behalf of patients beyond the hospital and direct patient management.[16] Within the hospital, CL psychologists share their expertise by serving on hospital committees and contributing to the development of care pathways for diseases they frequently help manage. This involvement ensures that both the physical and psychological needs of patient are addressed in system-level planning.

Outside the hospital, CL psychologists can serve as a bridge between admitted patients and the school system. This is especially important as many of the disease processes that CL psychologists help manage frequently lead to many missed days of school. CL psychologists can offer suggestions for Individualized Education Plans and Section-504 Plans to help minimize the negative impact of hospitalization on attendance and academic performance. In addition, they can coordinate with school personnel to help students reintegrate into the school environment when the time comes. CL psychologists also can help inform public policy regarding integrating mental and behavioral health into medical health care models and advocate for the public mental health needs.[16]

SUMMARY

Pediatric CL psychologists offer unique support as consultants to child patients, their caregivers, and medical providers by providing efficient, specific, and tailored psychological evaluation and intervention to hospitalized patients for a variety of presenting concerns. They help connect patients to services outside the hospital and promote return to usual functioning on discharge. In addition, they use research and clinical expertise to inform quality improvement initiatives within health care systems and provide advocacy for their child patients and the public health through community advocacy initiatives. Physicians are encouraged to request the involvement of pediatric CL psychologists whenever a patient is admitted to the hospital, as they can help promote healthy adjustment and psychological well-being and reduce distress. They support the medical team by offering insight into the motivation and behavior of patients with complex challenges and help the team operate effectively to best meet each patient's needs. Involving a pediatric CL psychologist in a patient's care early and often can help transform the experience of the care team and the patient.

CLINICS CARE POINTS

- Pediatric consultation-liaison (CL) psychologists are trained to offer brief and targeted psychological assessments and interventions to medically hospitalized children.
- Physicians are encouraged to request CL psychology involvement with their patients early, as this optimizes parent and child acceptance of the psychologist as a part of their care team and allows for early identification of psychological issues affecting admitting concerns.
- Assessment of a hospitalized child by a CL psychologist will typically include caregiver and child interviews focusing on psychological symptoms, current/past psychological/psychiatric interventions, biopsychosocial factors influencing medical condition, and behavioral observations.

- CL psychologists help manage a wide range of concerns including somatic/functional symptoms, acute/chronic pain, trauma, eating disorders, and adjustment to/coping with new medical diagnosis.
- Intervention provided by CL psychologists for hospitalized children often uses as practice elements approach and may include psychoeducation, biobehavioral (e.g., relaxation, biofeedback), cognitive behavioral therapy (e.g., exposure with response prevention, cognitive restructuring), and behavioral (e.g., schedule with reinforcers) strategies.

DISCLOSURE

The authors have nothing to disclose.

REFERENCES

1. Wright L. The pediatric psychologist: a role model. Am Psychol 1967;22(4):323–5.
2. Melamed BG, Meyer R, Gee C, et al. The influence of time and type of preparation on children's adjustement to hospitalization. J Pediatr Psychol 1976; 1(4):31–7.
3. Mesibov GB. Evolution of pediatric psychology: historical roots to future trends. J Pediatr Psychol 1984;9(1):3–11.
4. Carter BD, Kronenberger WG, Scott EL, et al. Inpatient pediatric consutation-liaison. In: Roberts MC, Steele RG, editors. Handbook of pediatric psychology. 5th edition. New York, NY: The Guilford Press; 2017. p. 105–18.
5. Palermo TM, Janicke DM, Beals-Erickson SE, et al. Training and competencies in pediatric psychology. In: Roberts MC, Steele RG, editors. Handbook of pediatric psychology. 5th edition. New York, NY: The Guilford Press; 2017. p. 56–66.
6. La Greca AM, Stone WL, Drotar D, et al. Training in pediatric psychology: survey results and recommendations. J Pediatr Psychol 1988;13(1):121–39.
7. Spirito A, Brown RT, D'Angelo E, et al. Society of pediatric psychology task force report: recommendations for the training of pediatric psychologists. J Pediatr Psychol 2003;28(2):85–98.
8. Palermo TM, Janicke DM, McQuaid EL, et al. Recommendations for training in pediatric psychology: defining core competencies across training levels. J Pediatr Psychol 2014;39(9):965–84.
9. Roberts MC, Carlson CI, Erickson MT, et al. A model for training psychologists to provide services for children and adolescents. Prof Psychol Res Pract 1998; 29(3):293–9.
10. Steele RG, Borner KB, Roberts MC. Commentary: finding the middle bowl: goldilocks' lessons on professional competencies in pediatric psychology. J Pediatr Psychol 2014;39(9):988–97.
11. Bowling AA, Bearman SK, Wang W, et al. Pediatric consultation-liaison: patient characteristics and considerations for training in evidence-based practices. J Clin Psychol Med Settings 2021;28(3):529–42.
12. Bronfenbrenner U. The ecology of human development: experiments by nature and design. Cambridge, MA: Harvard University Press; 1979.
13. Kazak A. Pediatric psychosocial preventative health model: research, practice, and collaboration in pediatric family systems medicine. Fam Syst Health 2006; 24:381–95.
14. Carter BD, von Weiss RT. Inpatient pediatric consultation-liaison: applied child health psychology. In: Steele RG, Roberts MC, editors. Handbook of mental

health services for children, adolescents, and families. Dordrecht, The Netherlands: Kluwer Academic/Plenum; 2005. p. 63–83.

15. Manguy A-M, Joubert L, Oakley E, et al. Psychosocial care models for families of critically Ill children in pediatric emergency department settings: a scoping review. J Pediatr Nurs 2018;38:46–52.

16. American Psychological Association. Guidelines for psychological practice in health care delivery systems. Am Psychol 2013;68(1):1–6.

17. Sharpe M, Carson A. "Unexplained" somatic symptoms, functional syndromes, and somatization: do we need a paradigm shift? Ann Intern Med 2001;134(9 Pt 2):926–30.

18. Williams SE, Zahka NE, Kullgren KA. Somatic Symptom and Related Disorders. In: Carter BD, Kullgren KA, editors. Clinical handbook of psychological consultation in pediatric medical settings. issues in clinical child psychology. Washington, DC: Springer International Publishing; 2020. p. 169–81.

19. Williams SE, Zahka NE. Treating somatic symptoms in children and adolescents. New York, NY: Guilford Press; 2017.

20. Walker LS, Garber J, Greene JW. Psychosocial correlates of recurrent childhood pain: a comparison of pediatric patients with recurrent abdominal pain, organic illness, and psychiatric disorders. J Abnorm Psychol 1993;102(2):248–58.

21. Ring A, Dowrick CF, Humphris GM, et al. The somatising effect of clinical consultation: what patients and doctors say and do not say when patients present medically unexplained physical symptoms. Soc Sci Med 2005;61(7):1505–15.

22. Salmon P, Peters S, Stanley I. Patients' perceptions of medical explanations for somatisation disorders: qualitative analysis. BMJ 1999;318(7180):372–6.

23. Tsang KK, Hayes LC, Bujoreanu S, et al. Characterization study of patients presenting to an acute care pediatric hospital identified with avoidant/restrictive food intake disorder. Hosp Pediatr 2020;10(7):600–7.

24. American Psychiatric Association. Diagnositic and statistical manual of mental disordrs. 5th Edition. Washington, DC: American Psychiatric Publishing; 2013. Available at: https://www.psychiatry.org/psychiatrists/practice/dsm. Accessed January 30, 2022.

25. Silverman AH. Behavioral management of feeding disorders of childhood. Ann Nutr Metab 2015;66(Suppl 5):33–42.

26. Tsang KK, Hayes LC, Cammarata C. Eating disorders and avoidant/restrictive food intake disorder. In: Carter BD, Kullgren KA, editors. Clinical handbook of psychological consultation in pediatric medical settings. issues in clinical child psychology. Cham, Switzerland: Springer International Publishing; 2020. p. 211–26.

27. MacKenzie NE, Tutelman PR, Chambers CT. The problem of pain: acute pain and procedures. In: Carter BD, Kullgren KA, editors. Clinical handbook of psychological consultation in pediatric medical settings. issues in clinical child psychology. Cham, Switzerland: Springer International Publishing; 2020. p. 139–53.

28. Birnie KA, Hundert AS, Lalloo C, et al. Recommendations for selection of self-report pain intensity measures in children and adolescents: a systematic review and quality assessment of measurement properties. Pain 2019;160(1):5–18.

29. Cascella M, Bimonte S, Saettini F, et al. The challenge of pain assessment in children with cognitive disabilities: Features and clinical applicability of different observational tools. J Paediatr Child Health 2019;55(2):129–35.

30. Breau LM, Finley GA, McGrath PJ, et al. Validation of the non-communicating children's pain checklist-postoperative version. Anesthesiology 2002;96(3):528–35.
31. McMurtry CM, Taddio A, Noel M, et al. Exposure-based Interventions for the management of individuals with high levels of needle fear across the lifespan: a clinical practice guideline and call for further research. Cogn Behav Ther 2016;45(3): 217–35.
32. Sanchez Cristal N, Staab J, Chatham R, et al. Child life reduces distress and pain and improves family satisfaction in the pediatric emergency department. Clin Pediatr (Phila) 2018;57(13):1567–75.
33. Caes L, Fisher E, Clinch J, et al. The role of pain-related anxiety in adolescents' disability and social impairment: ALSPAC data. Eur J Pain Lond Engl 2015;19(6): 842–51.
34. Simons LE, Kaczynski KJ. The Fear Avoidance model of chronic pain: examination for pediatric application. J Pain 2012;13(9):827–35.
35. Palermo TM, Chambers CT. Parent and family factors in pediatric chronic pain and disability: an integrative approach. Pain 2005;119(1–3):1–4.
36. Lewandowski AS, Palermo TM, Stinson J, et al. Systematic review of family functioning in families of children and adolescents with chronic pain. J Pain 2010; 11(11):1027–38.
37. Fisher E, Law E, Dudeney J, et al. Psychological therapies for the management of chronic and recurrent pain in children and adolescents. Cochrane Database Syst Rev 2018;9:CD003968.
38. Marsac ML, Meadows A, Kindler C, et al. Trauma and intensive care. In: Carter BD, Kullgren KA, editors. Clinical handbook of psychological consultation in pediatric medical settings. issues in clinical child psychology. Cham, Switzerland: Springer International Publishing; 2020. p. 239–50.
39. Treatment (US) C for SA. Understanding the impact of trauma. Washington, DC: Substance Abuse and Mental Health Services Administration (US); 2014. Available at: https://www.ncbi.nlm.nih.gov/books/NBK207191/. Accessed January 30, 2022.
40. Kazak A, Price J, Kassam-Adams N. Pediatric medical traumatic stress. In: Carter BD, Kullgren KA, editors. Clinical handbook of psychological consultation in pediatric medical settings. issues in clinical child psychology. Cham, Switzerland: Springer International Publishing; 2020. p. 179–90.
41. Whitehead-Pleaux AM, Zebrowski N, Baryza MJ, et al. Exploring the effects of music therapy on pediatric pain: phase 1. J Music Ther 2007;44(3): 217–41.
42. Landolt MA, Ystrom E, Sennhauser FH, et al. The mutual prospective influence of child and parental post-traumatic stress symptoms in pediatric patients. J Child Psychol Psychiatry 2012;53(7):767–74.
43. Roque ATF, Lasiuk GC, Radünz V, et al. Scoping review of the mental health of parents of infants in the NICU. J Obstet Gynecol Neonatal Nurs 2017;46(4): 576–87.
44. Hoffman C, Greene MM, Baughcum AE. Neonatal Intensive Care. In: Carter BD, Kullgren KA, editors. Clinical handbook of psychological consultation in pediatric medical settings. issues in clinical child psychology. Cham, Switzerland: Springer International Publishing; 2020. p. 277–94.
45. Smith LB, Liu X, Johnson SB, et al. Family adjustment to diabetes diagnosis in children: can participation in a study on type 1 diabetes genetic risk be helpful? Pediatr Diabetes 2018;19(5):1025–33.

46. Maddux M, Ricks S, Delurgio S, et al. A pilot study evaluating the impact of an adherence-promoting intervention among nonadherent youth with inflammatory bowel disease. J Pediatr Nurs 2017;35:72–7.

47. Hommel KA, Hente EA, Odell S, et al. Evaluation of a group-based behavioral intervention to promote adherence in adolescents with inflammatory bowel disease. Eur J Gastroenterol Hepatol 2012;24(1):64–9.

The Role of a Clinical Psychologist in Pediatric Nephrology

Vimal Master Sankar Raj, MD[a],*, Priyal Patel, BS[b]

KEYWORDS

- Chronic kidney disease (CKD) • End-stage renal disease (ESRD) • Dialysis
- Depression • Self-esteem

KEY POINTS

- Chronic kidney disease (CKD) is a progressive condition with decline in renal function.
- Assessment and management of the psychosocial and mental component of CKD.
- Family dynamics and parental stress in taking care of a child with CKD.
- Need for multidisciplinary approach and role of psychologist in maintaining the mental well-being in pediatric CKD.

INTRODUCTION

Chronic kidney disease (CKD) is a progressive and life-threatening condition with continuous loss of kidney function, manifesting with a myriad of symptoms including fluid retention, elevated blood pressures, anemia, electrolyte imbalances, and decreased ability to remove toxins from the body. CKD is classified into five stages based on the degree of glomerular filtration rate (GFR) with stage 5 (GFR $\leq$ 15 mL/min/1.73 m^2) labeled as an end-stage renal disease (ESRD), which is irreversible.[1] Dialysis or renal replacement therapy is required at the ESRD stage, as this is when about 85% to 90% of the kidney has lost its function and is close to failure. CKD is often diagnosed in both pediatric and adult patients, and it continues for many years. Many patients with CKD transit from pediatric to adult CKD care unit during their dialysis or treatment. This transition can often leave a lasting psychosocial impact on patients as few effective tools and programs have been developed for a smooth transition.[2] Usually, this transition involves a major change in the model of care provided to the patients by the health care professionals, which contains more self-directed management by the patients with chronic disease themselves.[3]

[a] Division of Pediatric Nephrology, University of Illinois College of Medicine, 420 Northeast Glen Oak Avenue, Suite 201, Peoria, IL 61603, USA; [b] Bradley University, Peoria, IL, USA
* Corresponding author.
E-mail address: vraj@uic.edu

Pediatr Clin N Am 69 (2022) 941–949
https://doi.org/10.1016/j.pcl.2022.05.007
0031-3955/22/© 2022 Elsevier Inc. All rights reserved.

ESRD is more commonly found in adult patients than pediatric patients, yet its symptoms, causes, and treatment options may vary among both groups of the population. Pediatric ESRD accounts for a tiny proportion of the total number of patients with ESRD in the United States.[4] In pediatric patients with CKD, factors such as "growth and development, nutrition, school attendance and performance, family dynamics, and psychosocial well-being of the child and family" play an important role in the modality and effectiveness of a specific treatment.[2] Etiology of pediatric ESRD is vastly different from that of adult ESRD with primary congenital nephrological conditions such as vesicoureteral reflux and renal dysplasia contributing to the majority of cases. For the better care and understanding of pediatric patients with other underlying primary illnesses, pediatric nephrologists often operate in multidisciplinary teams. These teams include, but are not limited to, "pediatric urologists, pediatric surgeons, renal dieticians, skilled pediatric nurses, social workers, child life specialists, and transplant coordinators."[2]

The treatment, but not the cure, of pediatric patients with CKD varies majorly depending on the age of the child. Components such as immigration status, race, and poverty also play an influential role in the decision about the choice of therapy in both pediatric and adult patients.[5] In pediatric patients with ESRD, a kidney transplant is generally the preferred modality of renal replacement therapy and has been shown to have a better survival rate and quality of life when compared with procedures such as dialysis.[4] Even though renal replacement therapy has a higher survival rate, it still remains about 30 times lower when compared with treatments of other pediatric diseases.[6] Though a preemptive transplant or a transplant performed before starting dialysis is a preferred therapy for pediatric patients with ESRD, unfortunately, this is not possible for every patient with ESRD. Factors such as availability of suitably matched transplant graft, age, the weight of the child, and other coexisting comorbidities could delay the transplant process needing the patients to be maintained on dialysis for a period of time. There are two modalities of dialysis used in patients with ESRD namely peritoneal and hemodialysis. Peritoneal dialysis is preferred in the pediatric population because of the difficulty with obtaining and maintaining vascular access in small children. Parents or caregivers are trained in peritoneal dialysis techniques, which allows them to perform dialysis at home daily and monitored monthly in dialysis clinic visits. According to data[4] from the North American Pediatric Renal Transplant Cooperative Study, more pediatric patients were maintained on peritoneal dialysis than being treated with hemodialysis. There have been studies utilizing different treatment options on adults, but when it comes to pediatric patients, not enough research has been conducted to evaluate the appropriate quality outcomes of other treatments. It has further been hard to take quality measures in adolescents because they are the least cooperative group of patients.[2]

Treatment of pediatric kidney disease is complicated and requires a multidisciplinary approach. However, the limitation of resources including the limited number of clinical pediatric nephrologists, dialysis facilities, pediatric trained dialysis nurses, social workers, and psychologists makes it a challenging proposition even in bigger academic centers.[2] A majority of pediatric nephrologists also work full-time as faculty members or hold other affiliations in various academic medical centers, which could limit them from devoting their time to clinical activities.[7] This further restricts access for pediatric patients with kidney diseases from receiving proper dialysis care and follow-up treatment options, which could lead to additional psychological and social stresses in the lives of both the pediatric patients and their families.

PSYCHOSOCIAL ISSUES IN CHRONIC KIDNEY DISEASE
Socioeconomic Issues

Pediatric patients with CKD, as well as their parents, come across various socioeconomic issues during their lengthened dialysis treatments and transplantation procedures. Because of the complicated nature of ESRD in pediatric patients, they may not be able to fulfill their long-term life goals.[8] Children with CKD typically face difficulties adapting to regular school life due to their prolonged dialysis that leads to frequent absences and poor academic performance in school. Furthermore, it influences the psychosocial development of children with CKDas they have a difficult time engaging in extracurricular activities and having a normal peer relationship with their classmates.[9] A cross-sectional research that was conducted on pediatric patients with CKD for 6 months on dialysis treatment examined their mental health and it was found that about 14.3% of the patients reported being extremely tired when performing activities they normally performed before the illness. This reveals how CKD takes a toll on both the patients' physical and mental health.[10] For these patients, homeschooling is also an option; however, oftentimes this leads to parents, mainly mothers, having to quit their jobs and run a "high-dependency unit" at home for their child.[11] This leaves the parents with more burden and stress on top of having to look after the financial impacts of having a child with CKD as well as attending to the needs and wants of other children in the household.[12]

A few additional financial burdens that parents have to face by having a child with CKD include dialysis treatment costs, medication prices, relocation expenses for traveling or moving closer to a dialysis center, and costs of hiring a special nurse to babysit.[12] One primary factor that contributes to parents' financial difficulties includes the inability to sustain employment at one place as most of the time parents of children with CKD have to focus on child care and their child's medical and nonmedical expenses on top of facing hardships accessing the government support.[13] Owing to the time commitment, responsibility, and high level of stress involved in taking care of a child with CKD, some parents end up having additional marital and family issues.[1] For example, if one parent becomes a caregiver for a child with CKD, it might reduce the amount of time they are available to spend with their other children and partner. This can lead to depression in the caregiver, causing the child with CKD to become the focus of negative emotions in the family and leading to the emergence of other psychosocial issues.[1] To minimize some of these major financial and psychosocial issues among parents, more domestic and government interventions are needed to take place and the accessibility of those resources needs to be easier for both the children with CKD and their families so that they can focus on having better health outcomes and quality of life when undergoing prolonged treatments.[13]

Psychosocial Issues

The continuous and unpredictable alterations in pediatric patients' lifestyle due to CKD can negatively affect their psychological well-being. This can lead to "anxiety, depression, and impaired quality of life."[1] The sex of pediatric patients with CKD correspondingly determines their quality of life depending on various factors. A cross-sectional study[14] conducted on Asian pediatric patients and their parents using PedsQL 4.0 Generic Core Scale Module in the KoreaN cohort study for Outcome in patients with Pediatric CKD cohort reported that male patients when compared with female patients had a better quality of life scores in the physical, emotional, and school functioning categories. This might be due to the attribute that female patients tend to be more concerned with their stature and weight than male patients in general.[9]

Likewise, CKD impairs the growth and development of pediatric patients due to various factors that include "metabolic acidosis, decreased caloric intake, metabolic bone disease, growth hormone resistance, and increased levels of Insulin like Growth factor-1 (IGF-1) binding proteins."[15] Because of developmental problems, pediatric patients living with CKD may encounter issues with their self-image and body image. This may negatively affect their self-esteem, hinder their overall quality of life, and lead to signs of depression.[9] A study conducted at seven pediatric nephrology centers in South Korea revealed that about 18% of patients with CKD exhibited short stature and about 24% of patients exhibited lower weight.[9] This is relevant because the short stature and lower weight pediatric patients displayed signs of having lower self-esteem and other emotional and behavioral problems.[9,16] However, the same study with pediatric patients with CKD recently found that an increase in height with the use of a growth hormone improved the patient's physical and social functioning overall.[9] This demonstrates how certain psychosocial adjustment problems can be resolved with proper dietary and hormonal interventions.

Another study investigated family environment, levels of parenting stress, and child behavioral problems in children who had one of the following kidney diseases for at least one year: steroid-sensitive nephrotic syndrome, chronic renal insufficiency, and ESRD.[17] They found that a positive family environment where expressing emotions is encouraged had lower rates of child behavior problems and parenting stress.[17] They also found that the variety of medications used to treat kidney disorders can elevate both internalizing and externalizing symptoms, furthermore affecting the emotional state of the pediatric patient and those around them.[17] For the purpose of this study, the externalizing behaviors were described as anger, aggression, hyperactivity, and inattentiveness. The internalizing behaviors were characterized as anxiety and depressive symptoms. It was found that externalizing behaviors were reported more commonly in children of 8 years of age and younger by their parents, as compared with school-aged and adolescent children whose parents reported them displaying more internalizing behaviors that were often paired with low motivation or poor attitudes toward academics.[17] Being a single parent also had an adverse impact on a child's externalizing behaviors, further raising the parenting stress and psychosocial issues in a single parent.[17]

A prevalent psychological disorder found among patients with ESRD is depression, which is caused due to a high level of stress during dialysis or after receiving transplantation.[18] In the lifetime of a general population, the prevalence of depression is nearly 16%.[1,18] In contrast, among the ESRD population, the prevalence of depression is approximately 20% to 30%.[1,18] A survey[19] conducted in the United States in 2005 discovered that the prevalence of major depression is about two times higher in people with hypertension, congestive heart disease, diabetes, cerebrovascular disease, and coronary heart disease; however, in a population with ESRD, major depression was found to be almost four times higher when compared with the general population without these medical conditions. Pediatric patients with CKD are also diagnosed with other psychiatric disorders than depression when compared with healthy age- and sex-matched controlled individuals.[20] A study found that about 40.9% of pediatric patients with CKD were diagnosed with a psychiatric disorder, whereas only about 16.2% of healthy age- and sex-matched controlled group were diagnosed with a psychiatric disorder.[20] Despite depression being the most common psychopathology in patients with ESRD, it is still underdiagnosed due its overlap of symptoms in patients.[18] Some typical symptoms seen in both depression and patients with ESRD include fatigue, appetite disturbance, loss of energy, lack of motivation, and cognitive impairments.[21] In addition, depressed youths with CKD score worse than nondepressed youths with CKD when examined in various neurocognitive domains such as "attention, visual memory, visual-spatial, visual working memory, and problem-solving."[16] Depression scores were also seen to be higher in pediatric patients on dialysis when compared with those with kidney transplants.[22] A reasonable explanation for this could be that pediatric patients on dialysis have a restricted lifestyle due to the frequent and lengthy dialysis sessions that further lessens their time for other activities.[23] Thus, to maximize their treatment-related outcomes and quality of life, it is necessary for pediatric patients and their families to have psychological and social support.[1]

Delivery of Psychosocial Care in Chronic Kidney Disease

When providing care for a child with CKD, it is crucial to receive a psychosocial prescription along with a medical and dietetic prescription.[12] This can be achieved by having social workers or specialist nurses moderating with other medical staff on the multidisciplinary team that is designed to care for pediatric patients with progressive CKD.[12] Social workers can also guide the parents of a child with CKD in finding support resources such as grants that are valuable because of the lifelong nature of the disease.[12] Having a social worker and a specialist nurse on the team who can visit the pediatric patients at home also puts the parents at ease; during this time, parents are able to ask and absorb information regarding the dialysis and treatment options in a more relaxed environment.[12] This is extremely beneficial because oftentimes parents think that they are not being thoroughly informed about their child's health and even if they are, they might have additional questions that they might have been afraid to ask at the hospital because of their fear of being labeled as an overprotective or troublesome parent.[24] The involvement of play therapists or child life specialists on the multidisciplinary team from earlier on in the treatment can aid in the management of children receiving renal replacement therapy as well. These team members can make the patients feel more comfortable with procedures that involve the use of needles and other equipment that can cause a procedural phobia.[12] Therefore, early interventions of social workers, play therapists, and family or systemic psychotherapists in combination with the medical staff can potentially prevent major stressors and trauma experienced in both children with CKD and their families.

Educational support and interventions for children with CKD can likewise prevent them from falling behind and having poor academic performance. For instance, having a teacher who can attend the clinic to teach the pediatric patients or provide additional education support during summer breaks and other holidays can deter children from falling behind in school.[12] A visit to the school by a dialysis nurse can also encourage the school staff and teachers to be up-to-date with the situation of the child with CKD.[12] Incorporating a few educational interventions similar to these can put the children with CKD at ease and uplift them by building up their self-esteem that could have been lower initially because of the lack of time spent on school work and activities.[12]

Home peritoneal dialysis and the use of portable automatic cyclers during vacations or holidays can also help children with CKD enjoy their time with family and friends, away from the hospital.[12] This also lessens the burden on parents because it gives them time off to focus on their partner and other children instead of being at the hospital regularly for dialysis. These treatments give children with CKD additional time to socialize with people other than their renal peers, medical treatment team, siblings, and parents.[12] This can also give children with CKD a self-esteem boost because during holiday time they can participate in activities that may be restricted during other times of the year when undergoing dialysis or transplantation procedures.[12]

As discussed earlier, the transition from pediatric to adult CKD care during dialysis or treatment can leave various other psychosocial impacts.[2] To manage and deal with this change, some hospitals employ youth workers to ensure that the self-esteem of children with CKD is not affected. Youth workers can assist and provide support to children to boost self-esteem, which is important during this transitional period before moving the adolescent to adult services.[12] Still, this is not enough support compared with the psychosocial issues and other stressors that children with CKD and their families have to go through during this chronic disease. A systematic review[25] that focused on looking at the transition stage indicated that about 50% of adolescents were not ready to be transferred at the time from the pediatric unit to the adult care unit. Both adolescents and parents felt anxious during the time of transfer due to an emotional attachment they had with the pediatric unit health care team.[25] Adolescents also felt unsure and overwhelmed around the older patients because of the lack of attention provided by the health care team in the adult care unit.[25] A possible initiative that can help ease this transition includes allowing adolescents to meet with the adult health professionals before the time of transfer and also letting them take part in pediatric consultation independently for the time being till they start feeling prepared and responsible.[25]

ROLE OF PSYCHOLOGIST IN CHRONIC KIDNEY DISEASE

As renal impairment progresses from the mild stage to ESRD, the need for psychological intervention becomes indispensable. This is when a clinical child psychologist coordinates with the multidisciplinary team that includes other medical staff and social workers. Again, the team approach not only helps the clinical psychologist to gain valuable information regarding the pediatric patient but also helps in reinforcing the total care of pediatric patients with CKD among other team members.[26] A clinical psychologist can specifically help children with CKD and their families to cope with problems such as "growth and development issues, which may lead to feelings of shame and embarrassment; the financial burden of dialysis therapy; the disruptive effects of moving closer to a dialysis center; overprotectiveness of guilt-ridden parents; the dependence on others, medication, and a machine for a sense of well-being; and marital and intrafamilial strife caused by the absence of a parent from the home or neglect of their spouse and other children."[27–29] A clinical psychologist can moreover help adolescents with CKD get involved in the informed decision-making process for their treatments. Children with CKD often act rebellious, vulnerable, and uncertain because they have little control over their treatment options and have to depend on their parents and health care personnel to make critical decisions for them.[30] Thus, involving children in the decision-making process will better prepare them both mentally and physically to undergo treatments and also to take collaborative and informed decisions when they are transferred to the adult care unit.[30]

Typically, the intervention of a clinical child psychologist is preferred from the beginning when the renal impairment is first diagnosed so that they can conduct psychological testing on children with CKD and their parents to access their premorbid personality traits.[29] By meeting with the pediatric patients with CKD and their parents regularly from the start, clinical psychologists can assist in dealing with existing problems promptly before they end up becoming major obstacles that can get in the way of effective therapy when ESRD further develops.[26] Once children reach the ESRD stage, a child psychologist conducts "supplemental psychological testing, behavior modification, interviewing, and counseling, as well as provides support for other members of the team."[26] A clinical psychologist can also work with the child's pediatrician to utilize and administer cost-efficient tools needed to identify psychosocial problems. For example, the Pediatric Quality of Life Inventory or the Childhood Depression Inventory can be used to determine the pediatric patients' and their parents' psychosocial well-being during recurring hospital appointments.[31] Using these types of inventories as an intervention early on during the treatments can reduce the negative impacts of CKD on both pediatric patients and their families and can allow the clinical psychologist to help them adapt valuable coping skills.

Going through anxiety-provoking dialysis and transplantation procedures can cause children to develop certain types of fears. However, with the help of a clinical child psychologist, those fears can be identified and brought to the attention of the entire ESRD team at an early stage.[26] To overcome the fears in children with ESRD, clinical psychologists often use behavior modification techniques: "Behavior modification has also been found to be extremely helpful in increasing child's acceptance of venipunctures, dietary and fluid restrictions, and the like."[26] Thus, major underlying psychosocial stressors both pretransplantation and posttransplantation, such as anxiety about the child's body possibly rejecting a transplanted kidney, can be resolved by clinical psychologists with the help of other professionals on a multidisciplinary team.[26]

The involvement of clinical child psychologists has similarly shown advantages for parents of children with CKD. For instance, a clinical psychologist can assist in coping with a number of parental problems: the guilt of neglecting aspects of their child's disease or blaming themselves for their child's health outcomes, showing overprotectiveness toward their child that further halts the child's emotional growth, feeling angry toward the health care team for placing their child on fluid or dietary restrictions, feeling blameworthy for having to neglect other children in the family, and sometimes having guilty feelings of neglecting the child with CKD because as a caretaker they might be feeling overwhelmed.[26] To handle these types of issues, a clinical psychologist can educate and teach parents coping skills that may be useful in solving individual or shared problems.[26]

Lastly, a clinical child psychologist can provide assistance and support to medical staff by having an "ear" available, especially for the nursing staff to vent out their feelings and emotions.[26] Even the health care staff can feel drained at the end of their shifts when treating patients with long-term illnesses such as CKD because of all the attention and time they are required to put in. Thus, a clinical psychologist aids in lifting the burden from the nursing staff by listening to their anger, frustration, and grief relating to patients with kidney diseases.[26] As an outcome, a stronger bond is formed between all personnel on the multidisciplinary team that is providing care to the pediatric patients with CKD.[26]

SUMMARY

Treatment of pediatric patients with CKD and ESRD is a complicated process that requires a multidisciplinary approach. CKD patients, like other pediatric patients with chronic disabilities, tend to have a lot of psychological issues that are often overlooked, in part caused by lack of awareness and nonavailability of specialist providers such as a child psychologist from the beginning of the treatment. It is imperative that pediatric ESRD programs around the country are aware of this important deficit and take measures and early interventions to address the mental health component of ESRD treatment.

CLINICS CARE POINTS

- Mental health stress in CKD is often overlooked and not recognized due to lack of specialist providers and awareness.

- Common psychiatric conditions such as depression is often misdiagnosed as fatigue, cognitived decline which is not uncommon in ESRD patients.
- The importance of having appropriate resources/providers to ease the mental health burden in CKD/dialysis patients cannot be overemphasized.

DISCLOSURE

No commercial or financial conflicts of interest to disclose.

REFERENCES

1. White C, McDonnell H. Psychological distress in patients with end-stage kidney disease. J Ren Care 2014;40(1):74–81.
2. Andreoli SP, Brewer ED, Watkins S, et al. American society of pediatric nephrology position paper on linking reimbursement to quality of care. J Am Soc Nephrol 2005;16(8):2263–9.
3. Ritchie AG, Clayton PA, Mackie FE, et al. Nationwide survey of adolescents and young adults with end-stage kidney disease. Nephrology 2012;17:539–44.
4. Pediatric end stage renal disease. United states renal data system's 2001 annual report. Am J Kidney Dis 2001;38(Suppl):S107–16.
5. Schoenmaker NJ, Tromp WF, van der Lee JH, et al. Disparities in dialysis treatment and outcomes for Dutch and Belgian children with immigrant parents. Pediatr Nephrol 2012;27:1369–79.
6. Harambat J, van Stralen KJ, Kim JJ, et al. Epidemiology of chronic kidney disease in children. Pediatr Nephrol 2012;27:363–73.
7. Ad Hoc committee on nephrology manpower needs: estimating workforce and training requirements for nephrologists through the year 2010. J Am Soc Nephrol 1997;8(Suppl9):1–32.
8. Cristóvão F. Stress, coping and quality of life among chronic hemodialysis patients. J Ren Care 2012;25(4):36–45.
9. Kang NR, Ahn YH, Park E, et al. Mental health and psychosocial adjustment in pediatric chronic kidney disease derived from the KNOW-Ped CKD study. Pediatr Nephrol 2019;34(10):1753–64.
10. Pereira BDS, Fernandes NDS, de Melo NP, et al. Beyond quality of life: a cross sectional study on the mental health of patients with chronic kidney disease undergoing dialysis and their caregivers. Health Qual Life Outcomes 2017;15(1):74.
11. Watson AR. Stress and burden of care in families with children commencing renal replacement therapy. Adv Perit Dial 1997;13:300–4.
12. Watson AR. Psychosocial support for children and families requiring renal replacement therapy. Pediatr Nephrol 2013;29(7):1169–74.
13. Medway M, Tong A, Craig JC, et al. Parental perspectives on the financial impact of caring for a child with CKD. Am J Kidney Dis 2015;65(3):384–93.
14. Baek HS, Kang HG, Choi HJ, et al. Health-related quality of life of children with pre-dialysis chronic kidney disease. Pediatr Nephrol 2017;32(11):2097–105.
15. Fine RN. Etiology and treatment of growth retardation in children with chronic kidney disease and end-stage renal disease: a historical perspective. Pediatr Nephrol 2010;25:725–32.
16. Kogon AJ, Kim JY, Laney N, et al. Depression and neurocognitive dysfunction in pediatric and young adult chronic kidney disease. Pediatr Nephrol 2019;34(9):1575–82.

17. Soliday E, Kool E, Lande M. Psychosocial adjustment in children with kidney disease. J Pediatr Psychol 2000;25(2):93–103.
18. Kimmel P, Petterson R. Depression in end-stage renal disease patients treated with haemodialysis: tools, correlates, outcomes and needs. Semin Dial 2005; 18:91–7.
19. Egede L, Nietert P, Zheng D. Depression and all-cause and coronary heart disease mortality among adults with and without diabetes. Diabetes Care 2005; 28(6):1339–45.
20. Senses Dinc G, Cak T, Cengel Kultur E, et al. Psychiatric morbidity and different treatment modalities in children with chronic kidney disease. Arch Pediatr 2019; 26(5):263–7.
21. Drayer RA, Piraino B, Reynolds CF, et al. Characteristics of depression in hemodialysis patients: symptoms, quality of life and mortality risk. Gen Hosp Psychiatry 2006;28(4):306–12.
22. Jofre R, Lopez-Gomez J, Moreno F, et al. Changes in quality of life after renal transplantation. Am J Kidney Dis 1998;32(1):93–100.
23. Al Nazly E, Ahmad M, Musil C, et al. Hemodialysis stressors and coping strategies among Jordanian patients on hemodialysis: a qualitative study. Nephrol Nurs J 2013;40(4):321–7 [quiz: 328].
24. Geense WW, van Gaal BGI, Knoll JL, et al. The support needs of parents having a child with a chronic kidney disease: a focus group study. Child Care Health Dev 2017;43(6):831–8.
25. Crawford K, Wilson C, Low JK, et al. Transitioning adolescents to adult nephrology care: a systematic review of the experiences of adolescents, parents, and health professionals. Pediatr Nephrol 2020;35(4):555–67.
26. Berger M. The role of the clinical child psychologist in an endstage renal disease program. J Clin Child Psychol 1978;7(1):17–8.
27. Raimbault G. Psychological aspects of chronic renal failure and haemodialysis. Nephron 1973;11:252–60.
28. Steinhauer PD, Mushin DN, Rae-Grant Q. Psychological aspects of chronic illness. Pediatr Clin North Am 1974;21:825–40.
29. Berger M, Ginn RJ, Travis LB. Pediatrics dialysis and its psychosocial implications. Pediatr Psychol 1975;3:17–20.
30. Gutman T, Hanson CS, Bernays S, et al. Child and Parental Perspectives on Communication and Decision Making in Pediatric CKD: A Focus Group Study. Am J Kidney Dis 2018;72(4):547–59.
31. Aier A, Pais P, Raman V. Psychosocial aspects of children with chronic kidney disease and their families. Clin Exp Pediatr 2021. https://doi.org/10.3345/cep.2021. 01004.

Psychologist's Unique Role in Improving Quality of Life of Children with Chronic Lung Diseases and Their Families

Mariam Ischander, MBChB[a],*, Sheryl Lozowski-Sullivan, MPH, PhD[b]

KEYWORDS

- Psychologist • Pediatric chronic lung diseases • Severe asthma • Cystic fibrosis
- Bronchopulmonary dysplasia • Home mechanical ventilation

KEY POINTS

- Clinical psychologists have a significant role in helping pediatric patients with chronic lung diseases and their caregivers coping with their chronic illness.
- Psychologists should be an integrated component of the multidisciplinary team caring for children with chronic lung diseases.
- Addressing Mental Health is essential for improving outcome of pediatric chronic lung diseases.

PEDIATRIC CHRONIC LUNG DISEASES

Pediatric chronic lung diseases not only affect the physical aspect of children's health but also the emotional health of children and their families. Understanding the role of physical–emotional or "body–mind" interaction will enable the medical team to support pediatric patients and their families to thrive during periods of uncertainty and struggle.

Severe Asthma

Approximately 3% to 10% of individuals with asthma have severe asthma. Severe asthma is defined per Global Initiative for Asthma (GINA) Strategy 2021 as asthma that is not controlled despite medium- to high-dose inhaled steroids/long-acting beta agonists and treatment of the confounding factors, or when decreasing the dose of treatment, leads to worsening of symptoms. Chronic psychosocial stress

[a] Department of Pediatric and Adolescent Medicine, Division of Pulmonology and Sleep Medicine, Western Michigan University, Homer Stryker MD School of Medicine, 1000 Oakland Drive, Kalamazoo, MI 49008, USA; [b] Department of Pediatric and Adolescent Medicine, Division of Psychology, Western Michigan University, Homer Stryker MD School of Medicine, 1000 Oakland Drive, Kalamazoo, MI 49008, USA
* Corresponding author.
E-mail address: mariam.ischander@med.wmich.edu

Pediatr Clin N Am 69 (2022) 951–963
https://doi.org/10.1016/j.pcl.2022.05.008
0031-3955/22/© 2022 Elsevier Inc. All rights reserved.

and nonadherence to therapy are known risk factors for poorly controlled asthma and acute asthma exacerbation. GINA guidelines also recommend referral of patients with severe asthma to support services and to help them deal with different burden of severe asthma and its management.[1]

Patients with severe asthma are more likely to be hospitalized to intensive care units (ICUs), intubated, and on mechanical ventilation which may contribute to post-intensive care syndrome with cognitive, psychological, and physical comorbidities. A collaboration between patients, families, physicians, and psychologists is recommended to provide timely intervention upon transition home for the pediatric ICU patients to reduce the long-term psychological impact.[2]

Duodeny and colleagues[3] concluded in an article published in 2017 that the prevalence of anxiety is three times higher in youth with asthma than normal youth. Booster and colleagues[4] reported increase prevalence of internalizing disorders such as anxiety and affective disorders in children with asthma as compared with general population with an estimate of this prevalence to be between 5% and 43% in children with asthma.

Blackman and Gurka[5] concluded that children with asthma, in particular severe asthma, are at elevated risk for developmental, emotional, and behavioral problems. The more severe the asthma, the higher the incidence of developmental and behavioral problems. The author also addressed in the same article that attention-deficit/hyperactivity disorder is more common in children with asthma especially in severe asthma. Consequently, physicians managing asthma should be aware of these associations and use whole-patient approach to address the developmental, emotional, and behavioral problems in patients with severe asthma and adopt the multidisciplinary team approach for management of children with severe asthma with the addition of a psychologist to the care team.

Booster and colleagues[6] reported that there is increase prevalence of depression and anxiety in parents of children with asthma in addition to increase parental demands to cope with the extensive care needed for children with asthma. Booster and colleagues then concluded that pediatric psychologists with specific expertise in psychosocial intervention will be a valuable addition to the medical team and communities. In the same article, the author reported that children from low income and urban households have increased exposure to tobacco smoke, polluted air, and environmental stressors such as dangerous neighborhood, family conflict, chronic family stress, and housing-related stress.

Avcil and colleagues[7] reported in a cross-sectional study published in 2018 that depression and anxiety scores were significantly higher in mothers of children with asthma and that increased emergency department visits were associated with increasing depression in children with asthma. This study revealed that asthma may negatively affect the lives of children with asthma, their mothers, and their relationship. Parental emotional stress leads to difficulty in adherence to asthma therapy and poor technique. Parents of the children between 18 months and 7 years reported challenges with administering medication as the main cause of treatment nonadherence. Crying and temper tantrums during medication administration can trigger breath holding and breathing difficulties.

Puranik and colleagues[8] reported that chronic toxic psychosocial stress increases morbidity from asthma via nonadherence, decreases response to bronchodilators through down-regulation of B2 adrenergic receptors, and decreases expression of glucocorticoid receptors and leukocytes in children with asthma.

Pak and Allen[9] in a integrative literature review indicated that maternal depression enhanced asthma morbidity and health care utilization and led to decrease self-efficiency in following the asthma medication regimen recommended by physicians. The author recommended periodic depression screening for mothers, providing more education about asthma and depression via coordination of care with frequent follow-up visits when depression is reported. The conclusion of this review article was that these measures will improve the quality of life for children and caregivers, decrease emergency department visits and hospitalizations, and decrease missed school and workdays.

Practitioners must be aware of the enormous psychosocial and economic burden faced by pediatric asthma patients and their families. Depression in caregivers is associated with depression in their children. Siblings of children with asthma may also feel angry or jealous due to the attention their siblings receive. Waters and colleagues[10] conducted a qualitative study published in 2017 by interviewing African American and Hispanic parents of children with asthma aiming at reducing stress among parents; the study revealed that the unpredictability of asthma and the burden of asthma care led to parental stress, and parents were interested in a multimodal stress reduction intervention that focused on building relationships, allowed for flexibility, and encouraged staff–parent communication. Ekim[11] concluded in a systematic review published in 2016 that caregivers of the children with asthma often experience anxiety, fear, disappointment, grief, physical distress, and low quality of life as the outcomes of the caregiving burden.

Adherence to treatment for severe asthma is lifesaving. Taking medications as prescribed results in fewer exacerbations, control of symptoms, and less likelihood that mechanical ventilation will be needed. Objective measures of adherence include prescription filling, and electronic inhaler monitoring, serum levels of prescribed medications provide an objective measure of its recent use, and directly observing a patient can be used for teaching accurate techniques (eg, inhaler) and for adherence. Other methods of measuring adherence include patient logs, phone apps, 24-h recall interviews, and the clinician impression.

Psychologist role

The role of the clinical pediatric psychologist as an integrated member of the multidisciplinary team caring for patients with severe asthma is crucial through assessment of anxiety and depression in children with asthma and their caregivers, and providing the intervention needed via counseling and/or referral as needed. Psychologist's role also includes offering participation in a support group to help families cope with the chronicity of asthma and accept it as a lifelong illness and improve their quality of life. Family education about time management, delegation of other responsibilities as needed, and working on a reduced schedule will help the caregivers to meet the needs of a child with chronic illness. Providing families with the financial assistance resources available is essential to meet their financial restraints due to working less hours. Low-income families can qualify for government insurance like Medicaid which will improve access to care. Stewart and colleagues[12] revealed in a study that low-income children, adolescents, and caregivers facing respiratory problems reported isolation and resource deficits with the suggestion of partnership with these children and families in providing education and social support. Sullivan and colleagues[13] reported in a study that parents of children with asthma and an exacerbation missed 1.2 times more workdays, whereas those with an emergency department visit missed 1.8 times more workdays than parents of children without asthma. Foronda and colleagues[14] reported that treating both patients and caregivers is especially important, assessing both family and social support is crucial, and educating and empowering the caregiver is essential. Educating caregivers to include the importance of communicating their questions and concerns to the physicians and to self-advocate for their children. Exploring advanced technology in education to improve child health outcome such as asthma apps, online support groups for caregivers, and after-hours advise lines was recommended by Foronda and colleagues. Finally, the author suggested in the same article that providers should adopt a patient- and family-centered care, and social support system like school-based asthma programs, extended family members, alternative caregivers, and support groups.

Cystic fibrosis

Cystic fibrosis (CF) is an autosomal recessive genetic disease with a chronic and progressive nature. CF is due to a defect in the CF transmembrane conductance regulator gene (CFTR) with resulting defective CFTR protein. CF affects multiple systems and leads to organ failure. The treatment burden of CF is enormous with great demands regarding nutrition, medications, extensive respiratory therapy and airway clearance, need to do blood tests, imaging studies, frequent lung function testing, need to receive immunization, and for painful procedures like insertion of a peripherally inserted central lines. The need for frequent hospitalizations for days or weeks for CF pulmonary exacerbations and the restrictions applied by the infectious control policies during the admission can lead to depression and feelings of loneliness and isolation. Despite advances in CF care and the recent discovery of the CFTR modulators since 2012 that led to a significant improvement in CF care, the treatment burden of CF care remains high. Daily, CF patients often have multiple medications, including digestive enzymes, multiple breathing treatments, and airway clearance sessions involving high-frequency chest wall oscillation therapy. In addition, CF patients may develop CF-related diabetes which adds another burden.

The psychological and psychosocial aspects of CF not only affect the patients but also their caregivers and lead to decrease body mass index, lower lung function, decrease adherence to therapy, more hospitalizations, lower quality of life, and increase health care cost.[15] The Cystic Fibrosis Foundation and the European Cystic Fibrosis Society recommend annual screening for both patients and parents for depression and anxiety using patient Health Questionnaire-9 and Generalized Anxiety Disorder-7 scales, and that the screening to be performed by mental health specialists like psychologist or psychiatrist.[15] The prevalence of depression among children and adolescents of CF ranges from 8% to 29%.[15,16] A multicenter study for CF patients and their parents by Quittner and colleagues[17] revealed increased symptoms of depression in 10% of adolescents, 37% of mothers, and 31% of fathers. In addition, the elevation of anxiety was also noted in 22% of adolescents, 48% of mothers, and 36% of fathers. COVID-19 pandemic exaggerated the mental health crisis in the United States and led to more shortage in mental health providers, yet we still live in a society where mental health stigma is a huge concern. To overcome these challenges, patients need a psychologist whom they can connect with, trust, and be more open with.

Masson and colleagues[18] indicated that pain may be an underestimated symptom by the multidisciplinary team in CF patients, and pain like headache, and abdominal and chest pain was encountered in 70% of children and adults with CF and it decreases the quality of life.

There is evidence of an increased prevalence of eating disorders in the CF population. Darukhanavala and colleagues concluded in their article published in 2021 that although it is assumed that the nutritional disorder in CF patients is related to CF and its effects, the differential diagnosis should still include poor weight gain because of the psychological burden of CF, eating disorders, and disturbed eating. In addition, the author advocated for effective eating disorder prevention programs, promoting positive body image, and development of appropriate screening tools.[19]

Psychologist role

Investing in the psychologist role in CF care has been a focus of the Cystic Fibrosis Foundation and European Cystic Fibrosis Society. The psychologist's role includes doing annual screening for depression and anxiety, providing preventive supportive measures and behavioral interventions as well as assessing the need for referral for pharmacological interventions.[20]

James[21] poster presentation revealed that in the annual CF patient psychological assessment, the most frequent difficulty was stress (43%), followed by anxiety or worry (33%), low mood (23%), and difficulty managing all their treatment (23%), patients also described their health goals for the coming year. Wynberg-Williams and colleagues[22] concluded that systematic use of interviewing by a pediatric psychologist during screening for pediatric lung transplant helps to enable the decision-making process.

Quittner and colleagues[15] referenced a study, which showed that individuals with CF and a diagnosis of depression were hospitalized more than three times more often than nondepressed patients. In addition, adolescents have reported that disclosing that they have CF and the stigmatization interfere with completing their treatment like taking their breathing treatment or taking their pancreatic enzymes replacement therapy before meals. Stigmatization was associated with higher symptoms of depression and anxiety, decreased lung function, and decreased quality of life. Chronic cough in CF patients led to sending them home due to the thought that they are contagious. Psychologist's role here includes educating patients about CF and its psychosocial impact, encouraging patients to be the expert on their condition, enhancing personalized care to improve adherence, promoting comfort with disclosing the diagnosis, and implementing cognitive-behavioral therapy.[23] Infection control policies that are applied in all settings inpatient and outpatient prevent face-to-face contact between CF patients and lead to socialization restrictions between CF patients, which leads to the feeling of loneliness and isolation. Psychologists need to find alternative options to connect CF patients such as text messages, phone calls, or virtual support groups. In addition, CF exacerbations lead to hospitalizations and missing frequent days from school which also makes it difficult to make friends.[24]

Muther and colleagues[24] also referred to an article published in 2018 that adherence in adolescents and young adults is at its lowest level. Adolescents are expected to develop independence for which they may not be ready. Teaching adolescents and young adults positive coping styles such as acceptance, maintaining social support, and planning leads to improvement in quality of life and self-management. In addition, teaching resilience and overcoming challenges with a positive attitude and problem-solving skills is crucial. Meditation, exercise program, yoga, and tai chi may provide stress relief, improve mood, and promote well-being. Grossoehme and colleagues[25] reported that spirituality has a positive link to treatment adherence in patients with CF.

Positive newborn screen for CF leads to significant parental stress and anxiety. Eighty-seven percent of mothers called the time between the positive newborn screen and learning the results (the scariest time of their lives); consequently, providers should communicate with parents in a way that minimizes stress.[26] Although communication of the results and their interpretation is usually undertaken by the pediatric pulmonologist, the presence of a psychologist on the care team will address other aspects of cystic fibrosis care.

Finally, facing challenges with resilience, the passion to defeat CF, and the determination to improve the health of CF patients and their families is the key to the psychologist's success in CF care.

Bronchopulmonary Dysplasia

Bronchopulmonary dysplasia (BPD) also known as neonatal chronic lung disease is defined as the need for oxygen at 28 postnatal days or at 36 weeks postmenstrual age. BPD occurs mainly in extreme preterm (less than 28 weeks of gestation), and its incidence increase with decreasing gestational age. BPD can be mild, moderate, or severe.[27] Supplemental oxygen, invasive mechanical ventilation, and neonatal sepsis are all risk factors for BPD.[28] Extreme preterm 10-year-old children with BPD were at increased risk for decreased cognitive, language and executive function, as well as academic achievement, and lower health-related quality of life as compared with those without BPD.[29] BPD is also a risk factor for cerebral palsy.[30]

BPD is the abnormal growth and development of the lung due to prematurity. With advances in the medical field, a reduction in mortality of extremely premature infants was achieved; however, morbidity increased in survivors. A database review study published by Jarjour[31] revealed that the mortality rate of extremely premature infants born at 22 to 25 weeks of gestation is high and estimated to be $\geq$ 50%, and severe neurodevelopmental disabilities on short term follow-up estimated to be 17% to 59%. The rate of survival with minimal or no impairment was 6% to 20% for live-born infants $\leq$25 weeks of gestation and <5% for infants born at 22 and 23 weeks of gestation. Long-term follow-up for extremely premature infants showed that the rate of intellectual disabilities is 5% to 36%, cerebral palsy 9% to 18%, blindness 0.7% to 9%, and deafness at 2% to 4%. Mild disabilities in learning, behavior, and cognition were also noted in growing preterm through young adulthood.

Sillers and colleagues[32] reported in a summary of current literature that very preterm infants with BPD are predisposed to respiratory complications, increased respiratory medications use, frequent re-hospitalization through early childhood, and increased susceptibility to early-onset chronic obstructive lung disease in adulthood

Brady and colleagues concluded in a study that parental perceived health-related quality of life for their child with severe BPD was lower than expected for premature and term children. In addition, an increased number of postnatal morbidities was associated with worse parent-perceived health-related quality of life.[33]

Bray and colleagues reported that having an oxygen-dependent baby negatively affected maternal well-being for years with ongoing sadness, hurt, social isolation, decrease self-esteem, and continued worry about future pregnancies. Stress and anxiety were reported in mothers 1 year after preterm labor. Children with chronic lung disease felt bullied and teased by peers in school because of their small size, respiratory symptoms, and fatigue leading to self-exclusion from social activities, social isolation and even moving to school. However, children and their parents reported improvement in competence and confidence over time to deal with the challenges and live with the long-term condition, yet parents felt frustrated when their expertise was ignored by health care professionals or schools and the author suggested that the medical team should integrate the parents' expertise in managing their children's condition.[34]

But the journey starts even earlier, at the birth of a premature baby. Neonatal intensive care unit (NICU) environment despite being a life saver is stressful for premature infants and their parents, with parents having an intense feelings of fear, sadness, guilt, worry, or being helpless and overwhelmed. In addition, sleep disruption in NICU babies is a common concern. Using music and massage therapy as optional interventions to improve the neurodevelopmental outcomes of premature babies during NICU stay has gained a momentum.

Liu and colleagues reported in a literature review article that promoting better strategies to support the neurodevelopment in infants in the NICU includes preservation of sleep, positioning, gentle touch, and sound/light exposure modulation. Sleep preservation can prevent disruption of the process of normal brain development.[35]

Khel and colleagues[36] in a pilot study revealed that creative music therapy with premature infants and their parents can support the infant–parent relationship, induce feelings of joy and relaxation in parents, and encourage profound infant–parent interactions.

Loewy and colleagues[37] concluded in a randomized multicenter clinical trial of premature infants that music therapy applied by a certified music therapist can influence cardiorespiratory function, improve feeding/sucking behavior, and increase awake/quiet time. Parent chosen live lullabies can promote bonding and consequently decrease stress in parents.

Feeley and colleagues revealed in a study for maternal caregivers of young children with BPD that maternal caregivers were chronically sleep-deprived with reported 5.8 h of sleep per night and emphasized the importance of discussing proper sleep hygiene by providers with maternal caregivers. Empowering mothers with education, training, and resources like respite care is essential for relieving stress and promoting a sense of comfort with the care.[38]

Sairankyzy and colleagues[39] concluded in a study that the social characteristics of a family of a child with BPD showed increased average age of parents, high incidence of smoking in fathers, poor housing, low socioeconomic status with the financial situation of the family raising a child with BPD worsen to a degree that the financial resources available were only enough for food.

Strategies to work on in the future include prevention of prematurity, individualizing the care of each infant and the support needed for each family, minimizing neurodevelopmental impairment in NICU, and for children with neurodevelopmental delay, and ensuring the availability of early intervention programs, special education school programs to maximize their potential.

Psychologist role

The model of the multidisciplinary team in managing BPD as inpatient then outpatient is the key to success, including a psychologist in the team is becoming a necessity. BPD children also are in need of other services such as physical therapy, occupational therapy, speech-language pathologist, social workers, music therapy, massage therapy, child life, and case management to optimize the physical and neurodevelopmental outcome. Outpatient follow-up with multiple specialists is needed and may include neonatology, pulmonology, nutrition, cardiology, and endocrinology, so collaboration and communication between providers are essential and the role of care management is critical.

Providing not only the best medical care but also the psychosocial support necessary for the infants and their parents during this stressful time is crucial. Psychologist should screen parents for depression/anxiety and provide counseling as needed, ensure that family received adequate training to be able to be comfortable with the care, work with parents on adherence to therapy melting barriers that interfere with adherence, help families to advocate for their children and share decision-making with providers, and provide resources to the family in conjunction with the social worker to decrease stress due to financial burden. Psychologist should also help with connecting families with a support group or other parents with chronic lung disease children.

Home Mechanical Ventilation

The advances in medical care in both neonatal and pediatric ICUs led to improvement in survival and a growing population on home mechanical ventilation (HMV) both invasive and noninvasive. The indication of HMV is chronic respiratory failure due to a diverse group of diseases. The complications of HMV are tremendous and include tracheal decannulation, mucous plugging of tracheostomy tube, bleeding from tracheostomy tube and bronchospasm with respiratory distress. The care needed for a home ventilator patient is extensive and requires at least two trained family care givers and professional caregivers before discharge home. The American Thoracic Society recommends an awake and trained caregiver to attend the care of the home ventilator child 24 h daily, 7 days a week. The surgeon general's report indicated that children with special health care need deserve to live at home with their families. The family needs support, financial and psychosocial, including insurance coverage, arranging for a safe transportation, educational, vocational, and recreational services, family support with assessment for stress, depression and anxiety and providing therapy as indicated to optimize the caregiver's function. The caregivers of mechanically ventilated children develop anxiety over time due to concern about sudden complications for their children in the context of lack of adequately trained home care workers to provide respite care for their children. National shortage of nursing all over the country led to parental stress, sleep deprivation, marital problems, and financial burden due to difficulty to work while caring for a home ventilator child, as well as poor physical and mental health of caregivers.[40]

Benscoter and colleagues noted that parents of technology-dependent children struggle with creating normalcy and routine. It starts with a long admission for the new tracheostomy and home mechanically ventilated child. In addition, tremendous coordination is needed to arrange for training for caregivers, availability of home nursing, home medical equipment, and outpatient follow-up with multiple providers. Transition to home could be a happy yet a scary moment for the parents, with the significant commitment needed to care for the mechanically ventilated child and the nationwide shortage of home nurses, the risk of hospital readmission, and the risk of respiratory complications and even death. Even when home nurses are secured, there are times when nurses are unavailable due to sickness or family emergencies. Financial burden is a struggle for the family of a mechanically ventilated child because of difficulties to secure a job with the long hours needed to care for the child; also home mechanically ventilated child needs to have his own room which adds a burden on the family to move to a bigger house to accommodate the child's medical equipment and home nurses, in addition, the need for home remodeling like availability of a ramp for home entry, a lift, and grounding of electricity. Screening caregivers for anxiety and depression is recommended using a tool like (National Insitutes of Health (NIH) Toolbox Perceived Stress). Providing family support via a provider family meeting and help with decision-making is recommended as parents know what is best for their child. Treatment of caregivers is also recommended as indicated including cognitive behavioral therapy and acceptance and commitment therapy. This treatment should start early in the hospital and appropriate referral on discharge to continue after that.[41]

Falkson and colleagues noted that children and adolescents on mechanical ventilation want to be perceived as an individual and for who they are and not just being ventilated or on a wheelchair but to care for the person on the chair. Adolescents prefer to have no nurse as nurses interferes with their independence and they feel being observed all the time and not able to be themselves. For parents also, having a nurse at home interferes with their privacy. It is important for mechanically ventilated children to go to school, and to be included in their community. The social activities of the family typically are reduced by having a child on mechanical ventilation and the need for extensive preparation before taking child outside home.[42]

Telemedicine can be a great tool for mechanically ventilated children. Casavant and colleagues[43] revealed in a study that telemedicine encounters supported clinician decision-making and produced elevated level of family confidence in clinical management when patients were ill with telemedicine preventing the need for 23 clinic visits, 3 emergency room visits, and 1 hospitalization. In addition, telemedicine is a great tool for home ventilator patients as it takes a significant effort to prepare technology-dependent children for a trip to the doctor's office; in addition, in case of severe weather it is safer for the disabled child to have a telemedicine visit.

Introduction of palliative care as early as possible to improve quality of life, help with decision-making, and provide support for the family is crucial.

Psychologist role

The role of the psychologist in helping technology-dependent children and their caregivers is instrumental in guiding and supporting them through the challenging road ahead from early on, providing a patient and family-centered care, helping them with decision-making and developing a clear communication style with the medical team, assessing patients and caregivers for depression and anxiety, and empowering families with knowledge and resources to be successful. Providing psychotherapy as needed is crucial for depression, anxiety as well as for pain and sleep deprivation or insomnia. Mechanically ventilated patients are a population with high morbidity and mortality rates; thus, preparing and supporting families are essential. When deterioration of medical condition becomes imminent, helping families connect with palliative care, chaplain, and child life to walk them through the end-of-life period becomes essential, guiding them on how to incorporate their goals, beliefs, and family values into the decision making. Supporting grieving families and siblings in case of a sudden unexpected event that took the child's life is compassionate and caring. On the other hand, the psychologist should support hope and empower families to enjoy their children with positive attitudes that never give up and fighting for their children to achieve their maximal potential. Psychologist also should encourage the caregivers to attend to their own health care needs and well-being via eating healthy, exercising, and avoiding sleep deprivation while providing care to their children with love and commitment.

CHALLENGES AND SUMMARY

The COVID-19 pandemic exaggerated the mental health crisis in the United States and led to an increased shortage of mental health providers. The stigma of mental health services remains a huge concern and barrier for many patients and families. The availability of a psychologist on the care team of children with chronic lung diseases is imperative to overcoming all these issues. Although it may take many months, the presence of the psychologist on the care team becomes another resource with whom they can connect, trust, and access when the need arises.

CLINICS CARE POINTS

- A detailed mental health screening is recommended for patients and caregivers with severe asthma.

- Annual screeing for depression and anxiety for cystic fibrosis patients 12 years and older using Patient Health Questionnaire-9 and Generalized Anxiety Disorder-7 is recommended by the Cystic Fibrosis Foundation and the European Cystic Fibrosis Society.
- Annual screening for at least one primary caregiver of a CF child 0-17 years of age is recomended by the Cystic Fibrosis Foundation and the European Cystic Fibrosis Society.

ACKNOWLEDGMENTS

The authors acknowledge the contribution of Jessica Ziccarello, a medical student at Western Michigan University, Homer Stryker MD School of Medicine for her contribution to this work via performing a literature review with a summary.

CONFLICTS OF INTEREST

The authors have no conflicts of interest relevant to this article to disclose; however, both authors were part of the Mental Health Coordinator Grant sponored by the Cystic Fibrosis Foundation (CFF), United States CF Fundamentals to One CF Learning and Leadership Collaborative (CF FUN to One CF LLC) Grant which was supported by the Dartmouth Institute Microsystem Academy and sponsored by the CFF. Both authors are part of the Cystic Fibrosis Foundation Care Center Grant sponsored by the CFF. In addition, Mariam Ischander was part of Implementation of Outpatient Clinical Pharmacy Services Grant as well sponsored by CFF.

REFERENCES

1. Global Initiative for Asthma Strategy 2021: Executive Summary and Rationale for Key Changes, Crossref DOI link: https://doi.org/10.1016/J.JAIP.2021.10.001
2. Herrup EA, Wieczorek B, Kudchadkar SR. Characteristics of postintensive care syndrome in survivors of pediatric critical illness: a systematic review. World J Crit Care Med 2017;6(2):124–34.
3. Dudeney J, Sharpe L, Jaffe A, et al. Anxiety in youth with asthma: a meta-analysis. Pediatr Pulmonol 2017;52(9):1121–9.
4. Booster GD, Oland AA, Bender BG, et al. Psychosocial factors in severe pediatric asthma. Immunol Allergy Clin N Am 2016;36(3):449–60. https://doi.org/10.1016/j.iac.2016.03.012.
5. Blackman JA, Gurka MJ. Developmental and behavioral comorbidities of asthma in children. J Dev Behav Pediatr 2007;28(2):92–9.
6. Booster GD, Oland AA, Bender BG. Treatment adherence in young children with asthma. Immunol Allergy Clin N Am 2019;39(2):233–42.
7. Avcil S, Uysal P, Demir F, et al. Mothers' emotional states and attitudes regarding their children with asthma. J Asthma 2019;56(6):618–26.
8. Puranik S, Forno E, Bush A, et al. Predicting severe asthma exacerbations in children. Am J Respir Crit Care Med 2017;195(7):854–9.
9. Pak L, Allen PJ. The impact of maternal depression on children with asthma. Pediatr Nurs 2012;38(1):11–9, 30. PMID: 22474854.
10. Waters DM, Olson AM, Fousheé N, et al. Perceptions of Stress, Coping, and Intervention Preferences among Caregivers of Disadvantaged Children with Asthma. J Child Fam Stud 2017;26:1622–34. https://doi.org/10.1007/s10826-017-0670-3.
11. Ekim A. OC29 - Caregiver burden in childhood asthma. Nurs Child Young People 2016;28(4):75.

12. Stewart M, Evans J, Letourneau N, et al. Low-income children, adolescents, and caregivers facing respiratory problems: support needs and preferences. J Pediatr Nurs 2016;31(3):319–29.
13. Sullivan PW, Ghushchyan V, Navaratnam P, et al. The national burden of poorly controlled asthma, school absence and parental work loss among school-aged children in the United States. J Asthma 2018;55(6):659–67.
14. Foronda CL, Kelley CN, Nadeau C, et al. Psychological and socioeconomic burdens faced by family caregivers of children with asthma: an integrative review. J Pediatr Health Care 2020;34(4):366–76.
15. Quittner AL, Abbott J, Georgiopoulos AM, et al. International committee on mental health in cystic fibrosis: Cystic Fibrosis Foundation and European Cystic Fibrosis Society consensus statements for screening and treating depression and anxiety. Thorax 2016;71(1):26–34.
16. Clearance.Smith BA, Modi AC, Quittner AL. Wood BL Depressive symptoms in children with cystic fibrosis and parents and its effects on adherence to airway. Pediatr Pulmonol 2010;45(8):756–63.
17. Quittner AL, Goldbeck L, Abbott J, et al. Prevalence of depression and anxiety in patients with cystic fibrosis and parent caregivers: results of The International Depression Epidemiological Study across nine countries. Thorax 2014;69(12):1090–7.
18. Masson A, Kirszenbaum M, Sermet-Gaudelus I. Pain is an underestimated symptom in cystic fibrosis. Curr Opin Pulm Med 2017;23(6):570–3.
19. Amy D, Merjaneh L, Mason K, et al. Eating disorders and body image in cystic fibrosis. J Clin Translational Endocrinol 2021;26. https://doi.org/10.1016/j.jcte.2021.100280.
20. Abbott J, Elborn JS, Georgiopoulos AM, et al. Cystic Fibrosis Foundation and European Cystic Fibrosis Society survey of cystic fibrosis mental health care delivery. J Cystic Fibrosis 2015;14(4):533–9. https://doi.org/10.1016/j.jcf.2014.12.015.
21. James S. Phillips,256 Understanding the psychological difficulties patients with cystic fibrosis share at annual review. J Cystic Fibrosis 2015;14(Supplement 1):S124. https://doi.org/10.1016/S1569-1993(15)304318.
22. Wynberg-Williams BJ, van der Hulst J, Rottier BL. 335 Screening for pediatric lung transplantation: the pediatric psychologist's role. J Cystic Fibrosis 2012;11(Supplement 1):S142. https://doi.org/10.1016/S1569-1993(12)60503-7.
23. Quittner AL, Saez-Flores E, Barton JD, et al. The psychological burden of cystic fibrosis. Curr Opin Pulm Med 2016;22(2):187–91. https://doi.org/10.1097/mcp.0000000000000244.
24. Muther EF, Polineni D, Sawicki GS, et al. Overcoming psychosocial challenges in cystic fibrosis: promoting resilience. Pediatr Pulmonol 2018;53(S3). https://doi.org/10.1002/ppul.24127.
25. Grossoehme DH, Szczesniak RD, Mrug S, et al. Adolescents' Spirituality and cystic fibrosis airway clearance treatment adherence: examining mediators. J Pediatr Psychol 2016;41(Issue 9):1022–32. https://doi.org/10.1093/jpepsy/jsw024.
26. Chudleigh J, Chinnery H. Psychological Impact of NBS for CF. Int J Neonatal Screen 2020;6(2):27. https://doi.org/10.3390/ijns6020027.
27. Eichenwald E.C., Strak A.R., Bronchopulmonary dysplasia: Definition, pathogenesis, and clinical features, Uptodate. Available at: www.uptodate.com/contents/bronchopulmonary-dysplasia-definition-pathogenesis-and-clinical-features#!, 2017.

28. Thébaud B, Goss KN, Laughon M, et al. Bronchopulmonary dysplasia (primer). Nature Reviews: Disease Primers. 2019. Available at: https://liblynxgateway.com/wmed?url=https://www.proquest.com/scholarly-journals/bronchopulmonary-dysplasia-primer/docview/2314540163/se-2?accountid=160899. Accessed November 14, 2019.

29. Sriram S, Schreiber MD, Msall ME, et al. Cognitive Development and Quality of Life Associated With BPD in 10-Year-Olds Born Preterm. Pediatrics 2018; 141(6):e20172719.

30. Gou X, Yang L, Pan L, et al. Association between bronchopulmonary dysplasia and cerebral palsy in children: a meta-analysis. BMJ Open 2018;8:e020735.

31. Jarjour I. Neurodevelopmental outcome after extreme prematurity: a review of the literature. Pediatr Neurol 2014;52. https://doi.org/10.1016/j.pediatrneurol.2014. 10.027.

32. Sillers L, Alexiou S, Jensen EA. A Lifelong pulmonary sequelae of bronchopulmonary dysplasia. Curr Opin Pediatr 2020;32(2):252–60.

33. Brady JM, Zhang H, Kirpalani H, et al. Living with severe bronchopulmonary dysplasia-parental views of their child's quality of life. J Pediatr 2019;207:117–22.

34. Bray L, Shaw NJ, Snodin J, et al. Living and managing with the long-term implications of neonatal chronic lung disease: the experiences and perspectives of children and their parents. Heart & Lung 2015;44(6):512–6. https://doi.org/10. 1016/j.hrtlng.2015.08.002.

35. Liu WF, Laudert S, Perkins B, et al. The development of potentially better practices to support the neurodevelopment of infants in the NICU. J Perinatol 2007; 27:S48–74. https://doi.org/10.1038/sj.jp.7211844. Available at: https:// liblynxgateway.com/wmed?url=https://www.proquest.com/scholarly-journals/development-potentially-better-practices-support/docview/220422012/se-2?accountid=160899.

36. Kehl SM, La Marca-Ghaemmaghami P, Haller M, et al. Creative music therapy with premature infants and their parents: a mixed-method pilot study on parents' anxiety, stress and depressive symptoms and parent-infant attachment. Int J Environ Res Public Health 2020;18(1):265.

37. Loewy J, Stewart K, Dassler A, et al. The effects of music therapy on vital signs, feeding, and sleep in premature infants. Pediatrics 2013;131(5):902–18. https://doi.org/10.1542/peds.2012-1367. Available at: https://liblynxgateway.com/wmed?url=https://www.proquest.com/scholarly-journals/effects-music-therapy-on-vital-signs-feeding/docview/1492672826/se-2.

38. Feeley CA, Turner-Henson A, Christian BJ, et al. Sleep quality, stress, caregiver burden, and quality of life in maternal caregivers of young children with bronchopulmonary dysplasia. J Pediatr Nurs 2014;29(1):29–38.

39. Sairankyzy S, Zhakanovna Seisebayeva R, Nurbakytovna Nurbakyt A, et al. Social portrait of families raising children with bronchopulmonary dysplasia. Curr Pediatr Res 2021;25(10):987–92.

40. Sterni LM, Collaco JM, Baker CD, et al. An official american thoracic society clinical practice guideline: Pediatric chronic home invasive ventilation. Am J Respir Crit Care Med 2016;193(8):E16–35. https://doi.org/10.1164/rccm.201602-0276ST. Available at: https://liblynxgateway.com/wmed?url=https://www.proquest.com/scholarly-journals/official-american-thoracic-society-clinical/docview/1782403669/se-2?accountid=160899.

41. Benscoter D, Borschuk A, Hart C, Voos K. Preparing families to care for ventilated infants at home. Semin Fetal Neonatal Med 2019;24(5):101042. https://doi.org/10.1016/j.siny.2019.101042.

42. Falkson S, Knecht C, Hellmers C, et al. The Perspective of Families with a Ventilator-Dependent Child at Home. A Literature Review. J Pediatr Nurs 2017; 36:213–24. https://doi.org/10.1016/j.pedn.2017.06.021.
43. Casavant DW, McManus ML, Parsons SK, et al. Trial of telemedicine for patients on home ventilator support: feasibility, confidence in clinical management and use in medical decision-making. J Telemed Telecare 2014;20(8):441–9.

The Role of Psychology in Pediatric Rheumatic Diseases

William S. Frye, PhD, BCB, ABPP[a],*, Diana Milojevic, MD[b]

KEYWORDS

• Pediatric psychology • Rheumatic disease • Juvenile arthritis • Interdisciplinary care

KEY POINTS

• Youth with pediatric rheumatic diseases (PRDs) experience a complex disease course, which can be difficult to manage and lead to psychosocial impairments and functional challenges.

• Pediatric psychologists are equipped to address many of the concerns seen within the management of PRDs.

• Integration of pediatric psychologists into PRD treatment or interdisciplinary clinics can be beneficial in overcoming barriers youth with PRDs experience and improving quality of life.

Pediatric rheumatic diseases (PRDs) are chronic conditions caused by disorders of the immune system and characterized by systemic inflammation (several organs in the body are affected) and/or local inflammation (only specific organs, frequently joints, are affected). Different rheumatic diseases are more prevalent in children at certain ages, although pediatric rheumatologists care for children from the first year of life through early adulthood. It has been estimated that more than 300,000 children in the United States have a chronic rheumatic disease.[1]

Inflammation seen in rheumatic conditions is caused by the immune system attacking its own body, which can be triggered by defects in either the specific immune system (ie, autoimmune diseases) or the nonspecific "primitive" or "naïve" immune system (ie, autoinflammatory diseases). Autoimmune diseases include systemic lupus erythematosus (SLE), most forms of juvenile idiopathic arthritis (JIA), juvenile

Disclosures.
Funding: No funding, grants, or other support were received for this study.
Conflicts of interest/Competing interests: Dr W.S. Frye serves as an expert panelist for the Juvenile Arthritis Foundation.
[a] Department of Psychology, Johns Hopkins All Children's Hospital, 880 6th Street South, Suite 460, St Petersburg, FL 33701, USA; [b] Department of Medicine, Johns Hopkins All Children's Hospital, 601 5th Street South, Suite 502, Street, St Petersburg, FL 33701, USA
* Corresponding author.
E-mail address: wfrye1@jhmi.edu

Pediatr Clin N Am 69 (2022) 965–974
https://doi.org/10.1016/j.pcl.2022.05.009
0031-3955/22/© 2022 Elsevier Inc. All rights reserved.

dermatomyositis, different types of scleroderma, and some types of vasculitis (blood vessel inflammation). Examples of autoinflammatory diseases include periodic fever syndromes, some types of vasculitis (eg, Behcet's disease), some types of systemic arthritis, macrophage activation syndrome, and several rare, more recently described genetic disorders characterized by chronic inflammation. Although these are classified as two distinct groups of diseases, most of the autoimmune and autoinflammatory diseases share pathologic features and symptoms.

Our understanding of these disorders and immune mechanisms has evolved tremendously over the last 20 years and brought a number of new autoimmune and autoinflammatory diseases to our attention. Some of these diseases have been poorly understood and inadequately treated in the past, whereas some were never seen by rheumatologists because of the disease causing early death in childhood. However, with advancements in knowledge of basic science immunology and genetics, as well as diagnostic tools (eg, laboratory tests, imaging), these conditions are now readily identified. These advancements have resulted in an explosion of new treatments including "biologicals," which, unlike past medications, decrease inflammation by attacking specific targets in the immune system rather than causing broad immunosuppression with potentially more severe side effects on the body. The scenes from the twentieth-century pediatric rheumatology clinics of children in wheelchairs with severe musculoskeletal deformities affecting basic activities of daily living are largely gone. Indeed, the diagnosis of a rheumatic disease in a child today is no longer a sentence to a life with a severe physical disability or an early death. What they still experience; however, is a life with a chronic disease, most commonly without a promise of a cure, often with an unpredictable disease course despite the patient's and providers' best efforts.

DIFFICULTIES FOR YOUTH WITH PEDIATRIC RHEUMATIC DISEASES

The chronic nature and unpredictability of rheumatic disease course are features of PRDs that can be difficult for both the patient and their family to accept and can cause significant life disruption. As the disease often affects more than one organ, numerous organ-specific specialists are involved in care, causing numerous hospital visits and disruption of school life for children and work for parents. Patients' and families' reactions to the diagnosis may differ over time, as the child grows and family dynamics change. There may be denial at the time of the diagnosis, which can potentially lead to unnecessary harm from delaying treatment or interventions. Later, there may be a feeling of "defeat" when treatments were followed correctly, but the disease relapsed nonetheless, which can be detrimental to the patient/physician relationship and future compliance. Throughout a youth's disease journey, there are several concerns that are commonly seen and can obstruct management of PRDs.

Pharmacotherapy and Adherence

One of the mainstays of treating rheumatic conditions is the use of long-term pharmacotherapy such as disease-modifying antirheumatic drugs, immunosuppressive agents, or biological drugs to ameliorate symptoms.[2] Although these pharmacotherapies can halt disease process, medications must be regularly taken to be effective. Nonadherence to medications can lead to deleterious health outcomes and uncontrolled disease process and can be especially challenging for this population. Specifically, studies reviewing adherence rates to pharmacotherapy for JIA and SLE have described overall treatment adherence as inadequate.[3] Although nonadherence to PRD medications can occur due to a host of known and unknown reasons, researchers often describe forgetting medication, medication refusal, complexity of regimen, unwanted side-effects, perceived disease severity, lack of perceived benefit or loss of medication effect over time, cost, and access to care as potential explanations.[4–6]

Cognitive Impairment

Cognitive impairment is a common comorbidity in PRDs, which has a potential impact upon executive functions, memory, and concentration.[7–9] The pathogenic mechanisms leading to cognitive decline in individuals with rheumatic disease are unknown; however, there are several proposed factors including chronic systemic inflammatory process of disease, long-term use of glucocorticoid steroids, or chemotherapy agents such as methotrexate that may also have effects on the developing brain.[10] Executive functions are a particularly important factor when considering one's ability to remain adherent to medications and medical regimen, as well as an adolescents' ability to academically perform or engage in functional behavior.[11,12]

Pain Management

Pain is a symptom accompanying many PRDs that can debilitate normal life functioning and lead to distressed mood. Approximately 86% of youth with PRDs such as JIA are reported to experience pain.[13,14] Acute pain in PRDs is often related to local inflammation as part of the disease process. Although many youth with PRDs experience acute pain as part of the sequalae of active disease, they may also experience continued pain after the acute process is gone. Such is the case with chronic pain syndromes including amplified musculoskeletal pain syndrome (AMPS), in which youth who are in disease remission continue to experience pain without the presence of inflammatory process. Regardless of pain's etiology, many youth find pain to be functionally impairing and emotionally distressing, especially when pharmacotherapy treatments for their acute disease process are unable to provide relief. In fact, many of the medications that assist with inflammation and active disease process, such as biological drugs and immunosuppressive agents, are ineffective for chronic pain syndromes.[15,16] This can be a distressing situation for both families and providers as these medications are requested by families given their previous benefit, but are not appropriate for chronic pain management. Uncontrolled chronic pain despite inactive disease process can also lead to confusion, disrupted mood, and decreased functioning.[17]

Functional Disability

Youth with PRDs commonly experience increased functional disability and reduced quality of life (QoL) compared with healthy peers.[18,19] Functioning is especially impacted in youth with PRDs experiencing pain, who are found to be less likely to attend school, engage in sports, be physically active, or socially engage with their peers.[20–22] Such functional changes can have a compounding impact on youth. Although social support and engagement in physical activity is recommended to buffer the deleterious effects of chronic illness, youth who are unable to regularly attend school or engage in sports, groups, or other peer activities will have less social contact and may see peer support diminish.[23] Reduced functional behavior and socialization can lead to social isolation and peer rejection,[24] which may further impact mood and reinforce avoidance of social activities. In addition, reduced functioning and decreased use of joints and muscles can result in deconditioning, which can increase pain scores when youth with PRDs become more active, furthering the cycle of functional disability and impaired mood.[25]

Mood

Within patients who have rheumatic conditions, increased rates of anxiety and depression have been found when compared with healthy controls throughout the lifespan.[26] This impact upon mental health is apparent in youth. According to the Arthritis Foundation, almost two-thirds of youth with JIA reported having issues with anxiety, and almost half reported struggling with depression.[27] This is consistent with findings across PRDs, in which adolescents show higher rates of mental health disorders such as depression and anxiety than healthy peers.[28,29] Unfortunately, as symptoms of depression or anxiety worsen, youth with PRDs experience decreased health-related QoL and functional disability.[30,31] This can create a negative loop in which patients engage in less activity, experience increased pain, and subsequently develop feelings of sadness and helplessness.[32,33]

Mood impairments in PRDs are not solely triggered by functional disability and pain. Researchers have posited many reasons for why mood may be disrupted including the psychological burden of chronic illness, physical effects from disease damage, treatment-related side effects, and unpredictability of symptoms and disease course.[28,33,34] Illness uncertainty in particular is common among chronic illnesses and has a negative impact on coping, anxiety, and emotional adjustment.[35,36] As part of typical disease course, youth with PRDs often experience unpredictability of symptom flares and periods of quiescence, which can lead to feelings of lacking control of one's disease or uncertainty regarding management and outcome.

Changes in mood and functioning can also have a profound impact on families of youth with PRDs. In qualitative studies examining parents of youth with JIA, parents endorse confusion, emotional turmoil, guilt, worries, anger, helplessness, and frustration related to the disease and the process of caring for a child with JIA.[34,37] These emotions were often related to not understanding JIA, difficulty managing the disease, and feeling sorrow for their child's discomfort. Parents in these studies described how diseases such as JIA can impact the entire family unit and leave everyone feeling physically and emotionally drained. Even siblings of patients with JIA were noted to have difficulty understanding the illness, having difficult seeing their sibling in pain, and feeling frustrated or angry due to having less attention from their parents or less time together as an entire family.

INCLUSION OF PSYCHOLOGY IN INTERDISCIPLINARY CARE

Given the strong relationships between rheumatic conditions, disordered mood, and reduced QoL, it has been recommended that physicians treating patients with rheumatologic conditions integrate assessment and treatment of mood concerns into regular clinical practice.[38] One way this is conducted in pediatric rheumatology clinics is through the inclusion of a psychologist as part of an interdisciplinary team. In fact, there are many ways psychology has been integrated into treating the multifaceted concerns of youth with chronic illness.

Psychology's Role in Adherence

Psychologists are providers that can assist in leading interventions to improve treatment adherence in youth with PRDs. A combination of behavioral (eg, problem-solving, parent training) and educational (eg, providing instruction or teaching related to illness or treatment) interventions to improve adherence is recommended, as these have provided better health outcomes for patients with chronic illness.[39] Interventions that include social support, social skills training, family therapy, or other psychosocial targets may also be beneficial in improving adherence.[40] Psychologists can use these multicomponent interventions to target adherence to medication, physical activity recommendations, or other aspects of interdisciplinary care. In addition to these interventions, motivational interviewing is a patient-centered approach which focuses upon the patient's intrinsic motivation to change and a collaborative interaction style to help the patient understand their goals, reasons for change, and barriers.[41] A recent review of the literature suggests motivational interviewing appears to be a promising intervention to address nonadherence and improve QoL, and is well received by adolescents and young adults.[42] Psychologists may consider using motivational interviewing techniques to form a collaborative relationship with patients that allows for intrinsic change to improve adherence. A review of helpful and unhelpful motivational interviewing questions to assess adherence can be found within the practice implications of Schaefer and Kavookjian.[42]

Psychology's Role in Cognitive Decline

Pediatric neuropsychologists are frequently embedded within hospital systems to provide brief or comprehensive evaluations and diagnose cognitive and behavioral concerns related to a child's neurological profile. One way they can serve youth with PRDs is by offering neuropsychology testing to determine how neurological functioning may be impacted. Much like testing for late effects in cancer, baseline and repeat neuropsychological testing at age of onset, repeated during grade school, and college, can help determine cognitive impact or decline.[43] By identifying and addressing cognitive concerns, these psychologists can assist families in obtaining school accommodations and provide recommendations to help youth functional behavior. Identifying and addressing cognitive concerns can also help resolve barriers to adherence, subsequently leading to better disease management and improved QoL.

Psychology's Role in Pain Management

An often-unrecognized area in which psychologists can aid patients with PRDs is pain management. Pain is defined as both an emotional and physical process, regardless of etiology. Our current understanding of pain neuroscience describes our pain experience as a culmination of several parts of the brain, including our limbic system and emotional state.[44] The influence of emotional state, fear of pain, and the belief that pain can be controlled or changed are all aspects of youth's pain experience in which psychologists can help intervene. In both acute and chronic pain processes, psychologists can assist youth in learning relaxation and coping skills that calm the body's response to pain and reduce pain perception. Skills may include teaching diaphragmatic breathing, progressive muscle relaxation, imagery, meditation, or mindfulness strategies. Although these skills can reduce pain perception, they are also intended to serve as strategies that increase patients' self-efficacy for returning to functional activities. In the case of chronic pain conditions such as AMPS, psychologists can play multiple roles. As part of treatment, psychologists can teach skills to help patients find comfort while in pain and adjust to changes that have occurred in their life. A component of building self-efficacy related to managing chronic pain is education on chronic pain versus acute pain. With the assistance of a rheumatologist or other provider assessing disease progression, psychologists can help provide education upon how pain can persist despite having no active rheumatic disease process. Specifically, explaining sensitization of the nervous system and how, even though a child may still experience pain, chronic pain is not indicative of danger or harmful to their body. This explanation may allow patients to believe they have the ability to control aspects of their pain, subsequently reducing fear of pain and pain experience. As part of this education, providers should note that disruptions in mood do not cause pain, however, can influence and maintain chronic pain. In many pain conditions without obvious visible symptoms, such as AMPS or juvenile fibromyalgia, well-meaning providers invalidate patients by stating that pain is due to anxiety or "in the child's head." Proper psychoeducation on the relationship between pain and mood may reconcile some of these incorrect and invalidating remarks.

Psychology's Role in Functional Behavior

Consistent with the treatment of pain, pediatric psychologists can assist in improving functional behaviors by teaching youth coping skills and increasing their self-efficacy to improve functioning. These skills are intended to improve youths' management of both pain and mood, allowing for increased functioning. As previously mentioned, improving adherence can lead to decreased disease activity, decreasing pain, and allowing youth to engage in more functional behaviors.

Throughout a child's disease journey, families may have difficulties as they balance protecting their child from the outcomes of poor disease management while allowing their child to build medical self-efficacy and autonomy as a young adult. Although support and supervision of a child's medical regimen is frequently required, too much enmeshment and protectiveness can lead to negative outcomes.[45] Psychologists have the ability to assess family structure and dynamics, provide interventions that involve the entire family unit, and help teach caregivers how to respond to their children in ways that allow for promotion of functioning and management of their disease, rather than fostering the child's dependence on their parents. These strategies can include rewarding adherence and functional behaviors or encouraging steps toward independent disease management.

As these youth grow to become young adults with rheumatic disease, they continue to face many of the same challenges as during their adolescence, though often with less support. Psychologists can serve as part of the team assisting in transitioning pediatric patients to adult care by having frank discussions with families about the transition process, assessing for barriers and progress toward transition, and connecting families with social work for assistance with vocational and educational planning.

In addition to adjusting to general changes in life, psychologists are also equipped to assist youth in changes that occur socially. Psychologists can serve as a support system and guide youth who are navigating social changes or attempting to reintegrate into school or other peer activities. Part of this work can occur through teaching coping skills or using cognitive-behavioral therapy (CBT) to address worried thoughts or fears youth may have when returning to functional activities. For youth who have been away from their peers for long periods or feel they generally lack interpersonal skills, psychologists can work with them to develop scripts to explain their condition or absence, role play worrisome interactions, or teach social skills that may improve confidence.

Psychology's Role in Mood and Coping

At its core, the field of psychology is known for the treatment of mood concerns. When working with youth with rheumatic conditions, psychologists often apply therapies such as CBT to challenge unhelpful thinking patterns and assist patients in improving mood and functioning.[46] Within PRDs, CBT often focuses upon restructuring unhelpful thoughts about physical illness, encourages social and other functional activities, and prevents learned helplessness that can occur from disease unpredictability and has shown positive effects on QoL and mood.[47] Given the chronicity of rheumatic conditions, psychologists can help youth with adjustment to symptoms at different developmental phases and teach coping strategies to improve mood or functioning. Although these skills may not be expected to remove all symptoms that limit function, they can teach youth ways to better control their pain and improve self-efficacy in their own disease management. In the case of illness uncertainty, families often cite the lack of information about PRDs and treatment options as major concerns.[48] These concerns may be ameliorated by providing information about the pathophysiology and treatment of PRDs in the early stages of the disease process, as well as having a trained professional, such as a psychologist, help treat the emotional aspects of illness uncertainty.

SUMMARY

PRDs are a heterogeneous group of diseases which have similar characteristics of chronic, episodic, and unpredictable disease course that can greatly impact the patient and patient's family life in multiple areas of mood and functioning. Providers should consider psychosocial complexities as part of managing active disease process when working with youth with PRDs. Pediatric psychologists are well-equipped to assess cognitive impairment and emotional distress, and provide empirically based interventions addressing adherence to treatment, pain management, improving functional disability, and regulating mood. These interventions can then be adjusted and adapted to the unique needs of patients with PRDs depending on their ever-changing psychosocial functioning and disease course. Referring patients with PRDs to psychology can be part of regular holistic practice. Providers may also choose to integrate a pediatric psychologist into an interdisciplinary rheumatology clinic, allowing them to assess psychosocial concerns, jointly develop a conceptualization and plan with a rheumatologist, and provide a targeted intervention. Providing this style of comprehensive disease management can address the complex needs of patients with PRDs, help obtain favorable disease outcomes, and deliver quality care.

CLINICS CARE POINTS

- Integration of pediatric psychologist into interdisciplinary care for youth with pediatric rheumatic diseases (PRDs) can assist in addressing psychosocial concerns and holistic disease management.

- Early involvement of pediatric psychologists in the care of youth with PRDs can allow for monitoring and intervention throughout disease course and address problems that may occur at different stages of development.

- Psychological interventions should be adapted to a patient's unique psychosocial needs, functional impairments, disease trajectory, and age.

REFERENCES

1. Arthritis Foundation. News Blog. Juvenile Arthritis (JA). Available at: https://www.arthritis.org/diseases/juvenile-arthritis. Accessed January 28, 2021.
2. Cavallo S, Brosseau L, Toupin-April K, et al. Ottawa panel evidence-based clinical practice guidelines for structured physical activity in the management of juvenile idiopathic arthritis. Arch Phys Med Rehabil 2017;98(5):1018–41.
3. De Achaval S, Suarez-Almazor ME. Treatment adherence to disease-modifying antirheumatic drugs in patients with rheumatoid arthritis and systemic lupus erythematosus. Int J Clin Rheumtol 2010;5(3):313.

4. Favier LA, Taylor J, Rich KL, et al. Barriers to adherence in juvenile idiopathic arthritis: a multicenter collaborative experience and preliminary results. J Rheumatol 2018;45(5):690–6.

5. Pelajo CF, Sgarlat CM, Lopez-Benitez JM, et al. Adherence to methotrexate in juvenile idiopathic arthritis. Rheumatol Int 2012;32(2):497–500.

6. Rapoff MA. Adherence to pediatric medical regimens. 2nd edition. London: Springer; 2010.

7. Meade T, Manolios N, Cumming SR, et al. Cognitive impairment in rheumatoid arthritis: a systematic review. Arthritis Care Res 2018;70(1):39–52.

8. Oláh C, Schwartz N, Denton C, et al. Cognitive dysfunction in autoimmune rheumatic diseases. Arthritis Res Ther 2020;22(1):78.

9. Sood A, Raji MA. Cognitive impairment in elderly patients with rheumatic disease and the effect of disease-modifying anti-rheumatic drugs. Clin Rheumatol 2020; 40(4):1221–31.

10. Katchamart W, Narongroeknawin P, Phutthinart N, et al. Disease activity is associated with cognitive impairment in patients with rheumatoid arthritis. Clin Rheumatol 2019;38(7):1851–6.

11. Bagner DM, Williams LB, Geffken GR, et al. Type 1diabetes in youth: the relationship between adherence and executive functioning. Child Health Care 2007; 36(2):169–79.

12. Cortés Pascual A, Moyano Muñoz N, Quilez Robres A. The relationship between executive functions and academic performance in primary education: Review and meta-analysis. Front Psychol 2019;10:1582.

13. Arnstad ED, Rypdal V, Peltoniemi S, et al. Early self-reported pain in juvenile idiopathic arthritis as related to long-term outcomes: results from the Nordic Juvenile Idiopathic Arthritis Cohort Study. Arthritis Care Res 2019;71(7):961–9.

14. Bromberg MH, Connelly M, Anthony KK, et al. Self-reported pain and disease symptoms persist in juvenile idiopathic arthritis despite treatment advances: an electronic diary study. Arthritis Rheumatol 2014;66(2):462–9.

15. Howard RF, Wiener S, Walker SM. Neuropathic pain in children. Arch Dis Child 2014;99(1):84–9.

16. Palermo TM, Eccleston C, Lewandowski AS, et al. Randomized controlled trials of psychological therapies for management of chronic pain in children and adolescents: an updated meta-analytic review. Pain 2010;148(3):387–97.

17. Liossi C, Howard RF. Pediatric chronic pain: biopsychosocial assessment and formulation. Pediatrics 2016;138(5):e20160331.

18. Jones JT, Cunningham N, Kashikar-Zuck S, et al. Pain, fatigue, and psychological impact on health-related quality of life in childhood-onset lupus. Arthritis Care Res 2016;68(1):73–80.

19. Müller-Godeffroy E, Lehmann H, Küster RM, et al. Quality of life and psychosocial adaptation in children and adolescents with juvenile idiopathic arthritis and reactive arthritis. Z Rheumatol 2005;64(3):177–87.

20. Milatz F, Klotsche J, Niewerth M, et al. Participation in school sports among children and adolescents with juvenile idiopathic arthritis in the German National Paediatric Rheumatologic Database, 2000–2015: results from a prospective observational cohort study. Pediatr Rheumatol Online J 2019;17(1):1.

21. Limenis E, Grosbein HA, Feldman BM. The relationship between physical activity levels and pain in children with juvenile idiopathic arthritis. J Rheumatol 2014; 41(2):345–51.

22. Rebane K, Ristolainen L, Relas H, et al. Disability and health-related quality of life are associated with restricted social participation in young adults with juvenile idiopathic arthritis. Scand J Rheumatol 2019;48(2):105–13.

23. Bailey R. Physical education and sport in schools: a review of benefits and outcomes. J Sch Health 2006;76(8):397–401.

24. Kashikar-Zuck S, Lynch AM, Graham TB, et al. Social functioning and peer relationships of adolescents with juvenile fibromyalgia syndrome. Arthritis Rheum 2007;57(3):474–80.

25. Gualano B, Bonfa E, Pereira RMR, et al. Physical activity for paediatric rheumatic diseases: standing up against old paradigms. Nat Rev Rheumatol 2017;13(6): 368–79.

26. McWilliams LA, Clara IP, Murphy PD, et al. Associations between arthritis and a broad range of psychiatric disorders: findings from a nationally representative sample. J Pain 2008;9(1):37–44.

27. Arthritis Foundation. News Blog. Improving Mental Health for Kids with Juvenile Arthritis. Available at: http://blog.arthritis.org/news/improving-mental-health-kids-juvenile-arthritis/. Accessed December 6, 2021.

28. Fair DC, Rodriguez M, Knight AM, et al. Depression and anxiety in patients with juvenile idiopathic arthritis: current insights and impact on quality of life, a systematic review. Open Access Rheumatol 2019;11:237–52.

29. Knight A, Weiss P, Morales K, et al. Depression and anxiety and their association with healthcare utilization in pediatric lupus and mixed connective tissue disease patients: a cross-sectional study. Pediatr Rheumatol Online J 2014;12:42.

30. Donnelly C, Cunningham N, Jones JT, et al. Fatigue and depression predict reduced health-related quality of life in childhood-onset lupus. Lupus 2018; 27(1):124–33.

31. Hoff AL, Palermo TM, Schluchter M, et al. Longitudinal relationships of depressive symptoms to pain intensity and functional disability among children with disease-related pain. J Pediatr Psychol 2006;31(10):1046–56. https://doi.org/10.1093/jpepsy/jsj076.

32. Tarakci E, Yeldan I, Mutlu EK, et al. The relationship between physical activity level, anxiety, depression, and functional ability in children and adolescents with juvenile idiopathic arthritis. Clin Rheumatol 2011;30(11):1415–20.

33. El-Najjar AR, Negm MG, El-Sayed WM. The relationship between depression, disease activity and physical function in juvenile idiopathic arthritis patients in Zagazig University Hospitals–Egypt. Egypt. Rheumatol 2014;36(3):145–50.

34. Gómez-Ramírez O, Gibbon M, Berard R, et al. A recurring rollercoaster ride: a qualitative study of the emotional experiences of parents of children with juvenile idiopathic arthritis. Pediatr Rheumatol Online J 2016;14(1):13.

35. Johnson LM, Zautra AJ, Davis MC. The role of illness uncertainty on coping with fibromyalgia symptoms. Health Psychol 2006;25(6):696.

36. Van Pelt JC, Mullins LL, Carpentier MY, et al. Brief report: illness uncertainty and dispositional self-focus in adolescents and young adults with childhood-onset asthma. J Pediatr Psychol 2006;31(8):840–5.

37. Yuwen W, Lewis FM, Walker AJ, et al. Struggling in the dark to help my child: parents' experience in caring for a young child with juvenile idiopathic arthritis. J Pediatr Nurs 2017;37:e23–9.

38. Anyfanti P, Gavriilaki E, Pyrpasopoulou A, et al. Depression, anxiety, and quality of life in a large cohort of patients with rheumatic diseases: common, yet undertreated. Clin Rheumatol 2016;35(3):733–9.

39. Graves MM, Roberts MC, Rapoff M, et al. The efficacy of adherence interventions for chronically ill children: a meta-analytic review. J Pediatr Psychol 2010;35(4): 368–82.

40. Kahana S, Drotar D, Frazier T. Meta-analysis of psychological interventions to promote adherence to treatment in pediatric chronic health conditions. J Pediatr Psychol 2008;33(6):590–611.

41. Miller WR, Rollnick S. Motivational interviewing. New York: Guilford Press; 1991.

42. Schaefer MR, Kavookjian J. The impact of motivational interviewing on adherence and symptom severity in adolescents and young adults with chronic illness: a systematic review. Patient Educ Couns 2017;100(12):2190–9.

43. Annett RD, Patel SK, Phipps S. Monitoring and assessment of neuropsychological outcomes as a standard of care in pediatric oncology. Pediatr Blood Cancer 2015;62(Suppl 5):S460–513.

44. Bushnell MC, Ceko M, Low LA. Cognitive and emotional control of pain and its disruption in chronic pain. Nat Rev Neurosci 2013;14(7):502–11.

45. Hann-Moorrison D. Maternal enmeshment: the chosen child. SAGE Open 2012; 2(4). https://doi.org/10.1177/2158244012470115.

46. Butler AC, Chapman JE, Forman EM, et al. The empirical status of cognitive-behavioral therapy: a review of meta-analyses. Clin Psychol Rev 2006;26(1): 17–31.

47. Rubinstein TB, Davis AM, Rodriguez M, et al. Addressing mental health in pediatric rheumatology. Curr Treat Options Rheum 2018;4(1):55–72.

48. Pearce C, Newman S, Mulligan K. Illness uncertainty in parents of children with juvenile idiopathic arthritis. ACR Open Rheumatol 2021;3(4):250–9.

The Role of Psychologists in Sport Medicine Practice

Judy Jasser, MBBS*, Dilip R. Patel, MBBS, MBA, MPH, Katherine T. Beenen, PhD

KEYWORDS

- Pediatrics • Sport medicine • Multidisciplinary • Psychology • Mental health
- Psychological disorders • Integration

KEY POINTS

- Generally, sport participation serves as a protective factor against some mental health problems but may put athletes at increased risk for the development of others.
- Sport-related psychological concerns may come to the attention of treating physicians in several ways.
- Integrating psychologists into sport medicine clinics confers several benefits to patients, such as improving psychological screenings, promoting healthy sport involvement, problem-solving related to health-related behaviors and treatment adherence, and provision of brief, problem-focused psychological intervention to young athletes.

INTRODUCTION

There has been increased awareness of athletes' mental health following media coverage of high-profile athletes who cited mental health concerns in their withdrawal from major sporting events as well as athletes who have described the long-term psychological effects after team doctors sexually abused them. Events like these underscore that even the most successful elite athletes are not immune from psychological distress. Athletes have a comparable risk of psychological disorders relative to that of the general population.[1] However, sport participation presents different stressors that may uniquely contribute to increased risk for mental health problems. For example, this risk is increased for athletes experiencing performance difficulty, sustained physical injury, or facing retirement from the sport.[2,3]

Unsurprisingly, better access to psychological services by athletes, coaches, trainers, and administrators facilitates athletes' engagement in these services.[4] One important way to improve access is the integration of psychologists into sport medicine clinics. There is strong evidence that integrating psychological and physical

Department of Pediatric and Adolescent Medicine, Western Michigan University, Homer Stryker M.D. School of Medicine, 1000 Oakland Drive, Kalamazoo, MI 49008, USA
* Corresponding author.
E-mail address: Judy.Jasser@med.wmich.edu

Pediatr Clin N Am 69 (2022) 975–988
https://doi.org/10.1016/j.pcl.2022.05.010
0031-3955/22/© 2022 Elsevier Inc. All rights reserved.
pediatric.theclinics.com

health care improves patient outcomes, but universal uptake is lacking.[5,6] Psychologists play an important role in multidisciplinary pediatric sport medicine teams in managing the mental health aspects of sport participation for youth, including identifying and treating psychological concerns and promoting health-related behaviors. The author first review some of the common behavioral issues that young athletes face, then discuss how physicians and psychologists may work together to manage these conditions.

PSYCHOLOGICAL AND BEHAVIORAL CONCERNS IN YOUTH SPORT PARTICIPATION
Internalizing Disorders (Anxiety, Depression, and Suicide)

The prevalence of anxiety disorders in adolescents ranges widely, from 6% to 20% of adolescents.[7] For young athletes, anxiety manifests differently based on an individual's characteristics and those of their chosen sport. For example, an athlete with underlying social anxiety may have a greater physical and mental health burden if they participate in a team sport or one with many spectators like basketball, as opposed to an individual event with fewer spectators like long-distance running. Young athletes may experience performance-related anxiety ranging from mild to severe, with or without accompanying functional impairment. In some cases, anxiety may even serve a facilitative effect by enhancing performance, such as increasing the likelihood the athlete will engage in preparatory activities before the performance and heightening their senses during the performance.

In the case of debilitative anxiety, young athletes may have maladaptive or negative thoughts before the competition about their ability to perform to some standard. In post-competition anxiety, an athlete experiences distressing thoughts related to their evaluation of their performance.[8] Most athletes seek help for anxiety when it impairs their performance. Post-performance anxiety, though potentially less likely to inhibit performance, is nevertheless distressing but rarely comes to clinical attention and, therefore, may go unaddressed.

There is a complex relationship between sport participation and depression. Participation may increase the risk for a major depressive disorder (MDD) but also can serve a protective role against its development.[9,10] The mechanism by which sport participation may increase the risk of depression and even suicidality is poorly understood but may be influenced by sport-related psychological stressors. In one study, being female, a freshman, or experiencing pain was associated with greater endorsement of depression. Furthermore, overtraining and experiencing sport-related injuries were additional correlates of depression, and, to a lesser extent, competitive failure, aging, and retirement from the sport.[11]

The mechanism for sport's protective role against MDD is better understood and relates to the increase in physical activity, social support, and self-esteem that can accompany participation.[12–15] On a biological level, physical activity increases the secretion of endogenous endorphins, neurotransmitters that act on the opioid receptors to increase feelings of pleasure and well-being and to reduce pain and discomfort. In nonathletes, exercise is often recommended as a treatment of MDD, along with psychotherapy and medication.[16]

For athletes experiencing depressive symptoms, assessment for suicidal ideation should be a routine practice. In Baum's review of athletes who have contemplated, attempted, or completed suicide, the high completion rate points to the importance of recognizing and managing mood disorders early on.[11,17] Participation specifically in football and basketball is associated with greater suicide risk, due in part to higher rates of injury in these sport. Other risk factors for suicide are listed in **Box 1**.[17]

Box 1
Risk factors for suicide in athletes

- Substance abuse
- Postretirement
- Eating disorders
- Sport-related injury (particularly if significant)
- Anabolic steroid use
- Family history of suicide
- Homosexuality and sexual abuse (including sexual abuse by coaches)

Use of Alcohol and Performance-Enhancing Agents

There is an increased rate of substance abuse in athletes compared with the general population. Athletes may use different substances to enhance their performance or help them cope with stress related to sport participation, whether it is due to overtraining, performance anxiety, or coping with a sport-related injury. A wide range of substances may be abused by athletes, with the most common being alcohol, anabolic steroid (ie, testosterone and its derivatives), growth hormone (GH), and stimulants (cocaine, amphetamine, and caffeine).[11,18–20]

It is important to address this topic because of its multiple consequences. In addition to its effect on the preservation of fair play and competition, its negative effects on health can put athletes at significant risk of danger. For example, excessive alcohol use can lead to loss of coordination that is essential in some sport like gymnastics. Other consequences of alcohol include its high association with other performance-enhancing drugs and psychiatric illness. Some athletes use anabolic steroids to increase their training performance and shorten recovery times.[21] Some athletes also use types of steroids (referred as "designer steroids") that are not identified by routine laboratory testing.[11] Anabolic steroids are associated with anxiety, manic symptoms, depression, and suicide.[22–25] GH improves the aerobic exercise capacity of the body.[26–28] GH increases the lean body mass and decreases the body fat contents.[28] Excessive use of GH can lead to hypertrophy of the bone and soft tissues of the face and tongue, causing abnormal facial characteristics and macroglossia.[28,29] It can also lead to edema and hypertrophy of the airways' soft tissue, which can lead to sleep apnea. Other systematic side effects of GH use include increased glucose and lipid levels. It can also induce hypertension and cause other cardiac effects, such as arrhythmias, valve disorders, and cardiomyopathy in severe cases.[28,29]

Overtraining Syndrome

Overtraining syndrome (OTS) is a chronic maladaptive condition resulting from excessive, prolonged training with no adequate recovery time.[30] The mechanism underlying OTS remains unknown; however, it has been postulated that OTS and MDD share similar etiology and manifestations in terms of signs and symptoms, neurotransmitter abnormalities, immune responses, and responsible endocrine pathways.[31–34] This shared similarity between OTS and MDD can often make it difficult to distinguish between the two.

Clinically, OTS and MDD may present with sleep disturbance, persistent fatigue, appetite and weight change, and decreased concentration.[11] The denial and stigmatization of mental illness in athletes might lead to a tendency to diagnose OTS in athletes who present with identical symptoms that would have been diagnosed as MDD in the nonathlete patient.[35-37]

Psychologists can help to distinguish between the two conditions through detailed history-taking and validated assessment measures. The main difference between OTS and MDD is the type of dysfunction present: social, cognitive, and work performance impairment in case of MDD, and athletic performance impairment in the case of OTS.[37] Furthermore, some of the physiological alterations that are present only in OTS include hormonal changes, increased blood pressure and heart rate, and muscle pain.[38,39] One of the main psychological differences is that temporary cessation of training usually leads to mood improvement in patients with OTS. However, training cessation, even if temporary, often leads to a worsening mood in those with MDD.

Eating Disorders

Eating disorders (EDs) are prevalent psychiatric disorders in the athletic population.[40] EDs are a group of psychiatric illnesses characterized by preoccupation with food and body weight or shape.[41] These preoccupations drive the patient to practice certain behaviors that help them temporarily alleviate their preoccupations. Behaviors may include excessive calorie restriction in anorexia nervosa and excessive exercising, inducement of vomiting, passive (eg, sauna, hot baths) or active dehydration (eg, exercise with sweat suits), or use of diuretics or laxatives in bulimia nervosa. With time, this has a serious impact on the physical, psychological, and social functioning of pediatric athletes.[42] EDs typically first emerge during adolescence and are more commonly identified in female patients.[43] EDs can affect athletic performance both physically and psychologically. For example, the electrolyte and other metabolic abnormalities seen in patients with anorexia nervosa prohibit them from participating in strenuous sport activities. In addition, the associated mood and anxiety symptoms often affect their ability to participate in sport. EDs are often comorbid with other psychiatric disorders.

Identifying athletes with abnormal eating behaviors and providing early intervention is crucial to preventing the progression of these behaviors to ED.[44] Nattiv and *colleagues* discussed the risk factors for the development of ED and classified them into three main categories: (1) predisposing factors that increase the risk for developing this disorder, (2) trigger factors that set off the disease in predisposed people, and (3) perpetuating factors that maintain these behaviors. **Table 1** includes some examples of these risk factors.[44]

The Female Athlete Triad

The female athlete triad (FAT) is common among young women participating in sport and is a condition that can have significant short-term and long-term sequelae on the

Table 1 Risk factors for development of eating disorders	
Predisposing Factors	Biological: Genetic, age, gender Psychological: Low self-esteem, body dissatisfaction, personality trait as perfectionism Sociocultural factors: Media influence and history of bullying
Trigger factors	Participation in a sport requiring leanness, sport-related injury, negative comments regarding body weight or shape by the coach
Perpetuating factors	Approval by the coach or team members, ability to achieve success with weight changes

well-being of youth. FAT consists of low energy availability (differentiating it from EDs), menstrual dysfunction, and decreased bone mineral density.[45] FAT can present along a continuum of symptom severity for each of these three components and is associated with negative health consequences.[45] Energy deficiency can be caused by an inability to provide the body with the caloric intake that is needed for the rigorous physical activities performed by athletes. This can be due to certain dietary lifestyles or behaviors such as food restriction, veganism, purging, or use of laxatives. It has recently been proposed that the term "Female Athlete Triad" be replaced with "Relative Energy Deficiency in Sport", a more comprehensive term that includes various impaired physiologic functions that can also be inclusive of male athletes.[46]

Sport-Related Injury

The protective relationship between sport participation and depression, anxiety, and suicidality is well-established. However, sport-related injury can affect the mental health of an athlete on the short-term and long-term level.[47,48] The psychological response to injury depends on many factors (**Box 2**).[49–54] Most children and adolescents cope well with sport-related injury and transient inability to continue participation in sport. Most realize that their injury heals in time, and they are able to resume sport participation. Some athletes may welcome the special attention given to them during rehabilitation; for example, some may take pride in having a cast signed by friends. However, a small percentage of children and adolescents may find it difficult to adjust and may manifest anger, frustration and a depressed mood following injury. Late adolescent athletes in highly competitive or elite level sport may go through emotional stages similar to other losses, beginning with disbelief, denial, and isolation, followed in succession by anger, bargaining, depression, and acceptance and resignation.[49–54] However, for most children and adolescents, the progression from denial to recovery is of short duration. For athletes who do not recover as expected, further assessment is indicated to find complicating factors such as underlying depression, fear and anxiety, secondary gain, or conflicts with parents.

Management of parental anxiety within the context of their injured child can be challenging. Parents should be helped to understand the implications of injury on future sport participation and the emotional reactions of the athlete. Pediatricians play an important role in helping athletes and parents during this period by recognizing potential problems, having realistic expectations, and not yielding to external pressures to

---

Box 2
Factors influencing psychological response to sport-related injury

Emotional maturity of the child or adolescent

Severity and type of the injury

Extent to which the injury will limit sport participation

Individual pain tolerance

Ability to cope

Personal motivation

One's place on the team

Seasonal timing

Context of the injury

Support from family and others

return athlete prematurely to sport. The pediatrician should consult a psychologist who can help the athlete with behavioral techniques during the rehabilitation process.

CLINICAL APPROACH TO PREVENTION AND EARLY IDENTIFICATION

Pre-participation physicals and well or health maintenance visits all present physicians and psychologists with an opportunity to present sport-related anticipatory guidance that will promote mental well-being and foster healthy competition. Potential topics are included in **Box 3**.[55–66]

Recent guidance from the National Collegiate Athletic Association stipulates that mental health screening should occur as early as pre-participation physicals.[67] Annual check-ups present another routine opportunity for screening, as do visits related to a specific presenting concern. For example, in the case of the patient coming to clinical attention for a sport-related injury, the team should consider the psychological burden that this event might induce. Screening for psychological distress should be done at the time of treating the primary event and during any follow-up visits. In this example, assessing whether there has been a change in the youth's psychological or behavioral functioning is crucial.

Box 3
Sport-related anticipatory guidance

- Readiness for competitive sport depends on a child's developmental stage, sociocultural environment, parental attitudes, as well as skills and demands required of a particular sport. The desire to compare skills to others develops by age 6 to 7 years; cognitive understanding of the social and competitive nature of sport is developed by age 8 to 9 years. Not all psychological skills needed for competitive sport may be achieved before age 11 or 12 years.

- It is difficult to identify specific athletic talents in a child with any certainty. Because of multiple variables (genetics, effects of growth, and development) involved, it is challenging to reliably predict future athletic excellence.

- Students who are involved in co-curricular activities, including sport (and others such as, debate, music, voluntary activities, and student governing), also generally do well in academics. Academic failure should not be the sole reason to not to allow the athlete to continue participation.

- Know the primary goal of the youth sport program before enrolling. Be sure it matches with the child's readiness as well as the purpose of participation.

- Be aware of the coaching style and philosophy. Win at all cost attitudes do not lead to the best outcome from sport. Be involved and do not abandon your parental role nor abdicate all control to the coach.

- Only a handful of children and adolescents ever make it to the elite or professional level. Nurture realistic expectations. Avoid the temptation of using sport to achieve other goals (for example, scholarships, financial gain, fame, and social status).

- Children and adolescents with chronic disease, and physically or mentally challenging conditions should be appropriately matched to sport activities they can participate in. This will have great physical and psychological benefits.

- Sport participation can be beneficial or detrimental depending up on the child's experience. Whether the experience is positive or negative depends on the involved adults and societal attitudes and goals.

- Early intensive participation in sport and sport specialization does not necessarily guarantee future athletic success. Exposure to multiple sport and activities is desirable and recommended.

After obtaining a routine psychosocial history and mental status examination, focused questions related to sport participation can be used (**Box 4**).[68–77] The overall goal of this assessment is to determine whether the problem is related to sport participation or there is an underlying concern presented in the context of athletic activity.

In addition to informal screening and considerations, there are several published and validated screening measures appropriate for the use with pediatric and collegiate-level athletes.[78] Psychologists are competent in the selection, administration, scoring, and interpretation of appropriate screeners for a chosen population.[79] Psychologists' involvement in psychosocial screenings at routine visits introduces them to the patient early and establishes their role as important team members to whom the patient (and parent) may turn in the future with specific concerns.

There are times when a comprehensive psychological evaluation by a psychologist may be appropriate. This may be the case if psychological symptoms are causing

---

Box 4
Sport-related psychosocial screening

Does the athlete or parents have a specific sport-related concern?

Does the athlete participate in organized sport or plays recreationally?

What is the level of participation? How many hours per week? Does the athlete often travel away from home for games or special training?

How is the athlete doing in school? Does he or she participate in any non-sport activities?

Does the athlete have any professional sport hero? Does the athlete aspire to be like him or her?

Do parents or the coach exert undue pressure on the athlete to participate or perform?

Who wants the athlete to participate and why?

Is sport the sole focus to the exclusion of other activities?

Do parents or the athlete perceive he or she is overinvolved or underinvolved in sport?

Why does the athlete want to participate in sport?

Why do parents want the athlete to participate in sport?

How important is winning to the athlete, the parents, and the coach?

How do athletes and parents handle a win or a loss?

What do the athlete and parents know about the philosophy of the coach, team, or the program in which the athlete participates?

Is the athlete exempted from other responsibilities because of his or her status as an athlete? Is he or she asked to share the expenses of sport participation?

Is the athlete compared with athletic siblings? Or is he or she the last hope for the family to achieve athletic success?

Do parents like to participate in sport? Were they involved as children? Have they expressed any unfulfilled wishes for athletic achievement?

What do parents think of the opposing team's coach? Parents? Fans?

Has a parent (or parents) been barred from attending the game? Have they been involved in fights with other parents or a coach?

Have parents made an excessive financial commitment to sport? Have they moved to a new location, or have the athlete moved to participate in sport?

significant distress and/or impairment to the young athlete, on or off the field (eg, to interpersonal relationships or academic performance). In addition, patients presenting with a concussion from a sport-related injury may experience changes to their psychosocial and neuropsychological functioning. Psychologists have expertise in clinical interviewing, administration of standardized assessment measures (eg, intellectual, educational, adaptive, personality, social-emotional, memory, and perception), case conceptualization, differential diagnosis, effective written and oral communication of findings, and provision of treatment recommendations. A psychologist serving on a sport medicine team may draw on any number of these competencies in their evaluation of patients and, in some more complex cases, may refer the patient to a provider with more advanced skills in neuropsychological assessment.

CLINICAL APPROACH TO MANAGEMENT

The NCAA, in its recent guidance, advised that mental health services be accessible to athletes.[67] Integrating psychology into a multidisciplinary team improves patients' access to effective interventions.[80] If psychologists have been actively involved in routine psychosocial screening, they will already be known to the patient. Thus, early involvement increases psychologists' visibility as core members of the treating team and reduces the stigma associated with seeking psychological services. This is important for athletes who may face unique barriers in their pursuit of mental health treatment from non-athletes. For example, those engaged in contact or individual sport are less likely to seek support, as are athletes with coaches who emphasize toughness and self-reliance. Moreland and *colleagues*[4] offer a full review of facilitators and barriers to college athletes' behaviors toward seeking mental health services.

Psychologists' more traditional role in treating psychological disorders is likely well-known to the reader. There are several evidence-based interventions that psychologists use with children and adolescents. Some of these are included in **Table 2**. Psychologists in these clinics should have expertise in adapting the underlying principles of evidence-based therapies to fit into a brief, problem-focused therapy model that fits into an integrated clinic. In the case of more severe or impairing psychological disorders (eg, EDs, suicidality), psychologists will help connect the athlete with appropriate referrals outside of the sport medicine clinic (eg, multidisciplinary EDs clinic, and partial hospitalization program). Psychologists may also serve a role in return-to-play guidance following a major psychological event.[80]

Importantly, the psychologist's role on a sport medicine team is not only limited to the identification and management of psychological disorders. Psychologists also have a crucial role in facilitating patient health-related behaviors to help in injury recovery and performance enhancement, as well as other issues pertaining to young athletes. This may include compliance to medical regimens through psychological interventions.[81]

For example, in the case of a sport-related injury, psychologists work with the patient to educate them on their condition and medical plan, if appropriate, work with the caregivers on age-appropriate expecations in the management of their condition and engage in problem-solving and individualized planning to promote the adherence to their physicians' treatment recommendations. They are also well-suited to delivering the brief cognitive-behavioral interventions identified in one recent meta-analysis as crucial to the prevention of injury or re-injury.[82]

Psychologists are well-versed in systemic considerations, operating from a biopsychosocial viewpoint. As such, they may advise athletes on other areas of functioning. For pediatric patients, one important area is educational functioning. To use

Table 2
Evidence-based interventions in the management of mental health concerns

Intervention	Description
Acceptance and Commitment Therapy	Teaches patients how to change the relationship between thoughts and feelings through mindfulness, acceptance, and commitment to values
Cognitive-Behavioral Therapy	Develops awareness of the interconnection between thoughts, behaviors, and feelings; skill-building approach to coping through changing unhelpful thoughts and behaviors
Dialectical Behavior Therapy	Skill building to reduce emotional and behavioral dysregulation through coping skills and problem-solving
Family Therapy	Improves communication among family members
Interpersonal Psychotherapy	Skill building to improve interpersonal relationships
Modeling and Exposure-Based Protocols	Therapist demonstrates a non-fearful response to the patient's anxiety-inducing stimuli; in exposures, the patient practices engaging with anxiety-inducing stimuli (often in a gradual manner) until anxiety reduces
Motivational Interviewing	Reduces ambivalence and improves motivation to acknowledge problems and engage in treatment
Organizational Skills Training	Teaches organization, time-management, and planning skills.

the concussion as an example, psychologists can have a role in creating a plan for school re-entry and educational accommodations. They may assist a physician in crafting a letter of academic accommodation and educating the patient and their caregiver on communicating with the school.[83] For the student-athlete struggling with academic performance and facing possible probation, a few sessions focusing on organization, study habits, and test-taking skills could be beneficial.

DISCUSSION

Awareness of the psychological issues facing young athletes is insufficient without access to detection and early intervention.[84] For many athletes experiencing mental health problems associated with sport participation, treatment by a qualified psychologist can help reduce distress and restore functioning on and off the field. Psychologists may offer short-term, targeted interventions specific to the challenges this population faces. Psychologists integrated into sport medicine clinics have specific proficiencies including, but not limited to, developmental and social issues related to sport participation, assessment and counseling for psychological issues related to participation, skills training for performance enhancement, and biobehavioral bases of sport and exercise.[85] Psychologists may furthermore draw on their general proficiencies in screening, detection, early intervention, and promotion of health-related behaviors to serve as important members of multidisciplinary sport medicine teams.

SUMMARY

In addition to maintaining physical wellness, there must also be attention to athletes' mental health to maintain productivity in their sport performance. Increasing awareness of sport-related psychological stressors and improving access to early screening, identification, and intervention are important for all young athletes. Failure to do so might lead to progressive negative impacts on multiple aspects of pediatric athletes. Sport psychology is an integral part of the medical management of such disorders and offers safe and effective non-pharmacologic measures.

CLINICS CARE POINTS

- Recognizing the occult signs of internalizing disorders (anxiety, depression, and suicide) and substance abuse in athletes is of extreme clinical significance. Continuous screening by the treating clinicians allows for early interventions that can prevent hazardous complications and maintain sport performance.
- The role of the psychologist in pediatrics sport clinics is complementary to the role of the treating clinician. Integration of sport-oriented psychology practice is of certain positive impact on patients' outcomes.

DISCLOSURE

The authors have nothing to disclose.

REFERENCES

1. Gouttebarge V, Castaldelli-Maia JM, Gorczynski P, et al. Occurrence of mental health symptoms and disorders in current and former elite athletes: a systematic review and meta-analysis. Br J Sports Med 2019;53(11):700–6.
2. Rice SM, Purcell R, De Silva S, et al. The mental health of elite athletes: a narrative systematic review. Sports Med 2016;46(9):1333–53.
3. Gouttebarge V, Jonkers R, Moen M, et al. The prevalence and risk indicators of symptoms of common mental disorders among current and former Dutch elite athletes. J SportsSci 2017;35(21):2148–56.
4. Moreland JJ, Coxe KA, Yang J. Collegiate athletes' mental health services utilization: A systematic review of conceptualizations, operationalizations, facilitators, and barriers. J SportHealthSci 2018;7(1):58–69.
5. Asarnow JR, et al. Integrated medical-behavioral care compared with usual primary care for child and adolescent behavioral health: a meta-analysis. JAMAPediatr 2015;169(10):929–37.
6. Kolko DJ, Campo J, Kilbourne AM, et al. Collaborative care outcomes for pediatric behavioral health problems: a cluster randomized trial. Pediatrics 2014;133(4):e981–92.
7. Beesdo K, Knappe S, Pine DS. Anxiety and anxiety disorders in children and adolescents: developmental issues and implications for DSM-V. PsychiatrClin North Am 2009;32(3):483–524.
8. Patel DR, Omar H, Terry M. Sport-related performance anxiety in young female athletes. J PediatrAdolescGynecol 2010;23(6):325–35.
9. Payne JM, Kirchner JT. Should you suspect the female athlete triad? J FamPract 2014;63(4):187–92.
10. Panza MJ, Graupensperger S, Agans JP, et al. Adolescent sport participation and symptoms of anxiety and depression: a systematic review and meta-analysis. J SportExercPsychol 2020;1(18):1–18.
11. Reardon CL, Factor RM. Sport psychiatry: a systematic review of diagnosis and medical treatment of mental illness in athletes. Sports Med 2010;40(11):961–80.

12. Babiss LA, Gangwisch JE. Sports participation as a protective factor against depression and suicidal ideation in adolescents as mediated by self-esteem and social support. J DevBehavPediatr 2009;30(5):376–84.

13. Paykel ES. Life events, social support and depression. ActaPsychiatrScandSuppl 1994;377:50–8.

14. Potts MK. Social support and depression among older adults living alone: the importance of friends within and outside of a retirement community. SocWork 1997;42(4):348–62.

15. Werner-Seidler A, Afzali MH, Chapman C, et al. The relationship between social support networks and depression in the 2007 National Survey of Mental Health and Well-being. SocPsychiatryPsychiatrEpidemiol 2017;52(12):1463–73.

16. Kvam S, Kleppe CL, Nordhus IH, et al. Exercise as a treatment for depression: a meta-analysis. J AffectDisord 2016;202:67–86.

17. Baum AL. Suicide in athletes: a review and commentary. ClinSports Med 2005; 24(4):853–69, ix.

18. Reyes-Vallejo L. Current use and abuse of anabolic steroids. ActasUrolEsp(Engl Ed) 2020;44(5):309–13.

19. Garner AA, Hansen AA, Baxley C, et al. The Use of stimulant medication to treat attention-deficit/hyperactivity disorder in elite athletes: a performance and health perspective. Sports Med 2018;48(3):507–12.

20. Jones AR, Pichot JT. Stimulant use in sports. Am J Addict 1998;7(4):243–55.

21. McDuff DR, Baron D. Substance use in athletics: a sports psychiatry perspective. ClinSports Med 2005;24(4):885–97, ix-x.

22. Franey DG, Espiridion ED. Anabolic steroid-induced Mania. Cureus 2018;10(8): e3163.

23. Kanayama G, Hudson JI, Pope HG Jr. Long-term psychiatric and medical consequences of anabolic-androgenic steroid abuse: a looming public health concern? Drug Alcohol Depend 2008;98(1–2):1–12.

24. Piacentino D, Kotzalidis GD, Del Casale A, et al. Anabolic-androgenic steroid use and psychopathology in athletes. A systematic review. CurrNeuropharmacol 2015;13(1):101–21.

25. Talih F, Fattal O, Malone D Jr. Anabolic steroid abuse: psychiatric and physical costs. CleveClin J Med 2007;74(5):341–4.

26. Holt RI. Detecting growth hormone abuse in athletes. Drug Test Anal 2009; 1(9–10):426–33.

27. Holt RIG, Ho KKY. The use and abuse of growth hormone in sports. Endocr Rev 2019;40(4):1163–85.

28. Siebert DM, Rao AL. The use and abuse of human growth hormone in sports. Sports Health 2018;10(5):419–26.

29. Vilar L, Vilar CF, Lyra R, et al. Acromegaly: clinical features at diagnosis. Pituitary 2017;20(1):22–32.

30. Armstrong LE, VanHeest JL. The unknown mechanism of the overtraining syndrome: clues from depression and psychoneuroimmunology. Sports Med 2002; 32(3):185–209.

31. Hanna EA. Potential sources of anxiety and depression associated with athletic competition. Can J ApplSportSci 1979;4(3):199–204.

32. Morgan WP, Brown DR, Raglin JS, et al. Psychological monitoring of overtraining and staleness. Br J Sports Med 1987;21(3):107–14.

33. O'Connor PJ, Morgan WP, Raglin JS. Psychobiologic effects of 3 d of increased training in female and male swimmers. Med SciSportsExerc 1991;23(9):1055–61.

34. Puffer JC, McShane JM. Depression and chronic fatigue in athletes. ClinSports Med 1992;11(2):327–38.
35. Noakes TD. Denial of mental illness in athletes. Br J Sports Med 2000;34(4):315.
36. Saks ER. Some thoughts on denial of mental illness. Am J Psychiatry 2009; 166(9):972–3.
37. Schwenk TL. The stigmatisation and denial of mental illness in athletes. Br J Sports Med 2000;34(1):4–5.
38. Callister R, Callister RJ, Callister R, et al. Physiological and performance responses to overtraining in elite judo athletes. Med Sci Sports Exerc 1990;22(6): 816–24.
39. Hackney AC, Pearman SN, Nowacki JM. Physiological profiles of overtrained and stale athletes: a review. J ApplSportPsychol 1990;2(1):21–33.
40. Bradley SL, Reardon CL. Bipolar disorder and eating disorders in sport: a case of comorbidity and review of treatment principles in an elite athlete. PhysSportsmed 2021;1–8.
41. Campbell K, Peebles R. Eating disorders in children and adolescents: state of the art review. Pediatrics 2014;134(3):582–92.
42. Martínez-Sánchez SM, Martínez-García C, Martínez-García TE, et al. Psychopathology, body image and quality of life in female children and adolescents with anorexia nervosa: a pilot study on the acceptability of a pilates program. Front Psychiatry 2020;11(503274).
43. Ranalli DN, Studen-Pavlovich D. Eating disorders in the adolescent patient. DentClin North Am 2021;65(4):689–703.
44. Bratland-Sanda S, Sundgot-Borgen J. Eating disorders in athletes: overview of prevalence, risk factors and recommendations for prevention and treatment. Eur J SportSci 2013;13(5):499–508.
45. Nazem TG, Ackerman KE. The female athlete triad. Sports Health 2012;4(4): 302–11.
46. Mountjoy M, Sundgot-Borgen J, Burke L, et al. The IOC consensus statement: beyond the Female Athlete Triad–Relative Energy Deficiency in Sport (RED-S). Br J Sports Med 2014;48(7):491–7.
47. Covassin T, Beidler E, Ostrowski J, et al. Psychosocial aspects of rehabilitation in sports. ClinSports Med 2015;34(2):199–212.
48. Leddy J, Baker JG, Haider MN, et al. A physiological approach to prolonged recovery from sport-related concussion. J Athl Train 2017;52(3):299–308.
49. Smith AD. Rehabilitation of children following sport and activity-related injuries. In: Bar-Or O, editor. The child and adolescent athlete. Cambridge, MA: Blackwell Science Ltd; 1996. p. 224–39.
50. Ahern DK, Lohr BA. Psychosocial factors in sports injury rehabilitation. ClinSports Med 1997;16(4):755–68.
51. Heil J. Psychology of sport injury. Psychology of sport injury. Champaign, IL, England: Human Kinetics Publishers; 1993. p. xiv, 338.
52. Putukian M. The psychological response to injury in student athletes: a narrative review with a focus on mental health. Br J Sports Med 2016;50(3):145–8.
53. Smith AM. Psychological impact of injuries in athletes. Sports Med 1996;22(6): 391–405.
54. Smoll F, Smith R. Competitive anxiety: sources, consequences, and intervention strategies. Child youth Sport ABiopsychosocial Perspective 1996;359–80.
55. Agel J, Post E. Early sport specialization. JBoneJointSurg Am 2021;103(20): 1948–57.

56. Begel D, Burton R. Sport psychiatry: theory and practice. New York: Norton Professional Books; 2000.
57. Brenner JS, LaBotz M, Sugimoto D, et al. The psychosocial implications of sport specialization in pediatric athletes. J Athl Train 2019;54(10):1021–9.
58. Ewing M, Seefeldt V, Brown T. Role of organized sport in the education and health of American children and youth. East Lansing: Michigan State University. Institute for the Study of Youth Sports; 1996.
59. Micheli L, et al. Sports and children: consensus statement on organised sports for children. Bull WorldHealth Organ 1998;76(5):445–7.
60. Patel DR, Greydanus DE. Sport participation by physically and cognitively challenged young athletes. PediatrClin 2010;57(3):795–817.
61. Patel DR, Greydanus DE, Pratt HD. Youth sports: more than sprains and strains. ContempPediatr 2001;18(3):45.
62. Patel DR, Luckstead EF. Sport participation, risk taking, and health risk behaviors. Adolesc Med 2000;11(1):141–55.
63. Patel DR, Pratt HD, Greydanus DE. Pediatric neurodevelopment and sports participation: When are children ready to play sports? PediatrClin 2002;49(3): 505–31.
64. Patel DR, Soares N, Wells K. Neurodevelopmental readiness of children for participation in sports. Translational Pediatr 2017;6(3):167.
65. Pratt HD PD, Greydanus DE. Child and adolescent neurodevelopment and sport participation. In: De Lee JC DD, Miller MD, editors. Orthopedic sports medicine. Philadelphia: W. B. Saunders; 2004. p. 624–42.
66. Sullivan JA. Care of the young athlete. Rosemont, IL: Amer Academy of Pediatrics; 2000.
67. NCAA. Inter-association consensus document: best practices for understanding and supporting student-athlete mental wellness. 2016. Available at: https://ncaaorg.s3.amazonaws.com/ssi/mental/SSI_MentalHealthBestPractices.pdf.
68. Hellstedt J. Invisible players: a family systems model. In: Murphy SM, editor. Sport psychology interventions, 5. Champaign: Human Kinetics; 1995.
69. Horn, T.S., Advances in sport psychology. 2008: Human kinetics.
70. Jellinek MS, Knapp PK, Drell MJ, et al. The "achievement by proxy" spectrum: Recognition and clinical response to pressured and high-achieving children and adolescents. J Am Acad Child AdolescPsychiatry 1999;38(2):213–6.
71. Libman S. Adult participation in youth sports: a developmental perspective. Child AdolescPsychiatrClin N Am 1998;7(4):725–44.
72. Lindquist CH, Reynolds KD, Goran MI. Sociocultural determinants of physical activity among children. Prev Med 1999;29(4):305–12.
73. Micheli LJ, Jenkins MD. Sportswise: an essential guide for young athletes, parents, and coaches. Boston: Houghton Mifflin Harcourt; 1990.
74. SM M. The cheers and the tears: healthy alternative to the dark side of youth sports today. San francisco, CA: Jossey-Bass, Inc; 1994.
75. Stryer BK, Tofler IR, Lapchick R. A developmental overview of child and youth sports in society. Child AdolescPsychiatrClin 1998;7(4):697–724.
76. Thornton JS. Springing young athletes from the parental pressure cooker. Physician and Sportsmedicine 1991;19(7):92–9.
77. Tofler IR, Stryer BK, Micheli LJ, et al. Physical and emotional problems of elite female gymnasts. Waltham, MA: Mass Medical Soc; 1996. p. 281–3.
78. Knapp J, Aerni G, Anderson J. Eating disorders in female athletes: use of screening tools. CurrSports Med Rep 2014;13(4):214–8.

79. Rodolfa E, Bent R, Eisman E, et al. A cube model for competency development: implications for psychology educators and regulators. Prof Psychol Res Pract 2005;36(4):347–54.
80. Sudano LE, Collins G, Miles CM. Reducing barriers to mental health care for student-athletes: an integrated care model. FamSystHealth 2017;35(1):77–84.
81. APA. American Psychological Association. Briefing series on the role of psychology in health care - primary care. 2014. Available at: https://www.apa.org/health/briefs/primary-care.pdf.
82. Li S-s, Wu Q, Chen Z. Effects of psychological interventions on the prevention of sports injuries: a meta-analysis. Orthopaedic J Sports Med 2020;8:1–9.
83. Popoli DM, Burns TG, Meehan WP, et al. CHOA concussion consensus:establishing a uniform policy for academic accommodations. ClinPediatr 2014;53(3):217–24.
84. Purcell R, Gwyther K, Rice SM. Mental health in elite athletes: increased awareness requires an early intervention framework to respond to athlete needs. Sports Med Open 2019;5(1):46.
85. APA. American Psychological Association. Society for sport, exercise, and performance psychology. Washington, DC: APA Sport Psychology Proficiency; 2012. Available at: https://www.apadivisions.org/division-47/about/sport-proficiency.

Role of Psychologists in Pediatric Sleep Medicine

Mark G. Goetting, MD, DBSM[a,b,*]

KEYWORDS

• Insomnia • Circadian rhythm disorder • Sleep hygiene

KEY POINTS

• Chronic sleep disorders are common and treatable in children and adolescents yet often are undiagnosed.
• These disorders have a bidirectional relationship with emotional and cognitive function.
• Consequences of dysfunctional sleep and the underlying disorder itself can be identified and managed best with a partnered approach that includes both medical and psychology professionals.

INTRODUCTION

Psychology and neuroscience often attracts students intrigued by profound concepts such the nature of consciousness and theory of mind. However, eventually some find themselves in the clinic being asked, "How can I get my baby to sleep through the night?" Fortunately, most practitioners match their natural gift of curiosity with a passion for patient care.

Adequate sleep is essential for normal growth and development, even survival itself.[1] Nonetheless, it is often unsatisfactory, and aberrant sleep patterns are disruptive to both the child and the family. The importance of the problem and the availability of solutions are reflected in the number of excellent textbooks on pediatric sleep medicine, some that deal exclusively with sleep psychology. In addition, there are thousands of journal publications on topic. Here are current references for the reader seeking practical clinical advice on the most common pediatric sleep complaints.[2–5]

Pediatric sleep problems may be transient and resolve without any specific intervention. Crossing multiple time zones or relationship turbulences can be examples. On the other extreme, sleep disorders may be chronic and even disabling. Primary-care providers can identify and manage some. Those others may be referred to a

[a] Department of Pediatric and Adolescent Medicine; [b] Department of Medicine, Center for Clinical Research, Western Michigan University Homer Stryker M.D. School of Medicine, Office 2627, 1000 Oakland Drive, Kalamazoo, MI 49008-8010, USA
* Corresponding author. Department of Pediatric and Adolescent Medicine, Western Michigan University Homer Stryker M.D. School of Medicine, Office 2627, 1000 Oakland Drive, Kalamazoo, MI 49008-8010.
E-mail address: mark.goetting@med.wmich.edu

Pediatr Clin N Am 69 (2022) 989–1002
https://doi.org/10.1016/j.pcl.2022.05.011
0031-3955/22/© 2022 Elsevier Inc. All rights reserved.

psychologist, a sleep medicine specialist, or a behavioral sleep medicine specialist. The patient on occasions calls on expertise from all 3 specialties.

There are several purposes to this article. The first purpose is to inform the primary-care provider that sleep disorders are common and important, not just for the individual child but to help keep the family functioning. The second purpose is to highlight the bidirectional relationship between sleep disorders and cognitive, mood, and thought health. The third is to emphasize that some patients are complex and do best with co-ordination of care, a key component being the psychologist. Finally, it is hoped that article also helps the mental health expert appreciate the overlap among mood, anxiety, and developmental disorders with sleep disorders. This is important because many of these conditions induce or aggravate mood, cognitive, and behavioral problems, thus providing an opportunity for improved patient outcomes when properly addressed.[6] Although data are lacking in pediatrics, treatment of chronic insomnia in adults with cognitive-behavioral therapy (CBT) prevents both new onset and recurrent major depression.[7] Moreover, some sleep-wake symptoms can be misinterpreted as psychopathology.

It should be said that some common problems respond to straightforward behavioral therapy but a fraction are multilayered and challenging. As a related example, CBT for chronic insomnia is a mainstream effective tool in adults. A recent report showed durability of its positive effect for a 10 year period.[8] This large cohort showed remission in two-thirds at both 1 year and 10 year follow-up. Although that is impressive in its effect and durability, it leaves another third still suffering with the condition and that need additional treatment of some sort.

Failure with first-line interventions in children and adolescents can also happen, especially with chronic insufficient sleep, chronic insomnia, and circadian rhythm disorders. Home environment and family dynamics may limit success with a behavioral intervention plan. Often it is the caretaker, not the patient, who seeks change, creating resistance in the patient. There can be sleep disorders that produce chronic insomnia and that remit to specific treatment, for example, restless legs syndrome but do not address the conditioned arousal created by frustration in sleep initiation, leaving the patient with psychophysiologic insomnia. Finally, some medical, neurological, and psychological conditions preclude a meaningful response to common treatments and require highly individualized therapy. As an example, only about 25% of children with autism and insomnia respond well to behavioral therapy and sleep hygiene.[9]

PREVALENCE OF SLEEP DISORDERS

Sleep disorders are common and under recognized. They contribute to loss of productivity, diminished quality of life and cognitive capacity, chronic physical and mental illnesses, and serious accidents.

	Pediatric	Adult
Chronic insufficient sleep	>50% middle and high schoolers	40%
Obstructive sleep apnea	9%–40%	9%–38%
Restless legs syndrome	2%–3%, higher in ADHD and autism	12%
Chronic insomnia	10%–20%	5%–8%
Excessive daytime sleepiness	29%	50%

Abbreviation: ADHD, attention deficit hyperactivity disorder.

A recent study of more than 2,000 adults using a questionnaire methodology showed about 40% had chronic insufficient sleep, getting less than 7 hours a sleep nightly.

About 12% had symptoms of restless legs syndrome weekly, and 5% to 8% had chronic insomnia, one or more parasomnias, sleep apnea, a circadian rhythm disorder, and excessive daytime sleepiness. About 12% had 2 or more conditions.[10] As an indicator, melatonin use by adults has increased 5-fold between 1999 and 2018.[11]

The prevalence in children is also high. Chronic insufficient sleep is seen in more than half of middle school and high school students.[12] Chronic insomnia in children and adolescents is about 10% to 20%.[13–16] Restless legs syndrome occurs in about 2% in otherwise healthy children but is much higher in those with autism and attention deficit hyperactivity disorder (ADHD).[17–19] Obstructive sleep apnea was noted in 9% of school age children and adolescents of normal weight and more than 40% of those obese and overweight.[20] Sleep terrors or sleep walking in children aged 6 to 11 years had a prevalence slightly less than 4%. Circadian rhythm disorders are seen in about 3%. Excessive daytime sleepiness is common, approaching 30%.[21]

A little closer to home perhaps, a recent study revealed that slightly more than half of health-care workers had abnormal daytime sleepiness.[22]

These above statistics are important because of the significant probability that the child being seen by the provider has an important sleep disorder, is being parented by someone who also has a sleep disorder, and may be evaluated by a sleep-impaired professional! This troubling scenario speaks to the commonness of sleep disorders.

TERMINOLOGY AND CONCEPTS

The reader may not be acquainted with some sleep–wake phenomena and their terms, as well as those that can be confused with them. These are briefly described to provide a sense of the richness and diversity of overlap symptoms of the 2 states often thought to be mutually exclusive: sleep and wake.

Clinophilia: Clino derives from the Greek word for bed. Clinophilia is the strong preference to stay in bed beyond sleep needs, generally for the comfort and pleasure of it. Clinomania is a lesser used synonym. Dysania is a related term but implies anxiety about leaving the bed.

Clinophobia: A strong anxiety about being in bed. This is rare.

Somnophilia: Somnos is Latin for sleep. The term somnophilia at one time suggested a love or desire for sleep but without excessive daytime sleepiness. It is implied that there is more of a want than a need. However, it now refers to a sexual paraphilia involving a sleeping or unconscious partner or victim.

Sleepability: The capability to fall asleep rapidly without other indications of excessive sleepiness.

Sleepiness resistance: The tolerance to sleep deprivation without significant performance impairment.

Hypnagogic: The transitional state from wake to sleep. It has also been called presomnia.

Hypnopompic: The reverse of hypnagogic because it is the transition to wake from sleep.

Induced hypnagogia: There are techniques to sustain a transitional state in which wake and sleep repeatedly interdigitate. This can be for pleasure, dream exploration, and therapy.

Transitional hallucinations: Sensory disturbances are common entering and leaving sleep. The feeling of falling with a body jerk is a vestibular phenomenon that inspired the saying "falling asleep." Simple and complex visions and sounds, vibratory and floating sensations, and out-of-body experiences can be experienced by normal children and adolescents. These should not be confused with dreams, which are generally more complex and thematic.

Nightmare: A dream anxiety event that culminates in waking.

Lucid dreaming: Being conscious of dreaming while in a dream and having knowledge that wakefulness will return. This can occur spontaneously or be learned.

Sleep paralysis: The persistence of rapid eye movement sleep (REM) sleep paralysis and dream-like activity into the emergence of waking. This is typically frightening and often associated with the perception of a nearby threatening person or creature.

Sleep inertia: The grogginess during the process of waking until achieving full alertness. When severe, it has been referred to as sleep drunkenness.

Sleep debt: The difference between optimal and actual sleep duration. The debt can be acute due to sleep deprivation over a short period of time, or it can go on much longer in chronic sleep insufficiency.

Excessive daytime sleepiness: The inability to maintain full alertness during the major waking periods of the day.

Hypersomnia: This can be recurrent episodes or persistent sense of sleepiness despite adequate nighttime sleep, or it can be the routine need for prolonged nighttime sleep for daytime alertness.

Sleep attacks: Waves of intense sleepiness that can be hard to resist. These can be brief and resolve without sleep.

Cataplexy: A sudden and brief loss of muscle tone usually brought on with an emotion, commonly laughter. This can be partial and involve buckling of the knees or facial or neck weakness or it can result in collapsing. Consciousness is preserved. This is a symptom of narcolepsy.

False or fake memories: Recollection of a wake event that never happened. It may be from a dream. These can cause embarrassment because the patient believes the memory is real and others were present. These very occasionally happen in the healthy but are much more frequent in narcolepsy.

Social jet lag: The difference between one's inherent circadian rhythm for sleep and the actual sleep–wake pattern that is due to social schedules. Early school start times can often induce this, leading to catch up sleep on the weekends.

RHYTHMS AND SLEEP

The transitioning from wake to sleep and back again depends on the interplay between sleep pressure and arousal. Sleep pressure emanates mostly from sleep deprivation, which can be just from being awake during the day. Sleep deprivation from extended waking, staying up all night for example, or from chronic insufficient sleep will drive the sleep pressure to the point of causing daytime sleepiness. So sleep pressure can be imagined to be similar to food and liquid fasting. That is, the longer the deprivation, the greater the pressure to satisfy the need.

The circadian arousal system can mask the sleep pressure until it subsides, usually in the evening, and sleepiness descends. This helps allow sustained alertness during the day.

The term circadian translates to "about a day," lining up with the rotation of the Earth. Rhythms faster than that are ultradian, and ones that are slower are infradian. Our biology has some of all of these.

The baseline arousal pattern usually has slumps in the day. This facilitates naps or siestas. There can be an additional arousal effect that is summoned in times of danger, opportunity, and environmental and social factors and is not related to a biological rhythm.

Infradian rhythms include hormonal changes in women, which can affect sleep. Seasonal and annual changes in sleep patterns exist but are driven by the environment more than inherent biology. However, there is recent support that the gravitation forces of the Earth, Moon, and Sun may affect human sleep.[23] Stay tuned!

Ultradian rhythms would include the peaks and troughs of the normal wake arousal system during the day. Sleep has such quick rhythms, too. Sleep goes through repeated stages during the night. The ascent into light sleep can result in nighttime wakings. The fastest cycling rhythm related to sleep may be memory processing.[24] Consolidation of waking experiences seem to be entrained to the rhythm of respirations, at least in a recent animal experiment.

Circadian and ultradian dynamics of the wake arousal system are heavily influenced by genetics.[25–27] Combined with culture, social, and family needs, the result is variability in sleep patterns, some of which may not be very flexible. The results have a majority able to comfortably sleep in the desired window. There are a sizable number who cannot. Some are programmed to sleep best much later than the average, whereas fewer are biologic "early birds." This creates hardships for the outliers that cannot be wished away or overcome by willfulness. Taking the view of the evolutionary biologist, this produces in a tribe that some will have peak alertness at any time to tend animals and the sick and to protect the sleeping from threats. Sleep continuity throughout the night has become more important due to modernity and the industrial revolution, where daytime sleeping is mostly forbidden. Many cultures previously embraced multiple sleep periods. Siestas and 2 periods of nighttime sleep are examples.[28] Scheduling rigidity for school and employment greatly curtailed this. However, not all adapt with great flexibility. Consider that there are 2 prescription medications approved by the Food and Drug Administration just for middle of the night wakings in adults, Intermezzo and Zolpimist.

Strategically dosed melatonin and light therapy can shift the circadian rhythm to some degree.[29,30] These interventions work best when properly timed and are ineffective or harmful when mistimed. The treatments should be put on a schedule that considers the patient's circadian rhythm that is hoped to be influenced.

SOME SPECIFIC SLEEP DISORDERS

These medical conditions can present with behavior, cognitive, thought and mood problems that may reflect the underlying sleep disorder or be worsened by psychiatric medications.

Obstructive Sleep Apnea

This disorder involves partial or complete collapse of the upper airway during sleep. This results in increased work of breathing, alteration in oxygen and carbon dioxide blood tensions, sympathetic activation, and sleep fragmentation. Snoring is usually present, and there can be gasping and restlessness. Risk factors include environmental allergies, adenotonsillar hypertrophy, and obesity. Certain craniofacial abnormalities, conditions in which muscle tone is reduced, a history of prematurity, and a family history of obstructive sleep apnea are additional risk factors.[31] Children with a body mass index less than 5th percentile are also at risk, particularly with tonsillar hypertrophy or nasal allergy symptoms.[32]

Problematic daytime behavior with aggression, impulsivity, and hyperactivity as well has symptoms of depression, anxiety, and academic struggle can be associated with this condition.

History and physical examination can help identify those at higher risk for obstructive sleep apnea (OSA) but cannot fully rule this out or in.[33] Polysomnography is the diagnostic tool of choice.

Treatment focuses on the maintenance of airway patency during sleep. This can be achieved by surgical, medical, behavioral, and dental approaches.

Restless Legs Syndrome

This sensorimotor condition usually manifest in the evening and at night. There is typically an irresistible urge to move, rub, or stretch the legs that is associated with difficult to describe sensations. The symptoms emerge during quiescence, such as sitting watching television or lying in bed, and disappear promptly with physical activity, such as walking.

This condition can present as bedtime resistance, sleep onset insomnia, and nighttime wakings. Some children will have nocturnal leg pains.

Iron insufficiency and a family history for restless leg syndrome are risk factors. Prevalence among children in Europe and in the United States is estimated to be between 2% and 8%. The condition is very common among those diagnosed with ADHD, with 18% or more being comorbid, and autism, with almost 40% of those presenting for sleep medicine consultation with insomnia also had restless legs syndrome.[18,19]

Certain medications can induce or aggravate restless legs syndrome (RLS). These often are used for autism comorbidities and include antidepressants, antipsychotics, and antihistamines. This is important to consider.

Polysomnography is generally not needed when the history is clear. However, in challenging cases, it can be useful in demonstrating restlessness in the transition to sleep with recurrence during middle of the night waking. It may also reveal periodic limb movements.[34]

Iron insufficiency is common in those with restless leg syndrome. The likelihood of responding to iron treatment is assessed by serum ferritin level less than 50 mcg/mL or a fasting iron saturation less than 20%. An alternative treatment is gabapentin.

Restless Sleep Disorder

This condition recently has been defined as a separate entity.[35,36] Sleep-related restlessness has been described as persistent or recurrent body movements, arousals, and brief awakenings that occurred in the course of sleep. This phenomenon usually observed by caregivers often can be due to underlying conditions such as obstructive sleep apnea, gastroesophageal reflux, restless leg syndrome, and eczema. Recently, an entity independent of these conditions has been defined. Polysomnography documents 5 or more large muscle movements per hour on average during the study without a clear alternative cause and is necessary for confidence in the diagnosis because other disorders can produce restlessness.

Daytime symptoms can include mood dysregulation, inattentiveness, hyperactivity, and cognitive dysfunction.

Assessment of iron status is similar to that of RLS. Most improve with proper iron therapy. Gabapentin is a second-line therapy.

Narcolepsy

This uncommon neurologic condition typically has an onset in adolescence or the third decade. However, about 10% of those diagnosed begin their symptoms by age 10 or so. The prevalence is about 1/1000 persons. The most consistent symptom is daytime sleepiness, seen in virtually all patients. Often this comes in brief waves during the day.

There can be significant weight gain or precocious puberty at onset in children. Cataplexy may occur. Other symptoms can include hyperactivity, inattentiveness, irritability, and depression. Occasionally there can be delusional and even psychotic symptoms.[37]

HOW TO PROMOTE SLEEP

When awake, we live in a wake centric world. That is, we focus on achievement and pleasure in events and objects of the waking world and treat sleep as a necessary means to achieve more wake. Therefore, promoting or "selling" sleep can be challenging. The typical approach is characterize sleep as an investment for better wakefulness later. Although there is truth there, delayed gratification may not compete well with the immediate form.

Motivating exercise for the sake of benefit outside of the gym could be a comparable. Those who really enjoy exercising in the gym do not need additional incentive. Others do despite being aware of health and wellbeing benefits outside the gym. The challenge is reaching that majority. In a recent article, a "megastudy" of behavioral interventions to improve gym attendance among already paying members was presented. This included more than 61,000 Americans with evaluation of 54 separate interventions during a 4 week period. Several of them produced small-to-moderate weekly visits. The 10 week postintervention monitoring showed almost no sustained benefit however.[38]

Teaching that respecting sleep can improve the waking life also commonly falls flat by itself. In a recent report, medical students completed multiple standardized questionnaires on their knowledge of sleep, their sleep quality, and their daytime sleepiness score. The group average poor sleep quality. They then attended a lecture on the physiology and importance of sleep. The questionnaires were repeated in 4 months. These demonstrated better awareness in the importance of sleep but no improvement in sleep.[39]

One direct and obvious way to increase sleep time is to align wake activities better with the circadian rhythm of the age group, particularly addressing early wake times.[40,41] Delaying school start times increase total sleep time, daytime alertness, and academic achievement.[42] It also decreases delinquency and substance use.[43] Interestingly, school closures with the transition to home schooling increased adolescent sleep times by about 75 minutes, another indicator of a previous widespread sleep debt in this age group.[44]

There are some potential incentives to delay gratification that are not as well-known and touted. Well-rested individuals seem more attractive, intelligent, and interesting.[45–49] They tend to be more slender.[50] Sports performance also improves with adequate sleep and can provide a competitive edge.[51]

Sleep tracking can be by daily diary or log, which subjectively estimates sleep–wake patterns.[52] Digital sleep trackers, typically actigraphy with an ankle (young children) or wrist device removes subjectivity but may overestimate or underestimate sleep compared with polysomnography.[53,54] Initial experience with tracking without professional guidance in adults did not improve sleep.[55] It seems that sleep tracking may be most useful when coupled with ongoing proper counseling.

Modern Western culture generally does not hold the sleeping state with the meaningfulness as other cultures in history. There is a viewpoint argued by few that wake is not the primary human state of being for which sleep exists to support. Rather, sleep is the important realm and wake is but a cruder platform necessary to sustain and generate more sleeping beings. Granted, this is an extreme position but may initiate pondering about what can be enjoyable about sleep aside from resolving sleepiness.

There are alternative approaches to muster enthusiasm for sleep as a state of being, not just an investment for the day. Hypnagogia can be sustained to stretch out the process of entering sleep. Some find this pleasurable. It can produce a dream-like state and hallucinations.[56] This can be used to enhance creative problem solving also.[57] Tibetan dream yoga is an ancient practice that involves sustained hypnagogia with a REM sleep focus for spiritual purposes.[58] Rosicrucianism, originated in seventeenth century Europe, also uses sleep consciousness for healing and spiritual purposes.[59]

Out-of-body experiences can be induced in many by intentional sleep fragmentation in the second half of the night, when REM sleep is more abundant. This also is an ancient practice used for entertainment, self-exploration, and spiritual purposes.[60] The neurophysiology of this altered state is a subject of ongoing study.[61] There are books for the general public on out-of-body induction and on astral projection. There are also Internet-based forums for discussion.[62]

Some find interest in dream journaling and interpretation.[63,64] There are forums to share information with and socialize.[65]

Lucid dreaming is the simultaneous experience of dreaming while being aware of being in a dream. Many spontaneously have this experience while others may learn it. It is a therapeutic option for nightmare disorder and chronic insomnia.[66,67] It also can be a tool to promote sleep for patients. The training first involves identifying "dream signs." These are indicators that one is asleep. There are rules for dreams that are different than in wakefulness. For example, reading text fluently is usually not possible in dreams. Trying to read is frustrating and confusing. Light switches commonly do not work. Time displays are erratic. Gravity has less effect in dreams generally so jumping up results in a gentler landing. There are many other dream signs. The patient chooses a couple. A dream sign is tested for at least every half hour in what it is called a reality check. For example, the person will ask whether he or she is sleeping. That could be testing by trying to read some text or turn a light switch off and on. That will confirm wakefulness. After several weeks for doing this routinely the dreamer will often remember to do a reality check. That will confirm the dream state and achieve lucidity. Then the person can do dream exploration with or without planned task. There are books on dream exploration as well as Internet forums.[65,68]

The question will naturally arise as to whether lucid dreaming and dream exploration can have a benefit outside of the treatment of nightmare disorder. For some, it puts a greater value on sleep for sleep's sake and may increase the total sleep time. Many are not interested. For those who pursue it, there does seem to be benefit.[69]

The family can perhaps change their messaging about sleep for the benefit of the child as well as the family as a whole. Sleep is disrespected when the child hears things such as, "You can stay up late if you're good," "You can stay up because it's a special occasion," and "You have to go to bed if you fight." Skipping the winding routine and allowing screen time at bedtime are likewise unhelpful.

There are positive messages as well. These include that sleep makes you bigger, stronger, and smarter. The parent can be there to tuck the child in and ask about what he or she wants to dream about then ask about the dreams at breakfast. Most importantly, parents can set a good example with their attitudes and actions about their own sleep.

SLEEP HYGIENE AND SCHEDULING

Behavioral approaches often include "sleep hygiene." These are changes in behaviors and attitudes during wakefulness that are intended to improve sleep. Interestingly, sleep hygiene has not been found to be effective in treating chronic insomnia in adults.[70] The results have been mixed in children.

Physical activity during the day did not improve nighttime sleep in children in a recent study. Surprisingly, it had a mild negative effect. Moreover, longer sleep did not predict more physical activity the next day.[71] Light expose an hour before bedtime in preschoolers suppresses melatonin in a dose–response pattern and is suggested to delay sleep onset time.[72] The wavelengths that inhibit melatonin release are in the blue part of the light spectrum. However, blue light blocking eyewear did not improve sleep in adults when worn in the evening.[73]

Cell phone use before bedtime can delay sleep. Electromagnetic irradiation likely has little or no effect on sleep. Use of the phone does have an adverse influence that can only be partially reduced by screen filtering.[74,75]

Not surprisingly, caffeine consumption delayed sleep onset and offset in teens. This was seen in those having a single beverage per day.[76]

Diet composition may play a role in sleep quality.[77,78] The mechanism may be the gut microbiota, even in infants.[79–81] The preferred diet is controversial with some support for the Mediterranean diet in children and teens.

Extensive video game use does seem to delay sleep onset and decrease sleep quality.[82] It is unclear whether it is due to the cognitive and emotional activation, sedentary effects, light exposure, of loss of the winding down routine.

One study did show that mindfulness helped improve sleep in adolescents with chronic sleeplessness when coupled with other interventions.[83]

A nighttime routine is important in children and adults.[84,85] This can begin with a "sleep alarm" in older children, adolescents, and adults. It is the reciprocal of a morning alarm in that it signals that it is time to start the winding down activities. Some find checklists helpful children as a means to engage them.

Sleep is not coma. There is some environmental monitoring for safety. Recent data in the rat show sleep adaptation to arouse more promptly if the odor of a predator is nearby.[86] Humans will have arousals in sleep only when a stranger says the same words compared to a familiar voice.[87] The implications are what common sense tells us: the bedroom should be quiet and boring. If sound is helpful, it should be bland and familiar.

Sleep inertia can be problematic. Melodic music once wakefulness appears can lessen the unpleasantness in the transition to full alertness.[88,89] However, in severe cases medications are justified.[90]

SUMMARY

We have seen dramatic changes in our understanding, appreciation, and management of pediatric sleep disorders. The rate of progress will increase during the next decade as we translate research into clinical action. The first hope is to prevent sleep disorders using what we already know. In failing that, the prompt recognition and treatment is a must. That will require in most cases behavioral prescriptions and often a large role for the clinical psychologist.

CLINICS CARE POINTS

- Children should be routinely screened for common sleep disorders. Children with developmental, cognitive and mood symptoms warrant a more detailed inquiry on their sleep and whether their sleep disturbances distress the family.

REFERENCES

1. Galván A. The Need for Sleep in the Adolescent Brain. Trends Cogn Sci 2020; 24(1):79–89.
2. Vriend J, Corkum P. Clinical management of behavioral insomnia of childhood. Psychol Res Behav Manag 2011;4:69–79.
3. Lunsford-Avery JR, Bidopia T, Jackson L, et al. Behavioral treatment of insomnia and sleep disturbances in school-aged children and adolescents. Child Adolesc Psychiatr Clin N Am 2021;30(1):101–16.
4. Meltzer LJ, Crabtree VML. Pediatric sleep problems: A clinician's guide to behavioral interventions. American Psychological Association; 2015.
5. Mindell JA, Owens JA. A clinical guide to pediatric sleep: diagnosis and management of sleep problems. Third. LWW; 2015.
6. Harvey AG, Author Allison Harvey CG, Buysse D, et al. Treating sleep and circadian problems to promote mental health: Perspectives on comorbidity, implementation science and behavior change. Sleep 2022. https://doi.org/10.1093/SLEEP/ZSAC026.
7. Irwin MR, Carrillo C, Sadeghi N, et al. Prevention of incident and recurrent major depression in older adults with insomnia a randomized clinical trial. JAMA Psychiatry 2022;79(1):33–41.
8. Jernelöv S, Blom K, Isacsson NH, et al. Very long-term outcome of cognitive behavioral therapy for insomnia: one-and ten-year follow-up of a randomized controlled trial. Cogn Behav Ther 2022. https://doi.org/10.1080/16506073.2021.2009019.
9. Schröder CM, Broquère MA, Claustrat B, et al. Approches thérapeutiques des troubles du sommeil et des rythmes chez l'enfant avec TSA. Encephale 2022. https://doi.org/10.1016/J.ENCEP.2021.08.005.
10. Kerkhof GA. Epidemiology of sleep and sleep disorders in The Netherlands. Sleep Med 2017;30:229–39.
11. Li J, Somers VK, Xu H, et al. Trends in use of melatonin supplementsamong US Adults, 1999-2018. JAMA 2022;327:483.
12. Wheaton AG, Cooper AC, Croft JB. Short sleep duration among middle school and high school students - United States, 2015. MMWR Morb Mortal Wkly Rep 2018;67(3):85–90.
13. Chung KF, Kan KKK, Yeung WF. Insomnia in adolescents: prevalence, help-seeking behaviors, and types of interventions. Child Adolesc Ment Health 2014;19(1):57–63.
14. Almaas MAJ, Heradstveit O, Askeland KG, et al. Sleep patterns and insomnia among adolescents receiving child welfare services: a population-based study. Sleep Heal 2021;000:5–11.
15. Gariepy G, Danna S, Gobiņa I, et al. How are adolescents sleeping? adolescent sleep patterns and sociodemographic differences in 24 European and North American Countries. J Adolesc Health 2020;66(6):S81–8.
16. Johnson EO, Roth T, Schultz L, et al. Epidemiology of DSM-IV insomnia in adolescence: Lifetime prevalence, chronicity, and an emergent gender difference. Pediatrics 2006;117(2):247–56.
17. Turkdogan D, Bekiroglu N, Zaimoglu S. A prevalence study of restless legs syndrome in Turkish children and adolescents. Sleep Med 2011;12(4):315–21.
18. Kanney ML, Durmer JS, Trotti LM, et al. Rethinking bedtime resistance in children with autism: is restless legs syndrome to blame? J Clin Sleep Med 2020;16(12):2029–35.

19. Sierra Montoya AC, Mesa Restrepo SC, Cuartas Arias JM, et al. Prevalencia y caracteristicas clínicas del síndrome de piernas inquietas (SPI) en pacientes diagnosticados con trastorno por déficit de atención con hiperactividad (TDAH) en antioquia. Int J Psychol Res 2018;11(1):58–69.

20. Andersen IG, Holm JC, Homøe P. Obstructive sleep apnea in children and adolescents with and without obesity. Eur Arch Otorhinolaryngol 2019;276(3):871–8.

21. Liu Y, Zhang J, Li SX, et al. Excessive daytime sleepiness among children and adolescents: prevalence, correlates, and pubertal effects. Sleep Med 2019; 53:1–8.

22. Pereira Carvalho V, Alves Barcelos K, Paula De Oliveira E, et al. Poor sleep quality and daytime sleepiness in health professionals: prevalence and associated factors. Int J Environ Res Public Heal 2021;18:6864.

23. de Mello Gallep C, Robert D. Are cyclic plant and animal behaviours driven by gravimetric mechanical forcing? J Exp Bot 2021. https://doi.org/10.1093/JXB/ERAB462.

24. Karalis N, Sirota A. Breathing coordinates cortico-hippocampal dynamics in mice during offline states. Nat Commun 2022;13(1):467.

25. Mainieri G, Montini A, Nicotera A, et al. The genetics of sleep disorders in children: a narrative review. Brain Sci 2021;11(10). https://doi.org/10.3390/brainsci11101259.

26. Vitaterna MH, Shimomura K, Jiang P. Genetics of circadian rhythms. Neurol Clin 2019;37(3):487–504.

27. Arns M, JJS Kooij, Coogan AN. Review: identification and management of circadian rhythm sleep disorders as a transdiagnostic feature in child and adolescent psychiatry. J Am Acad Child Adolesc Psychiatry 2021;60(9):1085–95.

28. Jackson M, Banks S. Did we used to have two sleeps rather than one? Should we again? theconversation.com. Available at: https://theconversation.com/did-we-used-to-have-two-sleeps-rather-than-one-should-we-again-57806. Accessed June 20, 2022.

29. Sletten TL, Magee M, Murray JM, et al. Efficacy of melatonin with behavioural sleep-wake scheduling for delayed sleep-wake phase disorder: a double-blind, randomised clinical trial. PLoS Med 2018;15(6):1–24.

30. Richardson C, Cain N, Bartel K, et al. A randomised controlled trial of bright light therapy and morning activity for adolescents and young adults with Delayed Sleep-Wake Phase Disorder. Sleep Med 2018;45:114–23.

31. Oros M, Baranga L, Plaiasu V, et al. Obstructing sleep apnea in children with genetic disorders-a special need for early multidisciplinary diagnosis and treatment. J Clin Med 2021;10(10). https://doi.org/10.3390/JCM10102156.

32. Johnson C, Leavitt T, Daram SP, et al. Obstructive Sleep Apnea in Underweight Children. Otolaryngol Head Neck Surg (United States) 2021. https://doi.org/10.1177/01945998211058722.

33. Brietzke SE, Katz ES, Roberson DW. Can history and physical examination reliably diagnose pediatric obstructive sleep apnea/hypopnea syndrome? A systematic review of the literature. Otolaryngol Head Neck Surg 2004;131(6):827–32.

34. Drakatos P, Olaithe M, Verma D, et al. Periodic limb movements during sleep: a narrative review. J Thorac Dis 2021;13(11):6476–94.

35. DelRosso LM, Picchietti DL, Spruyt K, et al. Restless sleep in children: a systematic review. Sleep Med Rev 2021;56. https://doi.org/10.1016/j.smrv.2020.101406.

36. Liu WK, Dye TJ, Horn P, Patterson C, Garner D, Simakajornboon N. Large body movements on video polysomnography are associated with daytime dysfunction in children with restless sleep disorder. Sleep 2022;45(4):zsac005.

37. Hanin C, Arnulf I, Maranci JB, et al. Narcolepsy and psychosis: a systematic review. Acta Psychiatr Scand 2021;144(1):28–41.
38. Milkman KL, Gromet D, Ho H, et al. Megastudies improve the impact of applied behavioural science. Nature 2021;600(7889):478–83.
39. Mazar D, Gilleles-Hilel A, Reiter J. Sleep education improves knowledge but not sleep quality among medical students. J Clin Sleep Med 2021;17(6):1211–5.
40. Meltzer LJ, Wahlstrom KL, Plog AE, et al. Changing school start times: Impact on sleep in primary and secondary school students. Sleep 2021;44(7):1–14.
41. Watson NF, Martin JL, Wise MS, et al. Delaying middle school and high school start times promotes student health and performance: an American academy of sleep medicine position statement. J Clin Sleep Med 2017;13(4):623–5.
42. Meltzer LJ, Saletin JM, Honaker SM, et al. COVID-19 instructional approaches (in-person, online, hybrid), school start times, and sleep in over 5,000 U.S. adolescents. Sleep 2021;44(12). https://doi.org/10.1093/sleep/zsab180.
43. Semenza DC, Meldrum RC, Jackson DB, et al. School start times, delinquency, and substance use: a criminological perspective. Crime Delinq 2020;66(2):163–93. https://doi.org/10.1177/0011128719845147.
44. Albrecht JN, Werner H, Rieger N, et al. Association between Homeschooling and adolescent sleep duration and health during COVID-19 pandemic high school closures. JAMA Netw Open 2022;5(1):1–12.
45. Sundelin T, Lekander M, Sorjonen K, et al. Negative effects of restricted sleep on facial appearance and social appeal. R Soc Open Sci 2017;4(5). https://doi.org/10.1098/rsos.160918.
46. Holding BC, Sundelin T, Cairns P, et al. The effect of sleep deprivation on objective and subjective measures of facial appearance. J Sleep Res 2019;28(6). https://doi.org/10.1111/jsr.12860.
47. Léger D, Gauriau C, Etzi C, et al. "You look sleepy…" The impact of sleep restriction on skin parameters and facial appearance of 24 women. Sleep Med 2022;89:97–103.
48. Whitmore NW, Bassard AM, Paller KA. Targeted memory reactivation of face-name learning depends on ample and undisturbed slow-wave sleep. NPJ Sci Learn 2022;7(1):1.
49. Talamas SN, Mavor KI, Sundelin T, et al. Eyelid-Openness and mouth curvature influence perceived intelligence beyond attractiveness. J Exp Psychol Gen 2016;145(5):603–20.
50. Okoli A, Hanlon EC, Brady MJ. The relationship between sleep, obesity, and metabolic health in adolescents: a review. Curr Opin Endocr Metab Res 2021;17:15–9.
51. Watson AM. Sleep and athletic performance. Current Sports Medicine Reports 2017;16(6):413–8. Available at: www.acsm-csmr.org. Accessed June 20, 2022.
52. Van Meter AR, Anderson EA. Evidence Base Update on Assessing Sleep in Youth. J Clin Child Adolesc Psychol 2020;49(6):701–36. https://doi.org/10.1080/15374416.2020.1802735.
53. Danzig R, Wang M, Shah A, et al. The wrist is not the brain: Estimation of sleep by clinical and consumer wearable actigraphy devices is impacted by multiple patient- and device-specific factors. J Sleep Res 2020;29(1). https://doi.org/10.1111/jsr.12926.
54. Chee NIYN, Ghorbani S, Golkashani HA, et al. Multi-night validation of a sleep tracking ring in adolescents compared with a research actigraph and polysomnography. Nat Sci Sleep 2021;13:177–90.

55. Liang Z, Ploderer B. Sleep tracking in the real world: a qualitative study into barriers for improving sleep. Proc 28th Aust Comput Interact Conf Ozchi 2016;537–41. https://doi.org/10.1145/3010915.3010988.

56. Bless JJ, Hugdahl K, Kråkvik B, et al. In the twilight zone: an epidemiological study of sleep-related hallucinations. Compr Psychiatry 2021;108:0–5.

57. Lacaux C, Andrillon T, Bastoul C, et al. Sleep onset is a creative sweet spot. Sci Adv 2021;7(50):1–10.

58. Mota-Rolim SA, Bulkeley K, Campanelli S, et al. The Dream of God: How Do Religion and Science See Lucid Dreaming and Other Conscious States During Sleep? Front Psychol 2020;(11):1–9. https://doi.org/10.3389/fpsyg.2020.555731.

59. Vickers B. Frances Yates and the Writing of History. J Mod Hist 1979;51(2): 287–316.

60. Raduga M, Kuyava O, Sevcenko N. Is there a relation among REM sleep dissociated phenomena, like lucid dreaming, sleep paralysis, out-of-body experiences, and false awakening? Med Hypotheses 2020;144(April):110169.

61. Blanke O, Metzinger T. Full-body illusions and minimal phenomenal selfhood. Trends Cogn Sci 2009;13(1):7–13.

62. Lucid Dreaming and Out-of-Body Experience. Available at: https://www.remspace.net. Accessed June 20, 2022.

63. Schredl M, Göritz AS. Dream journaling: stability and relation to personality factors. Dreaming 2020;30(3):278–86.

64. Schredl M. Dream recording frequency in psychology students. Int J Dream Res 2020;13(2):306–8.

65. Dream Views. Available at: https://www.dreamviews.com/forum.php/. Accessed June 20, 2022.

66. Vanek J, Prasko J, Ociskova M, et al. Nightmares and their treatment. Neuro Endocrinol Lett 2020;41(2):86–101. Available at: https://pubmed.ncbi.nlm.nih.gov/33185995/. Accessed February 7, 2022.

67. Ellis JG, De Koninck J, Bastien CH. Managing insomnia using lucid dreaming training: a pilot study. Behav Sleep Med 2021;19(2):273–83.

68. International Association for the Study of Dreams. Available at: https://www.asdreams.org/. Accessed June 20, 2022.

69. Konkoly K, Burke CT. Can learning to lucid dream promote personal growth? Dreaming 2019;29(2):113–26.

70. Edinger JD, Arnedt JT, Bertisch SM, et al. Behavioral and psychological treatments for chronic insomnia disorder in adults: an American Academy of Sleep Medicine clinical practice guideline. J Clin Sleep Med 2021;17(2):255–62.

71. St. Laurent CW, Andre C, Holmes JF, et al. Temporal relationships between device-derived sedentary behavior, physical activity, and sleep in early childhood. Sleep 2022;(January):1–11. https://doi.org/10.1093/sleep/zsac008.

72. Hartstein LE, Behn CD, Akacem LD, et al. High sensitivity of melatonin suppression response to evening light in preschool-aged children. J Pineal Res 2022;1–10. https://doi.org/10.1111/jpi.12780.

73. Bigalke JA, Greenlund IM, Nicevski JR, et al. Effect of evening blue light blocking glasses on subjective and objective sleep in healthy adults: a randomized control trial. Sleep Heal 2021;7(4):485–90.

74. Höhn C, Schmid SR, Plamberger CP, et al. Preliminary results: the impact of smartphone use and short-wavelength light during the evening on circadian rhythm, sleep and alertness. Clocks & Sleep 2021;3(1):66–86.

75. Lowden A, Nagai R, Åkerstedt T, et al. Effects of evening exposure to electromagnetic fields emitted by 3G mobile phones on health and night sleep EEG architecture. J Sleep Res 2019;28(4):1–9.

76. Mathew GM, Reichenberger DA, Master L, et al. Too jittery to sleep? Temporal associations of actigraphic sleep and caffeine in adolescents. Nutrients 2022; 14(1):1–18.

77. Wilson K, St-Onge M-P, Tasali E. Diet composition and objectively assessed sleep quality: a narrative review. J Acad Nutr Diet 2022. https://doi.org/10.1016/j.jand.2022.01.007.

78. Yaghtin Z, Yuzbashian E, Ghayour-Mobarhan M, Khayyatzadeh SS. More Adherence To A Mediterranean Dietary Pattern is Associated With A Lower Insomnia Score. https://doi.org/10.21203/rs.3.rs-1073572/v1. Accessed June 20, 2022

79. Schoch SF, Castro-Mejía JL, Krych L, et al. From Alpha Diversity to Zzz: Interactions among sleep, the brain, and gut microbiota in the first year of life. Prog Neurobiol 2022;209:102208. https://doi.org/10.1016/j.pneurobio.2021.102208.

80. Wang Y, Van De Wouw M, Drogos L, et al. Sleep and the gut microbiota in preschool aged children. doi:10.1093/sleep/zsac020/6509073.

81. Han M, Yuan S, Zhang J. The interplay between sleep and gut microbiota. Brain Res Bull 2022;180(November 2021):131–46.

82. Peracchia S, Curcio G. Exposure to video games: effects on sleep and on post-sleep cognitive abilities. A systematic review of experimental evidences. Sleep Sci 2018;11(4):302–14.

83. de Bruin EJ, Meijer AM, Bögels SM. The contribution of a body scan mindfulness meditation to effectiveness of internet-delivered CBT for insomnia in adolescents. Mindfulness (N Y) 2020;11(4):872–82.

84. Mindell JA, Williamson AA. Benefits of a bedtime routine in young children: Sleep, development, and beyond. Sleep Med Rev 2018;40:93–108.

85. Arlinghaus KR, Johnston CA. The importance of creating habits and routine. Am J Lifestyle Med 2019;13(2):142–4.

86. Tseng Y-T, Zhao B, Chen S, et al. The subthalamic corticotropin-releasing hormone neurons mediate adaptive REM-sleep responses to threat. Neuron 2022. https://doi.org/10.1016/j.neuron.2021.12.033.

87. Ameen MS, Heib DP, Blume C, et al. The brain selectively tunes to unfamiliar voices during sleep. J Neurosci 2022. https://doi.org/10.1523/JNEUROSCI.2524-20.2021. JN-RM-2524-20.

88. McFarlane SJ, Garcia JE, Verhagen DS, et al. Auditory countermeasures for sleep inertia: exploring the effect of melody and rhythm in an ecological context. Clocks & Sleep 2020;2(2):208–24.

89. McFarlane SJ, Garcia JE, Verhagen DS, et al. Alarm tones, music and their elements: analysis of reported waking sounds to counteract sleep inertia. PLoS One 2020;15(1). https://doi.org/10.1371/journal.pone.0215788.

90. Schenck CH, Golden EC, Millman P. Treatment of severe morning sleep inertia with bedtime long-acting bupropion and/or long-acting methylphenidate in a series of 4 patients. J Clin Sleep Med 2021;17(4):653–7.

Role of Psychologists in Pediatric Metabolic Disorders

Shibani Kanungo, MD, MPH[a,b,]*, Katherine T. Beenen, PhD[a]

KEYWORDS

- IEMs or metabolic disorders
- Neurodevelopmental disorders (NDD)
- Behavioral disorders
- Psychological assessment
- Biopsychosocial lens

KEY POINTS

- IEMs have a wide range of neurodevelopmental and behavioral presentations.
- Age, clinical management, or stressors from common childhood/intercurrent illnesses/procedures/interventions can affect behavioral presentation in children with metabolic disorders.
- Clinical Psychologists can play a role in the diagnosis, management, and outcomes of metabolic disorders.

Historically, in the early 1900s, "Inborn Errors of Metabolism" (IEM) was coined by Sir Archibald Garrod after his understanding of Alkaptonuria to be a result of "alternative course of metabolism, harmless and usually congenital and lifelong."[1] For over a century, our understanding of IEMs has grown significantly and these once considered rare disorders (1 in 100,000 or more), with the onset of newborn screening (NBS) seem to be as common as approximately 1in 3234.[2] Currently, NBS programs help identify 35 core conditions (**Table 1**) and 26 secondary conditions (**Table 2**) listed in the Recommended Universal Screening Panel (RUSP), in almost 4 million newborns born annually in the United States.[3,4] **Table 3** lists other NBS conditions that are not part of RUSP. Initially considered harmless, as in case of Alkaptonuria, understanding the behavioral changes or how these IEMs can impact a patient's behavior and daily life along with improved classification in DSM criteria,[5] has helped expand our

Funding: None.

[a] Department of Pediatric and Adolescent Medicine, Western Michigan University Homer Stryker MD School of Medicine, 1000 Oakland Drive, Kalamazoo MI 49008, USA; [b] Department of Medical Ethics, Humanities and Law, Western Michigan University Homer Stryker MD School of Medicine, 1000 Oakland Drive, Kalamazoo MI 49008, USA

* Corresponding author. Department of Pediatric and Adolescent Medicine, Western Michigan University Homer Stryker MD School of Medicine, 1000 Oakland Drive, Kalamazoo MI 49008.

E-mail address: Shibani.Kanungo@med.wmich.edu

Table 1 Newborn screening RUSP "core conditions"		
Core Conditions Category	**Core Conditions Sub-category**	**Core Conditions/Abbreviation ([a])**
Metabolic Disorder	Organic acid disorders (OA)	[a][PA, MMA(mut), MMA(cbl), IVA, 3-MCC, HMG Co-A, HCS, BKT, GA1]
	Fatty acid oxidation Disorders (FAO)	[a][CUD, MCAD, VLCAD, LCHAD, TFP]
	Amino acid disorders (AA)	[a][ASS, CIT1, MSUD, HCY, PKU, TYR1]
Endocrine Disorder		[b][CH, CAH]
Hemoglobin Disorder		[c][SSD, ß-thal, SCD]
Other Disorder		Biotinidase deficiency (BIOT) Classic galactosemia (GALT) Glycogen Storage Disease Type II (Pompe) Mucopolysaccharidosis Type 1 (MPS I) X-linked Adrenoleukodystrophy (X-ALD) Severe combined Immunodeficiencies (SCID) Cystic fibrosis (CF) Hearing loss (HL) Critical congenital heart disease (CCHD) Spinal Muscular Atrophy due to the homozygous deletion of exon 7 in SMN1 (SMA)

[a] [Metabolic Disorders: PA - Propionic acidemia; MMA(mut) - Methylmalonic acidemia (methylmalonyl-CoA mutase); MMA(cbl) - Methylmalonic acidemia (cobalamin disorders); IVA - Isovaleric acidemia; 3-MCC - 3-Methylcrotonyl-CoA carboxylase deficiency; HMGCoA - 3-Hydroxy-3-methyglutaric aciduria; HCS - Holocarboxylase synthase deficiency; BKT - ß-Ketothiolase deficiency; GA1 - Glutaric acidemia type I; CUD - Carnitine uptake defect/carnitine transport defect; MCAD - Medium-chain acyl-CoA dehydrogenase deficiency; VLCAD - Very long-chain acyl-CoA dehydrogenase deficiency; LCHAD - Long-chain L-3 hydroxyacyl-CoA dehydrogenase deficiency; TFP - Trifunctional protein deficiency; ASS - Argininosuccinic aciduria; CIT1 - Citrullinemia, type I; MSUD - Maple syrup urine disease; HCY – Homocystinuria; PKU - Classic phenylketonuria; TYR1- Tyrosinemia, type I].
[b] [Endocrine Disorders: CH - Primary congenital hypothyroidism; CAH - Congenital adrenal hyperplasia].
[c] [Hemoglobin Disorders: SSD - S,S disease (Sickle cell anemia); ß-thal - S, βeta-thalassemia; SCD - S,C disease].

understanding of various phenotypes associated with IEMs. IEMs have heterogeneous and a wide scope of presenting symptoms[6] including neurodevelopmental and behavioral presentations. These can vary with age and/or management or stressors from common childhood/intercurrent illnesses/procedures/interventions. While most of the known IEMS are identified in children, some can emerge in adolescence or adulthood.[7]

INBORN ERRORS OF METABOLISMS OR METABOLIC DISORDERS

Inborn errors of metabolisms, commonly known as metabolic disorders are inherited biochemical genetic disorders.

These result from various enzyme defects in the various biochemical pathways of major nutrient groups helping our growth and survival through cellular metabolism. As a species, human growth and survival are dependent on food as a fuel source, which can be categorized into major nutrient groups, carbohydrates, proteins, fats,

Table 2		
Newborn screening RUSP "secondary conditions"		
Secondary Conditions Category	**Secondary Conditions Sub-category**	**Secondary Conditions/Abbreviation ([a])**
Metabolic Disorder	Organic acid disorders (OA)	[a][Cbl C,D; MAL; IBG; 2 MBG; 2M3HBA; 3MGA]
	Fatty acid oxidation Disorders (FAO)	[a][SCAD, M/SCHAD, GA2, MACT, DE RED, CPT IA, CPT II, CACT]
	Amino acid disorders (AA)	[a][ARG, CIT II,MET, H-PHE, BIOPT (BS), BIOPT (REG), TYR II, TYR III]
Hemoglobin Disorder		Other hemoglobinopathies (Var Hb)
Other Disorder		Galactoepimerase deficiency (GALE)
		Galactokinase deficiency (GALK)
		T-cell-related lymphocyte deficiencies

[a] [Metabolic Disorders: Cbl C,D - Methylmalonic acidemia with homocystinuria; MAL - Malonic acidemia; IBG - Isobutyrylglycinuria; 2 MBG - 2-Methylbutyrylglycinuria; 3MGA - 3-Methylglutaconic aciduria; 2M3HBA - 2-Methyl-3-hydroxybutyric aciduria; SCAD - Short-chain acyl-CoA dehydrogenase deficiency; M/SCHAD - Medium/short-chain L-3-hydroxyacyl-CoA dehydrogenase deficiency; GA2 - Glutaric acidemia type II; MACT - Medium-chain ketoacyl-CoA thiolase deficiency; DE RED - 2,4-Dienoyl-CoA reductase deficiency; CPT IA - Carnitine palmitoyltransferase type I deficiency; CPT II - Carnitine palmitoyltransferase type II deficiency; CACT - Carnitine acylcarnitine translocase deficiency; ARG – Argininemia; CIT II - Citrullinemia, type II; MET – Hypermethioninemia; H-PHE - Benign hyperphenylalaninemia; BIOPT (BS) - Biopterin defect in cofactor biosynthesis; BIOPT (REG) - Biopterin defect in cofactor regeneration; TYR II - Tyrosinemia, type II; TYR III -Tyrosinemia, type III].

vitamins, and minerals. These major nutrients are, respectively, broken down through a multitude of biochemical pathways using an enzyme at each step, into glucose or some other sugar form, amino acids, fatty acids, and cofactors. The function of each enzyme at each step is determined by the specific gene that encodes it. There are approximately 30,000 genes in the human genome (www.genome.gov), and we know that each gene consists of 4 nucleic acids often known by their first letters A (adenine), T (thymine), G (guanine), C (cytosine), in a specific spelling or sequence. Thus, any misspelling, also known as a mutation, can impair the genetic code and affect the encoded protein or enzyme function. Knowing how severely an enzyme function is affected, can often help determine and understand the clinical presentation and or the age of presentation of a specific IEM. Thus, IEM disorders can be categorized by the nutrient group affected as:

- Protein metabolism disorders – include inborn errors of amino acid, organic acid, urea cycle, creatine, and nucleic acid metabolism.
- Carbohydrate metabolism disorders – include inborn errors of glucose and glycogen, galactose, and fructose metabolism.
- Fat/lipid metabolism disorders – include inborn errors of mitochondrial beta-oxidation of fatty acids, lipoprotein, sterols, bile acids, and phospholipid metabolism, and mitochondrial disorders.
- Complex molecules – include inborn errors of lysosomal storage, peroxisomal, glycosylation, neurotransmitters, metals, and vitamin metabolism.

Textbooks such as GeneReviews, Saudubray Inborn Metabolic Diseases, Rudolph's Pediatrics 23e, Scriver's OMMBID, OMIM.org can be good resources for detailed information on each individual IEM.

Table 3	
Other newborn screening secondary conditions not included in RUSP	
Other Conditions Category	**Other Conditions/Abbreviation ([a])**
Organic acid disorders (OA)	[a][Cbl D-var1; Cbl E, CblG]
Amino acid disorders(AA)	[a][MTHFR]
Lysosomal Storage Disorder	Fabry, Gaucher, Niemann-pick type A and type B, Krabbe
Other Disorder	[a][BFP, PBD] [a][GAMT] [a][G6PD]

[a] Cbl D-var1 - Methylmalonic acidemia and homocystinuria, cbl D type; Cbl E - Homocystinuria-megaloblastic anemia, cbl E type; CblG - Homocystinuria-megaloblastic anemia, cbl G type; MTHFR - Homocystinuria due to MTHFR deficiency; BFP - D-bifunctional protein deficiency; PBD - Peroxisome biogenesis disorders (Zellweger spectrum disorders); GAMT - Guanidinoacetate methyltransferase deficiency; G6PD - Glucose-6-phosphate dehydrogenase (G6PD) deficiency.

Medical and Psychosocial Integration

Nearly 50 years ago, Engel argued in his influential article that the predominant biomedical model of disease was incomplete without consideration for the psychological and social determinants of health and illness behaviors.[8] In a rejection of reductionism and mind-body dualism, Engel proposed a new biopsychosocial model for explaining disease processes and outcomes that take individuals' social, psychological, and behavioral factors into account. As its initial conception, currently there is sufficient evidence of the validity and utility of this model's application to chronic illness.[9]

Even before this new model of disease, the field of pediatric psychology was emerging with an emphasis on, among other things, health promotion through prevention, identification, and intervention.[10] Today, pediatric psychologists serve in a range of medical settings, including primary care and specialty clinics. When providing care for patients with chronic medical conditions, psychologists apply the biopsychosocial framework in their assessment and intervention roles.[11] In IEMs (as in other chronic conditions), this includes patients' social, psychological, economic, educational, language, and cultural factors.[12] For patients with IEM, there should be an additional consideration for developmental factors, given the high prevalence of developmental disability within this population.

Neurodevelopmental and behavioral presentation and metabolic disorders

Neurodevelopmental and behavioral disorders are common presentations in children with IEM/metabolic disorders. The American Psychiatric Association's Diagnostic and Statistical Manual of Mental Disorders (DSM-5) diagnostic criteria help differentiate neurodevelopmental disorders (NDD) and behavioral disorders diagnosis.[13] NDD include intellectual disabilities, which are further categorized into:

- Intellectual disability (ID) or intellectual developmental disorder (IDD)
- Global developmental delay (GDD), and
- Unspecified ID

Intellectual disability (ID/IDD) includes the impairment of intellectual and adaptive functioning, with an onset typically seen before 18 years of age and is assessed by standardized testing. GDD is a diagnosis applicable to children under 5 years of age, when a child fails to meet expected developmental milestones, is unable to undergo intellectual assessment and or too young for such standardized assessment. Unspecified ID is applicable to children over 5 years of age, who are unable to undergo intellectual assessment due to physical disability and co-occurring mental illnesses. Standardized testing basically helps evaluate intellectual functions such as reasoning, problem-solving, planning, abstract thinking, judgment, academic learning, and learning from experience and adaptive functions such as communication, social participation, and independent living activities.[13] Other NDDs include autism spectrum disorders (ASD), attention-deficit/hyperactivity disorder (ADHD), learning disorders, motor disorders such as developmental coordination disorder such as childhood dyspraxia; Stereotypic movement disorders ± self-injurious behavior and Tic disorders. Some of the standardized testing tools used in IEMs include Wechsler Abbreviated Scale of Intelligence (WASI), Kaufman Brief Intelligence Test (K-BIT2), Test of Nonverbal Intelligence (TONI-4) and Leiter International Performance Scale, Third Edition (Leiter-3), Vineland Adaptive Behavior Scales, the Diagnostic Adaptive Behavior Scale, the Adaptive Behavior Assessment System (ABAS-III) and others[14,15] are noted in **Table 4**.

About 1% to 3% of the world's population are affected by ID and there are at least 116 easily treatable IEMs that are known to cause IDs if undiagnosed.[16] There are also many other IEMs associated with ID, other NDD, and behavioral disorders[15–18] and an extensive review of any individual disorder is beyond the scope of this article. As IEMs are multi-systemic disorders, findings of any NDD or behavioral presentation in isolation are rare. Most IEMs can present with multi-organ system involvement with feeding, growth, neurologic, gastrointestinal, cardiac, and dysmorphic features apart from NDD or behavioral presentations.

Almost all IEMS if untreated can present with developmental delay in early childhood and some can be transient such as Duarte Galactosemia.[19] Very few IEMs present in later childhood as isolated ID and should raise suspicion of L-2-Hydroxyglutaric aciduria, succinic semialdehyde dehydrogenase deficiency, 4-hydroxybutyric aciduria; X-linked creatine transporter deficiency syndromes (SLC6A), Sanfilippo disease type B and A (mucopolysaccharidosis type IIIB/A), cerebrotendinous xanthomatosis.[20]

Autism spectrum disorders can be seen with creatine deficiency disorders such as AGAT deficiency, GAMT deficiency; adenylosuccinate lyase deficiency; Sanfilippo disease type A (mucopolysaccharidosis type IIIA); Walker -Warburg Syndrome (POMGNT1-related); Smith Lemli Opitz syndrome; succinic semialdehyde dehydrogenase deficiency; mitochondrial disorders; metachromatic leukodystrophy; urea cycle disorders; phenylketonuria.[21–23]

Stereotypic bicycling movements can be seen with maple syrup urine disease.[24]

Self -injurious behavior can be seen with Lesch Nyhan syndrome, argininosuccinate lyase, deficiency and untreated PKU.

Psychiatric or behavioral presentations such as delusion, agitation, depression, and anxiety can be seen with hyperammonemia in organic acid disorder or urea cycle disorders,[25,26] homocystinuria[27] and can result from lack of diagnosis, poor metabolic management compliance postdiagnosis or metabolic decompensation with any common illnesses or fasting with planned intervention/procedures. Psychotic features such as hallucinations and disorganized behavior have also been reported. Psychiatric emergencies such as delirium can be seen with urea cycle defects, acute psychosis with late-onset Tay-Sachs, Fabry disease, and recurrent psychotic attacks with Wilson disease, lysosomal storage disease, and homocystinuria.[21]

Table 4	
Measures useful for pediatric patients with IEM	
Adaptive Functioning	Adaptive Behavior Assessment System, Third Edition
	Diagnostic Adaptive Behavior Scale
	Vineland Adaptive Behavior Scales, Third Edition
Attention Deficit/Hyperactivity Disorder	Brown Executive Function/Attention Scales
	Brown Attention-Deficit Disorder Scales
	Clinical Assessment of Attention Deficit
	Conners Continuous Performance Test, Third Edition
	Conners Continuous Auditory Test of Attention
	Conners, Third Edition
	Test of Variables of Attention
Autism Spectrum Disorder	M-CHAT -R/F
	Autism Diagnostic Observation Schedule, Second Edition
	Autism Diagnostic Interview – Revised
	Autism Spectrum Rating Scales
	Gilliam Autism Rating Scale, Third Edition
	Social Communication Questionnaire
Behavioral, Social, and Emotional	Achenbach System of Empirically Based Assessment
	Behavior Assessment System for Children, Third Edition
	Behavior Rating Inventory of Executive Function
	Beck Anxiety Inventory
	Beck Depression Inventory, Second Edition
	Children's Depression Inventory, Second Edition
	Eyberg Child Behavior Inventory
	Multidimensional Anxiety Scale for Children, Second Edition
	Sutter-Eyberg Student Behavior Inventory – Revised
Educational Achievement	Kaufman Test of Educational Achievement, Third Edition
	Wechsler Individual Achievement Test, Fourth Edition
	Wide Range Achievement Test, Fifth Edition
Intellectual	Comprehensive Test of Nonverbal Intelligence, Second Edition
	Kaufman Assessment Battery for Children, Second Edition Normative Update
	Kaufman Brief Intelligence Test, Second Edition
	Leiter International Performance Scale, Third Edition
	Primary Test of Nonverbal Intelligence
	Stanford-Binet Intelligence Scales, Fifth Edition
	Test of Nonverbal Intelligence, Fourth Edition
	Universal Nonverbal Intelligence Test, Second Edition
	Wechsler Abbreviated Scale of Intelligence
	Wechsler Adult Intelligence Scale, Fourth Edition
	Wechsler Intelligence Scale for Children, Fifth Edition
	Wechsler Preschool and Primary Scale of Intelligence, Fourth Edition

Though DSM-5 is of immense value and use for all clinicians including psychologists to address cognitive and behavioral aspects of mental health care in metabolic disorders, it can also provide tools for metabolic disorder clinicians subspecialty trained in biochemical genetics to understand and successfully engage mental health care providers in addressing comorbidities and potentially improving long-term morbidity and outcomes. Patients with metabolic disorders can best benefit from integrating behavioral health services, from collaborative and coordinated health care models especially when available in the same location. In clinical genetic services, genetic counselors often provide support to families and counseling for treatment adherence, and so forth. Clinical psychologists, also further help evaluate baseline functioning and help with behavioral therapies to ensure treatment adherence and promote health beliefs in children with metabolic disorders.

Psychologists' Role in Inborn Errors of Metabolisms

Psychologists could play an important role in children with metabolic disorders as cognitive and socio-emotional problems are commonly underdiagnosed or inadequately treated due to the lack of access to behavioral health providers.[28] This is especially relevant with more IEMs being detected by NBS. Successful long-term outcomes are dependent not only on early detection but on the successful management of each condition within the framework of the medical home of these pediatric patients. Regardless of the significant heterogeneity among IEMs' manifestation at a molecular, cellular, or organ system level, the developmental and psychological considerations are less limited to any individual disorder and can be understood to occur with some regularity in any individuals with IEMs. Thus, assessments of developmental and psychological functioning are crucial to the management of pediatric patients with IEM and are useful to establish a baseline of functioning, elicit DSM-V diagnosis, monitor treatment, and access educational, therapeutic, and financial resources. Psychologists are trained in the selection, administration, and interpretation of several measures that pertain to this population and in differential diagnosis and the communication of results to referring physicians and caregivers.[11] There are several measures that psychologists can select when completing a comprehensive evaluation of patients with IEM (see **Table 4**). Tests are selected for their applicability to pediatric and young adult populations and their relevance to common concerns among patients with IEMs. In the context of a comprehensive psychological evaluation, psychologists would individualize the test battery and also carefully consider the technical adequacy properties of selected measures, such as the inclusion of children with disabilities in the normative sample.

Intellectual measures include language-loaded, language-reduced, and language-free (nonverbal) measures. The latter 2 categories of intellectual assessment are important tools to consider, given some preliminary data to suggest that children with IEMs may be more likely to present with communication disorders.[29] Nonverbal tests also have utility for children with severe developmental disabilities. Adaptive measures provide data on functioning in conceptual, social, and practical domains, and aid in making a diagnosis of ID. In the behavioral and social/emotional domain, broad-band measures were selected over several narrow-band measures to assess a range of concerns in a single measure, but some narrow-band measures were also included. Some of the featured measures are ideally administered by psychologists (eg, intellectual assessments), but others may be administered by nonpsychologists trained in test administration, scoring, and interpretation.

Routine psychosocial screening

In addition to comprehensive assessment, there is a significant role for psychologists to conduct routine psychosocial screenings. Pediatric patients exist within interacting spheres of influence, including family, school, and the health care setting (eg, Bronfrenbrenner's 1979 ecological model[30]). For young patients with chronic illness, careful consideration must be made to the intersection of individual health (medical and behavioral) and family functioning. In addition to the typical parenting stressors, caregivers of children with IEMs are faced with the additional stressors of managing their child's chronic medical condition and their child's developmental and psychological needs that may be specific to their IEM. Therefore, the role of psychologists in screening for broader psychosocial concerns and caregiver distress is an important one. With routine screening, problems may be addressed early through appropriate support and referrals to minimize detrimental outcomes to health and family functioning.

For measuring the psychosocial risk of the family system, the Psychosocial Assessment Tool (PAT) is validated for chronically ill pediatric patients.[31] Most of the literature focuses on this tool's use in patients with pediatric cancer, but it has also been extended to other chronic illness populations. It screens families' risk and resilience factors and reliably predicts future psychosocial issues.[32] In addition to identifying risk, this tool is also useful for guiding treatment recommendations.

For measuring caregiver stress, the Parenting Stress Index, Fourth Edition (PSI-4) is a standardized assessment of stress in the parent–child relationship.[33] While it was not created for use with chronic illness populations specifically, there is a wealth of literature on its application to this population in research and clinical settings. It has also been applied to measuring stress in parents of children with IEMs.[34,35] There is also the Pediatric Inventory for Parents[36] which measures parenting stress specific to caring for a child with chronic illness and has been used in studies looking at parenting stress in managing IEMs.[37,38]

Psychologists' Role in Intervention

Psychologists in medical specialty settings focus on the promotion of health-related behaviors to improve treatment outcomes and support psychosocial well-being. Unfortunately, there are no best-practice standards for psychosocial treatment of patients with IEM specifically, and often genetic counselors will fill this gap.[39] In this review, we highlight 3 areas in which psychologists can make significant contributions to treatment: adherence, illness coping, and caregiver support/educational advocacy.

Treatment adherence

Medical treatment of IEMs is crucial not only to manage disease progression but also to limit detrimental developmental outcomes. As in the management of any disease, patients and caregivers may present with nonadherence to medical recommendations. Parents of young children with PKU may struggle to follow the strict dietary recommendations, blood testing frequency, and specialist visit frequency.[40] By focusing on modifiable factors in adherence, psychologists play an important role on the treatment team.

For example, in the case of dietary adherence for patients with PKU, several barriers may exist that psychologists can help manage. One barrier is poor knowledge of the disease and poor insight into treatment recommendations. A practical solution to this is patient and caregiver education.[28] While the mechanisms of IEMs are complex, as in other chronic illnesses it is nonetheless important for patients and their families to be presented with appropriate teaching about their disease. The complexities of IEM can be communicated successfully to school-aged children, adolescents, and caregivers through pictures and transparent language.[41] Psychologists' understanding of the construction of developmentally appropriate teaching tools makes them well-suited to participate in patient education.

Another barrier to adherence is low motivation to change unhelpful behaviors in illness management.[28] Psychologists can draw from motivational interviewing strategies to elicit behavioral change, thus improving treatment adherence. Motivational interviewing addresses patients' and/or caregivers' ambivalence and possible resistance toward change through discussion of values.[42] The goal is to lead them to engage in "change talk," stating their motivation for change in their own terms. It has numerous applications for adult patients managing chronic illness[43] as well as pediatric patients managing IEMs.[44]

Many psychologists may approach treatment adherence from a behavioral perspective. Coaching caregivers on the use of prompts and positive reinforcement for adherence behaviors represents another practical solution for improving adherence.[28] Some behavioral psychological interventions may even be time-limited, such as teaching children to swallow oral medications through a pill-swallowing protocol to improve their compliance.[45] Psychologists can also apply this to feeding/eating behaviors, such as accepting medical foods for IEM. These protocols rely heavily on behavioral components as the active ingredients, including positive reinforcement for successive approximations of the target behavior.

Psychologists can also discuss realistic developmental expectations with families based on the functional level and chronologic age. For example, adolescence is known to be a time of decreased adherence for patients with IEMs and other chronic conditions. Adolescents and young adults with PKU are known to have greater noncompliance with their recommended diet, thus resulting in higher blood phenylalanine concentrations.[46] In their role in treating patients with IEMs, psychologists can lead families through setting appropriate expectations such as finding a balance between fostering independence in adolescents while still providing some oversight to their medical management.

Illness coping

Successful management of IEMs includes the use of metabolic formula and medical food supplementations; parenteral drug, enzyme, and gene therapy; hematopoietic stem cell transplantation, liver $\pm$ kidney transplantation, apart from recurrent hospitalization with metabolic decompensation. This confronts many pediatric patients and their families with strict metabolic nutritional adherence, avoidance of childhood or family enjoyed fun foods, constraining management, and initiating emergency/acute illness protocols and potentially painful procedures (eg, needle pokes for infusion therapy or laboratory specimen collection). Coping with the physical symptoms of the IEMs themselves, such as the potential for chronic pain associated with some IEMs, is also an important consideration. Psychologists can develop specific competencies in psychological interventions for pain management, such as relaxation exercises, activity pacing, and mindfulness.

The psychosocial aspects of coping with IEMs are numerous. Patients with IEMs and their caregivers experience a significant burden of disease due to factors such as adherence to strict dietary regimens, danger imposed by common illness, social isolation, developmental and psychological impacts, and transition periods.[47] Strict dietary control can make holidays and other celebrations challenging to navigate. Children may face questions from peers and teachers about their invisible disability. For the parent, there can be an adjustment phase to the new diagnosis and accompanying grief; parents may also experience guilt and shame regarding their carrier status.[47] Psychologists have a unique role relative to other health professionals in providing guidance and psychological treatment to the patient and family on these issues.

Caregiver support and educational advocacy

Disease-related caregiving stress is associated with both poorer psychological and health outcomes.[48] In parents of children with medical conditions and disability, positive appraisals, access to resources, problem-solving ability, and use of positive coping strategies increase resiliency.[49] Thus, ensuring access to adequate supportive resources is one area of intervention that should be emphasized. Additionally, cognitive-behavioral and solution-focused interventions help parents improve problem-solving and reduce cognitive distortions regarding their child's condition.

Psychological parenting interventions have been shown to improve parenting behavior in some chronic illness populations[50]; however, the large-scale reviews do not include children with IEMs. Parenting interventions for chronic illness populations include psychoeducation, effective illness management, and effective parenting strategies include the ability to deliver these interventions in the context of the child's medical treatment. In other words, such interventions are applicable to multiple conditions, and ensure interventions are responsive to families' individual characteristics.[51] We posit that these conditions can be met through embedding a psychologist within the clinical team.

The educational setting is another important consideration for intervention. Given the rate of NDDs in many IEMs, ensuring adequate educational support will be a consideration for many of these patients. Psychologists may provide counsel to families on obtaining educational accommodations through a 504 Plan (Rehabilitation Act of 1973), or special education programs and services through an Individualized Education Plan (Individuals with Disabilities Education Act). Additionally, psychologists can provide communication and education to schools, describing the common behavioral and developmental manifestations of a patient's IEM, and providing recommendations for psychoeducational support.

Thoughts On Transition/Lifespan Considerations For Patients With Inborn Errors of Metabolism

a. Most of the board-certified biochemical (metabolic) geneticists aka subspecialty providers for IEMs, are also board-certified in Pediatrics and are likely to see patients through their lifespan. This can help lessen transitioning of IEM medical care but in a colocation model, a psychologist can also help with other life transitions of patients with IEM.
b. It is estimated that in the United States and Canada, only one-third of PKU clinics follow patients past 18 years of age[52]; which may improve with more IEM providers with primary care board certification in Pediatrics and Internal Medicine, and with increasing adult IEM interests and clinics emerging.
c. In women with pregnant PKU, with potential teratogenic effects of maternal PKU; or men with PKU or Urea Cycle disorders with potential conduct disordered behavior; ongoing interim follow-up with psychologists can prevent such adverse outcomes.
d. Parental/family support is needed during pediatric IEM patient transitions into school, adolescence, and with social/future vocational challenges[53]

Physicians of patients with IEMs know all too well the psychological toll these disorders can take on patients and their families. Thus, the role of psychological and social factors in disease manifestation, disease progression, and outcome is known in any chronic illness. Pediatric psychologists can apply their knowledge of these factors to promote the mental and physical health of young patients with chronic illnesses.

Psychologists who work with patients with IEMs put a greater focus on the screening and assessment of developmental outcomes (ie, cognitive and adaptive functioning) than psychologists working with other chronically ill populations.

Future developments in IEM management should continue to view these disorders through the biopsychosocial lens. Embedding psychologists within IEM clinics can provide holistic patient-centered care and be a medical home for patients with IEM throughout their lifespan.

CLINICS CARE POINTS

- Children identified with IEMs through NBS or clinically can benefit from optimal neurodevelopmental and behavioral outcomes in collaboration wth pediatric clinical psychologists.

- Clinical psychologist can utilize various measures to determine optimal neurodevelopmental and behavioral outcomes and diagnose any co-morbid neurodevelopmental and or behavioral disorders.

- Clinical psychologists can help families utilize various resources available through the educational system to promote individualized learning plans to improve long-term neurodevelopmental and behavioral outcomes.

DISCLOSURE

The authors have nothing to disclose.

REFERENCES

1. AE G. Inborn errors of metabolism. 2nd Edition. Oxford University Press; 1923. Available at: http://www.esp.org/books/garrod/inborn-errors/facsimile/.
2. Grand Rounds CDC. Newborn screening and improved outcomes. Available at: https://www.cdc.gov/mmwr/preview/mmwrhtml/mm6121a2.htm.   Accessed September 26, 2019.
3. Kanungo S, Patel DR, Neelakantan M, et al. Newborn screening and changing face of inborn errors of metabolism in the United States. Ann Transl Med 2018; 6(24):468.
4. Recommended uniform screening panel | official web site of the u.s. health resources & services administration. Available at: https://www.hrsa.gov/advisory-committees/heritable-disorders/rusp/index.html. Accessed January 29, 2022.
5. Psychiatric Association American. Diagnostic and statistical manual of mental disorders (DSM-5). Washington, D.C.: American Psychiatric Pub; 2013.
6. Saudubray JM. Clinical approach to inborn errors of metabolism in paediatrics. In: Inborn metabolic diseases: diagnosis and treatment. 2012. p. 3–54. https://doi.org/10.1007/978-3-642-15720-2_1.
7. Sedel F, Baumann N, Turpin JC, et al. Psychiatric manifestations revealing inborn errors of metabolism in adolescents and adults. J Inherit Metab Dis 2007;30(5): 631–41.
8. Engel GL. The need for a new medical model: a challenge for biomedicine. Science 1977;196(4286):129–36.
9. Wade DT, Halligan PW. The biopsychosocial model of illness: a model whose time has come. Clin Rehabil 2017;31(8):995–1004.
10. Genik LM, Yen J, McMurtry CM. Historical analysis in pediatric psychology: the influence of societal and professional conditions on two early pediatric psychology articles and the field's subsequent development. J Pediatr Psychol 2015; 40(2):167–74.
11. Palermo TM, Janicke DM, McQuaid EL, et al. Recommendations for training in pediatric psychology: defining core competencies across training levels. J Pediatr Psychol 2014;39(9):965–84.
12. Stockler S, Moeslinger D, Herle M, et al. Cultural aspects in the management of inborn errors of metabolism. J Inherit Metab Dis 2012;35(6):1147–52.

13. Psychiatric Association American. Diagnostic and statistical mental disorders. DSM 5); 2013.
14. Soares N, Apple RW, Kanungo S. The role of integrated behavioral health in caring for patients with metabolic disorders. Ann Transl Med 2018;6(24):478.
15. Waisbren S, White DA. Screening for cognitive and social-emotional problems in individuals with PKU: tools for use in the metabolic clinic. Mol Genet Metab 2010; 99(Suppl 1):S96–9. https://doi.org/10.1016/J.YMGME.2009.10.006.
16. Hoytema van Konijnenburg EMM, Wortmann SB, Koelewijn MJ, et al. Treatable inherited metabolic disorders causing intellectual disability: 2021 review and digital app. Orphanet J Rare Dis 2021;16(1). https://doi.org/10.1186/S13023-021-01727-2.
17. Van Karnebeek CDM, Shevell M, Zschocke J, et al. The metabolic evaluation of the child with an intellectual developmental disorder: Diagnostic algorithm for identification of treatable causes and new digital resource. Mol Genet Metab 2014;111(4):428–38.
18. Shapiro E, Bernstein J, Adams HR, et al. Neurocognitive clinical outcome assessments for inborn errors of metabolism and other rare conditions. Mol Genet Metab 2016;118(2):65–9.
19. Waisbren SE, Tran C, Demirbas D, et al. Transient developmental delays in infants with Duarte-2 variant galactosemia. Mol Genet Metab 2021;134(1–2):132–8.
20. García-Cazorla A, Wolf NI, Serrano M, et al. Mental retardation and inborn errors of metabolism. J Inherit Metab Dis 2009;32(5):597–608.
21. Simons A, Eyskens F, Glazemakers I, et al. Can psychiatric childhood disorders be due to inborn errors of metabolism? Eur Child Adolesc Psychiatry 2017;26(2): 143–54.
22. Marin SE, Saneto RP. Neuropsychiatric Features in Primary Mitochondrial Disease. Neurol Clin 2016;34(1):247–94.
23. Haas RH. Autism and mitochondrial disease. Dev Disabil Res Rev 2010;16(2): 144–53. https://doi.org/10.1002/ddrr.112.
24. Strauss KA, Puffenberger EG, Morton DH. Maple syrup urine disease. University of Washington, Seattle; 1993. Available at: http://www.ncbi.nlm.nih.gov/pubmed/20301495. Accessed December 4, 2018.
25. Waisbren SE, Stefanatos AK, Kok TMY, et al. Neuropsychological attributes of urea cycle disorders: A systematic review of the literature. J Inherit Metab Dis 2019;42(6):1176–91.
26. Waisbren SE, Cuthbertson D, Burgard P, et al. Biochemical markers and neuropsychological functioning in distal urea cycle disorders. J Inherit Metab Dis 2018;41(4):657.
27. Almuqbil MA, Waisbren SE, Levy HL, et al. Revising the Psychiatric Phenotype of Homocystinuria. Genet Med 2019;21(8):1827–31.
28. MacDonald A, Gokmen-Ozel H, van Rijn M, et al. The reality of dietary compliance in the management of phenylketonuria. J Inherit Metab Dis 2010;33(6): 665–70.
29. Tiwari S, Kallianpur D, DeSilva KA. Communication Impairments in Children with Inborn Errors of Metabolism: A Preliminary Study. Indian J Psychol Med 2017; 39(2):146–51.
30. Bronfenbrenner U. Referenced the ecology of human development. Harvard University Press; 1979. Available at: https://books.google.mu/books?hl=en&lr=&id=. Accessed March 31, 2022.
31. Kazak AE, Barakat LP, Ditaranto S, et al. Screening for psychosocial risk at pediatric cancer diagnosis: the psychosocial assessment tool. J Pediatr Hematol Oncol 2011;33(4):289–94.

32. Alderfer MA, Mougianis I, Barakat LP, et al. Family psychosocial risk, distress, and service utilization in pediatric cancer: predictive validity of the Psychosocial Assessment Tool. Cancer 2009;115(18 Suppl):4339–49.
33. Abidin RR. Parenting stress index 4th edition. Par. 2012. Available at: https://www.parinc.com/products/pkey/333. Accessed March 31, 2022.
34. Waisbren SE, Albers S, Amato S, et al. Effect of expanded newborn screening for biochemical genetic disorders on child outcomes and parental stress. JAMA 2003;290(19):2564–72.
35. Waisbren SE, Rones M, Read CY, et al. Brief report: Predictors of parenting stress among parents of children with biochemical genetic disorders. J Pediatr Psychol 2004;29(7):565–70.
36. Streisand R, Braniecki S, Tercyak KP, et al. Childhood illness-related parenting stress: the pediatric inventory for parents. J Pediatr Psychol 2001;26(3):155–62.
37. Sadat R, Hall PL, Wittenauer AL, et al. Increased parental anxiety and a benign clinical course: Infants identified with short-chain acyl-CoA dehydrogenase deficiency and isobutyryl-CoA dehydrogenase deficiency through newborn screening in Georgia. Mol Genet Metab 2020;129(1):20–5.
38. Dimitrova N, Glaus J, Urben S, et al. The impact of disease severity on the psychological well-being of youth affected by an inborn error of metabolism and their families: A one-year longitudinal study. Mol Genet Metab 2021;29. https://doi.org/10.1016/J.YMGMR.2021.100795.
39. Weber SL, Segal S, Packman W. Inborn errors of metabolism: psychosocial challenges and proposed family systems model of intervention. Mol Genet Metab 2012;105(4):537–41.
40. Walkowiak D, Bukowska-Posadzy A, Ł Kałuzny, et al. Therapy compliance in children with phenylketonuria younger than 5 years: A cohort study. Adv Clin Exp Med 2019;28(10):1385–91.
41. Zeltner NA, Welsink-Karssies MM, Landolt MA, et al. Reducing complexity: explaining inborn errors of metabolism and their treatment to children and adolescents. Orphanet J Rare Dis 2019;14(1). https://doi.org/10.1186/S13023-019-1236-9.
42. Rollnick S, Miller WR. What is Motivational Interviewing? Behav Cogn Psychother 1995;23(4):325–34.
43. Lundahl B, Moleni T, Burke BL, et al. Motivational interviewing in medical care settings: a systematic review and meta-analysis of randomized controlled trials. Patient Educ Couns 2013;93(2):157–68.
44. Viau KS, Jones JL, Murtaugh MA, et al. Phone-based motivational interviewing to increase self-efficacy in individuals with phenylketonuria. Mol Genet Metab 2016;6:27–33.
45. Babbitt RL, Parrish JM, Brierley PE, et al. Teaching developmentally disabled children with chronic illness to swallow prescribed capsules. J Dev Behav Pediatr 1991;12(4):229–35.
46. Walter JH, White FJ, Hall SK, et al. How practical are recommendations for dietary control in phenylketonuria? Lancet (London, England) 2002;360(9326):55–7.
47. Beck N, Applegate C. Elements of genetic counseling for inborn errors of metabolism. Transl Sci Rare Dis 2019;4(3–4):197–208.
48. Cousino MK, Hazen RA. Parenting stress among caregivers of children with chronic illness: a systematic review. J Pediatr Psychol 2013;38(8):809–28.
49. Hall HR, Neely-Barnes SL, Graff JC, et al. Parental stress in families of children with a genetic disorder/disability and the resiliency model of family stress, adjustment, and adaptation. Issues Compr Pediatr Nurs 2012;35(1):24–44.

50. Law E, Fisher E, Eccleston C, et al. Psychological interventions for parents of children and adolescents with chronic illness. Cochrane Database Syst Rev 2019; 3(3). https://doi.org/10.1002/14651858.CD009660.

51. Morawska A, Calam R, Fraser J. Parenting interventions for childhood chronic illness: a review and recommendations for intervention design and delivery. J Child Health Care 2015;19(1):5–17.

52. Fisch RO, Matalon R, Weisberg S, et al. Phenylketonuria: current dietary treatment practices in the United States and Canada. J Am Coll Nutr 1997;16(2): 147–51.

53. Khangura SD, Tingley K, Chakraborty P, et al. Child and family experiences with inborn errors of metabolism: a qualitative interview study with representatives of patient groups. J Inherit Metab Dis 2016;39(1):139–47.

UNITED STATES POSTAL SERVICE ®

Statement of Ownership, Management, and Circulation
(All Periodicals Publications Except Requester Publications)

1. Publication Title	2. Publication Number	3. Filing Date
PEDIATRIC CLINICS OF NORTH AMERICA	424 – 66	9/18/2022

4. Issue Frequency	5. Number of Issues Published Annually	6. Annual Subscription Price
FEB, APR, JUN, AUG, OCT, DEC	6	$263.00

7. Complete Mailing Address of Known Office of Publication (Not printer) (Street, city, county, state, and ZIP+4®)

ELSEVIER INC.
230 Park Avenue, Suite 800
New York, NY 10169

Contact Person
Malathi Samayan

Telephone (Include area code)
91-44-4299-4507

8. Complete Mailing Address of Headquarters or General Business Office of Publisher (Not printer)

ELSEVIER INC.
230 Park Avenue, Suite 800
New York, NY 10169

9. Full Names and Complete Mailing Addresses of Publisher, Editor, and Managing Editor (Do not leave blank)

Publisher (Name and complete mailing address)

KERRY Holland, ELSEVIER INC.
1600 JOHN F KENNEDY BLVD. SUITE 1800
PHILADELPHIA, PA 19103-2899

Editor (Name and complete mailing address)

KERRY HOLLAND, ELSEVIER INC.
1600 JOHN F KENNEDY BLVD. SUITE 1800
PHILADELPHIA, PA 19103-2899

Managing Editor (Name and complete mailing address)

PATRICK MANLEY, ELSEVIER INC.
1600 JOHN F KENNEDY BLVD. SUITE 1800
PHILADELPHIA, PA 19103-2899

10. Owner (Do not leave blank. If the publication is owned by a corporation, give the name and address of the corporation immediately followed by the names and addresses of all stockholders owning or holding 1 percent or more of the total amount of stock. If not owned by a corporation, give the names and addresses of the individual owners. If owned by a partnership or other unincorporated firm, give its name and address as well as those of each individual owner. If the publication is published by a nonprofit organization, give its name and address.)

Full Name	Complete Mailing Address
WHOLLY OWNED SUBSIDIARY OF REED/ELSEVIER, US HOLDINGS	1600 JOHN F KENNEDY BLVD. SUITE 1800 PHILADELPHIA, PA 19103-2899

11. Known Bondholders, Mortgagees, and Other Security Holders Owning or Holding 1 Percent or More of Total Amount of Bonds, Mortgages, or Other Securities. If none, check box ▶ ☐ None

Full Name	Complete Mailing Address
N/A	

12. Tax Status (For completion by nonprofit organizations authorized to mail at nonprofit rates) (Check one)
The purpose, function, and nonprofit status of this organization and the exempt status for federal income tax purposes:
☒ Has Not Changed During Preceding 12 Months
☐ Has Changed During Preceding 12 Months (Publisher must submit explanation of change with this statement)

PS Form **3526**, July 2014 [Page 1 of 4 (see instructions page 4)] PSN: 7530-01-000-9931 PRIVACY NOTICE: See our privacy policy on www.usps.com

---

13. Publication Title	14. Issue Date for Circulation Data Below
PEDIATRIC CLINICS OF NORTH AMERICA	JUNE 2022

15. Extent and Nature of Circulation

			Average No. Copies Each Issue During Preceding 12 Months	No. Copies of Single Issue Published Nearest to Filing Date
a. Total Number of Copies (Net press run)			568	483
b. Paid Circulation (By Mail and Outside the Mail)	(1)	Mailed Outside-County Paid Subscriptions Stated on PS Form 3541 (Include paid distribution above nominal rate, advertiser's proof copies, and exchange copies)	276	264
	(2)	Mailed In-County Paid Subscriptions Stated on PS Form 3541 (Include paid distribution above nominal rate, advertiser's proof copies, and exchange copies)	0	0
	(3)	Paid Distribution Outside the Mails Including Sales Through Dealers and Carriers, Street Vendors, Counter Sales, and Other Paid Distribution Outside USPS®	220	180
	(4)	Paid Distribution by Other Classes of Mail Through the USPS (e.g., First-Class Mail®)	0	0
c. Total Paid Distribution (Sum of 15b (1), (2), (3), and (4))		▶	496	444
d. Free or Nominal Rate Distribution (By Mail and Outside the Mail)	(1)	Free or Nominal Rate Outside-County Copies included on PS Form 3541	51	22
	(2)	Free or Nominal Rate In-County Copies included on PS Form 3541	0	0
	(3)	Free or Nominal Rate Copies Mailed at Other Classes Through the USPS (e.g., First-Class Mail)	0	0
	(4)	Free or Nominal Rate Distribution Outside the Mail (Carriers or other means)	0	0
e. Total Free or Nominal Rate Distribution (Sum of 15d (1), (2), (3) and (4))		▶	51	22
f. Total Distribution (Sum of 15c and 15e)		▶	547	466
g. Copies not Distributed (See Instructions to Publishers #4 (page #3))		▶	21	17
h. Total (Sum of 15f and g)		▶	568	483
i. Percent Paid (15c divided by 15f times 100)		▶	90.67%	95.27%

* If you are claiming electronic copies, go to line 16 on page 3. If you are not claiming electronic copies, skip to line 17 on page 3.

PS Form **3526**, July 2014 (Page 2 of 4)

16. Electronic Copy Circulation		Average No. Copies Each Issue During Preceding 12 Months	No. Copies of Single Issue Published Nearest to Filing Date
a. Paid Electronic Copies	▶		
b. Total Paid Print Copies (Line 15c) + Paid Electronic Copies (Line 16a)	▶		
c. Total Print Distribution (Line 15f) + Paid Electronic Copies (Line 16a)	▶		
d. Percent Paid (Both Print & Electronic Copies) (16b divided by 16c × 100)	▶		

☒ I certify that 50% of all my distributed copies (electronic and print) are paid above a nominal price.

17. Publication of Statement of Ownership

☒ If the publication is a general publication, publication of this statement is required. Will be printed   ☐ Publication not required.
in the   OCTOBER 2022   issue of this publication.

18. Signature and Title of Editor, Publisher, Business Manager, or Owner	Date
Malathi Samayan - Distribution Controller *Malathi Samayan*	9/18/2022

I certify that all information furnished on this form is true and complete. I understand that anyone who furnishes false or misleading information on this form or who omits material or information requested on the form may be subject to criminal sanctions (including fines and imprisonment) and/or civil sanctions (including civil penalties).

PS Form **3526**, July 2014 (Page 3 of 4)   PRIVACY NOTICE: See our privacy policy on www.usps.com